Breast Cancer Global Quality Care

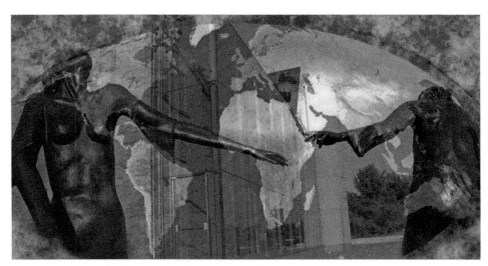

Phographic poetry - Robert Paridaens (with permission)

Breast Cancer Global Quality Care

Edited by

DIDIER VERHOEVEN

Medical Oncologist
Guest Professor, University of Antwerp, Belgium
Chair, Breast Clinic Voorkempen, AZ KLINA, Belgium

CARY S. KAUFMAN

Breast Surgeon
Associate Clinical Professor of Surgery, University of Washington, USA
Past Chairman, National Accreditation Program for Breast Centers, USA
Past President, National Consortium of Breast Centers, USA

ROBERT MANSEL

Breast Surgeon
Professor Emeritus of Surgery, University of Cardiff School of Medicine, UK
Chair of the Quality Assurance Committee of the ECIBC
Past President EUSOMA

SABINE SIESLING

Clinical Epidemiologist
Professor of Outcomes Research and Personalized Cancer Care,
University of Twente, The Netherlands,
Senior Researcher, Netherlands Comprehensive Cancer Organisation (IKNL)
Past General Secretary of the International Association of Cancer Registries (IACR)

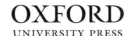

OXFORD
UNIVERSITY PRESS

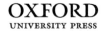

OXFORD

UNIVERSITY PRESS

Great Clarendon Street, Oxford, OX2 6DP,
United Kingdom

Oxford University Press is a department of the University of Oxford.
It furthers the University's objective of excellence in research, scholarship,
and education by publishing worldwide. Oxford is a registered trade mark of
Oxford University Press in the UK and in certain other countries

First Edition published in 2020

Impression: 2

Published in the United States of America by Oxford University Press
198 Madison Avenue, New York, NY 10016, United States of America

British Library Cataloguing in Publication Data

Data available

Library of Congress Control Number: 2019951488

ISBN 978–0–19–883924–8

Printed in Great Britain by
Ashford Colour Press Ltd, Gosport, Hampshire

Preface

This book is the result of a project addressing a global approach to the quality of breast cancer care which began ten years ago in Paris. Since 2010, meetings have been organized in Paris, Antwerp, and Aachen as well as during several international breast conferences devoted to quality management, organization of breast cancer care, breast centre quality, guidelines, and the influence of local economics and resources in breast care. In 2012, during the 2nd International Congress of Breast Disease Centres, our group of experts joined others to draft the Paris statement which was later approved by the Chairs of EUSOMA (European Society of Breast Cancer Specialists), NAPBC (National Accreditation Program for Breast Centers), and SIS (Senologic International Society) and endorsed by the President of UICC (Union for International Cancer Control). We were unified in support of the Paris Statement that said 'All women across the world should have access to fully equipped, quality assured, dedicated breast centers/units, that provide competent and comprehensive care.' We joined forces with the Chairs of these organizations and added a large network of highly motivated experts to make this statement a reality.

During the last three years, a faculty of 115 experts from five continents and 25 different countries communicated during expert meetings, mailings, Skype conferences and telephone conversations to form a collaborative vision on defining quality breast cancer care. We have collected the insights and perspectives of leading experts including physicians, epidemiologists, economists, pharmacists, psychologists, nurses, patient advocates, journalists, and academics. Our project focuses on the melding of high-quality breast care influenced by local economics and personnel resources affecting breast centres in all countries. This book is not the endpoint, rather it serves as the foundation for further innovations on organization and integration of breast cancer care for all women.

We believe this book has value for everyone working in the field of integrated breast cancer care. Whereas established breast care experts will find value in the topic-oriented chapters of this book, non-experts, such as those new to the field or caregivers focusing on other types of diseases/cancers which demand a multidisciplinary approach, will be interested in the general overview provided by the book as a whole. Individuals involved in forming breast centres will find valuable and practical information to include into the foundations of their new centres. Policymakers will have special interest in the social, financial, and political integration in the total scope of breast cancer care as the book leads the reader through the labyrinth of organizations and modalities. Whereas the Breast Health Global Initiative focuses on low- and lower-middle income countries, this book is applicable to all regions.

Although the basics in diagnosis and treatment are well known, we have focused on providing, monitoring, and assessing the quality of breast care and the challenges these may bring. The authors provide thorough descriptions of high-quality breast care, define benchmarks to strive for, methods to assess one's care, and ideas on how to improve within one's resources. Hallmarks of innovation, communication, and patient-centred multidisciplinary care are reported with budget considerations to guide specific recommendations. A comprehensive overview takes into account global and local considerations and guides the reader on how to optimally organize high-quality 'integrated' breast cancer care. In successive chapters, each component of the whole care pathway (e.g. imaging, surgery, systemic treatment, genetic assessment, role of general practitioner, etc.) is discussed from both theoretical and practical aspects. Each discipline identifies a desired level of care which is possible, and balances it with the local resources that define what is achievable. The choice of a final recommendation for each component of care is facilitated by the rational and practical approaches laid out at each step by this knowledgeable group of experts.

Beyond discussions on how to integrate the different breast care disciplines into a coordinated breast unit, the book provides practical considerations regarding accreditation and certification as well as discussions about the influence of budget on value of treatment. Finally, it demonstrates how best practices may be altered by emerging technologies and transitions of future societal values.

The editors thank the contributors from around the globe who lent their expertise in breast cancer care to the writing of this book. We give special thanks for the outstanding secretarial support of Sofie Pauwels and medical writing support of John Bean (without whom the work would not have been possible). We thank AZ KLINA, Brasschaat, where Didier Verhoeven practices medicine, and the legacies of two of their patients with cancer who supported this project financially. Also, thanks go to Robert Paridaens for providing photographic poetry. Finally, the lead editor, Didier Verhoeven, thanks and dedicates this work to his lovely wife, Jana, and his two supportive children, Michaël and Sophie.

Didier Verhoeven, lead editor

Cary S. Kaufman, Robert Mansel, and Sabine Siesling, co-editors

Contents

Abbreviations

ABSI	Association of Breast Surgeons of India
ACOSOG	American College of Surgeons Oncology Group
ACP	Advanced Care Planning
ACS	American Cancer Society
ADM	Acellular Dermal Matrix
AGREE II	Appraisal of Guidelines for Research and Evaluation II
AIOM	Italian Association of Medical Oncology
ALND	Axillary Lymph Node Dissection
ANZBCTG	Australia–New Zealand Breast Cancer Trials Group
ASCO	American Society for Clinical Oncology
ASTRO	American Society for Radiation Oncology
BcCert	Breast Centre Certification
BCN	Breast Care Nurse
BCS	Breast-Conserving Surgery
BCT	Breast-Conserving Therapy
BHGI	Breast Health Global Initiative
BIA	Budget Impact Analysis
BIG	Breast International Group
BRENDA	Breast Cancer Care under Evidence-Based Guidelines Cohort
BreastSurgANZ	Breast Surgeons of Australia and New Zealand
BQA	BreastSurgANZ Quality Audit
CANCON	Commission Expert Group on Cancer Control
CEA	Cost-Effectiveness Analysis
CME	Continuing Medical Education
CN	Consultant Nurses
CNB	Core Needle Biopsy
CNS	Clinical Nurse Specialist
COI	Cost of Illness
CP	Computerized Prescription
CPG	Clinical Practice Guidelines
CUA	Cost Utility Analysis
CUP	Cancer of Unknown Primary
DCE	Discrete Choice Experiment
DCIS	Ductal Carcinoma In Situ
DCISM	Ductal Carcinoma In Situ with Microinvasion
DG SANTE	Directorate General of Health and Food Safety
DICA	Dutch Surgical Colorectal Audit
DLT	Dose-Limiting Toxicity
EACCME	European Accreditation Council for Continuing Medical Education
EBCTCG	Early Breast Cancer Trialists' Collaborative Group
EC	European Commission
ECIBC	European Commission Initiative on Breast Cancer

EEA	European Economic Area
EGFR	Epidermal Growth Factor Receptor
EGP	Educational Group Programme
EHR	Electronic Health Record
ENBDC	European Network of Breast Development and Cancer Laboratories
ENCR	European Network of Cancer Registries
EORTC	European Organisation for Research and Treatment of Cancer
EPAAC	European Partnership for Action Against Cancer
ER	Oestrogen Receptor
ESMO	European Society of Medical Oncology
ESO	European School of Oncology
ESTRO	European Society for Therapeutic Radiotherapy and Oncology
ESSO	European Society of Surgical Oncology
EUROCARE	European Cancer Registry-based study on survival and care of cancer patients
EUROCHIP	European Cancer Health Indicator Project
EUROCOURSE	Europe Against Cancer: Optimisation of the Use of Registries for Scientific Excellence research
European QA scheme	European Quality Assurance Scheme for Breast Cancer Services
EUSOMA	European Society of Breast Cancer Specialists
EU	European Union
FNA	Fine-Needle Aspirates
FNAB	Fine-Needle Aspiration Biopsy
GDP	Gross Domestic Product
GP	General Practitioner
GPS	Glasgow Prognostic Score
GTFRCC	Global Task Force on Radiation Therapy for Cancer Control
HIC	High-Income Countries
HIV	Human Immunodeficiency Virus
HRQoL	Health Related Quality of Life
HRT	Hormonal Replacement Therapy
IARC	International Agency for Research in Cancer
IBIS	International Breast Cancer Intervention Study
IBSCG	International Breast Cancer Study Group
ICER	Incremental Cost-Effectiveness Ratio
ICHOM	International Consortium for Health Outcomes Measurement
ICT	Information and Communications Technologies
IKNL	Comprehensive Cancer Organisation the Netherlands
IMI	Innovative Medicines Initiative
IPOS	International Psycho-Oncology Society
Italcert	Italian Certification Body
JBCRG	Japan Breast Cancer Research Group
JBCS	Japanese Breast Cancer Society
JRC	European Commission's Joint Research Centre
LABC	Locally Advanced Breast Cancer
LACs	Latin American Countries
LACOG	Latin American Cooperative Group
LMICs	Low- and Middle-Income Countries
MA	Meta-Analysis
MBC	Multidisciplinary Breast Conference

MDC	Multidisciplinary Breast Clinic
MDM	Multidisciplinary Meeting
MDT	Multidisciplinary Tumour Decision Team
MEA	Managed Entry Agreement
MIPS	Merit-Based Incentive Payment System
MRI	Magnetic Resonance Imaging
MJC	Multidisciplinary Joint Committee
MRM	Modified Radical Mastectomy
MTB	Molecular Tumour Board
MU	Mastology Unit
NAACCR	North American Association of Central Cancer Registries
NABCG	North American Breast Cancer Groups
NABON	National Breast Cancer Organisation Netherlands
NAC	Nipple–Areola Complex
NAPBC	National Accreditation Program for Breast Centers
NBCA	NABON Breast Cancer Audit (Netherlands)
NBCA	National Breast Cancer Audit (Australia and New Zealand)
NBCC	National Breast Cancer Coalition
NCCP	National Cancer Control Programmes
NCDB	National Cancer Database
NCCN	National Comprehensive Cancer Network
NCI	National Cancer Institute
NGS	Next Generation Sequencing
NHS	National Health Service
NICE	National Institute for Health and Clinical Excellence
NP	Nurse Practitioners
NQMBC	National Quality Measures for Breast Centers
NSABP	National Surgical Adjuvant Breast and Bowel Project
PALGA	Pathologisch-Anatomisch Landelijk Geautomatiseerd Archief
PARP	Poly ADP Ribose Polymerase
PBCR	Population-Based Cancer Registries
PBI	Partial Breast Irradiation
PC	Palliative Care
PCP	Primary Care Physician
PCR	Polymerase Chain Reaction
PDCA	Plan–Do–Check–Act cycle
PDQ	Physician Data Query
PEBC	Program in Evidence-Based Care
PPI	Palliative Prognostic Index
PPP	Purchasing Power Parity
PPS	Palliative Prognostic Score
PQRS	Physician Quality Reporting System
PREMs	Patient-Reported Experience Measures
PROMs	Patient-Reported Outcome Measures
PRS	Polygenic Risk Score
PST	Primary Systemic Treatment
QA	Quality Assurance
QALYs	Quality-Adjusted Life-Years
QASDG	Quality Assurance Scheme Development Group
QI	Quality Indicator

QLQ	Quality of Life Questionnaire
QoL	Quality of Life
RACS	Royal Australasian College of Surgeons
RT	Radiation Therapy
SA	South Africa
SAM	Sociedad Argentina de Mastología
SCP	Survivorship Care Plan
SIS	Senologic International Society
SLNB	Sentinel Lymph Node Biopsy
SNPs	Single Nucleotide Polymorphisms
SOC	Standard Oncological Care
SPICT™	Supportive and Palliative Care Indicators Tool
SR	Systematic Review
TKI	Tyrosine Kinase Inhibitor
TNBC	Triple-Negative Breast Cancer
TNEH	Total National Expenditure on Health
UEMS	Union of European Medical Specialists
UICC	Union for International Cancer Control
UK	United Kingdom
USA	United States of America
USPSTF	US Preventive Services Task Force
VNPI	Van Nuys Prognostic Index
VUS	Variants of Unknown Clinical Significance
WHO	World Health Organization

List of contributors

Philippe Aftimos, Medical Oncologist, Bordet Institute, Brussels, Belgium

Claudia Allemani, Associate Professor of Cancer Epidemiology, Cancer Survival Group, London School of Hygiene and Tropical Medicine, London, UK

Benjamin O. Anderson, Chair, Breast Health Global Initiative (BHGI); Professor of Surgery and Global Health Medicine, University of Washington, Seattle, WA, USA

Kwanele Asante-Shongwe, Health Lawyer and Bioethicist, University of the Witwatersrand, Johannesburg, South Africa; Patient Advocate, African Organization for Research and Training in Cancer

Deanna J. Attai, Assistant Clinical Professor of Surgery, David Geffen School of Medicine, University of California, Los Angeles, CA, USA

Ahmad Awada, Professor of Medical Oncology, Bordet Institute, Brussels, Belgium

Benjamin Baelus, Former Advisor to Lieve Wierinck MEP, Belgium

Carol Benn, Professor of Surgery, University of the Witwatersrand and Helen Joseph Hospital, Johannesburg, South Africa

Annette J. Berendsen, Assistant Professor of Primary Care, University of Groningen, University Medical Center Groningen, Groningen, The Netherlands

Nirmala Bhoo-Pathy, Associate Professor of Epidemiology, University of Malaya, Malaysia

Liesbeth Boersma, Professor of Radiation Oncology, Maastro Clinic, Maastricht, The Netherlands

Carole Bouleuc, Head, Department of Supportive Care, Curie Institute, Paris, France

Etienne Brain, Professor of Medical Oncology, Curie Institute, Hopital René Huguenin, Paris, France

Freddie Bray, Head, Section of Cancer Surveillance, International Agency for Research on Cancer, Lyon, France

Sara Y. Brucker, Executive Medical Director, Department of Women's Health, University of Tubingen, Germany

Wolfgang Buchberger, Head of Institute of Quality and Efficiency in Medicine, UMIT Privat University for Health Sciences, Medical Informatics and Technology, Hall in Tirol, Austria

Barry D. Bultz, Professor and Head, Division of Psychosocial Oncology, Daniel Family Leadership Chair in Psychosocial Oncology, Cumming School of Medicine, University of Calgary, Alberta, Canada

Ornella Campanella, Breast Nurse, Patient Advocate Organization aBRCAdabra, Italy

Fatima Cardoso, Director Breast Unit, Champalimaud Clinical Centre, Champalimaud Foundation, Lisbon, Portugal

Luigi Cataliotti, Professor of Surgery, President Breast Centres Certification, Florence, Italy

Eduardo L. Cazap, President, Latin-American & Caribbean Society of Medical Oncology (SLACOM); Past President and Board Member Union for International Cancer Control (UICC), Buenos Aires, Argentina

AnneMarie Mercurio, Independent Patient Advocate, New York, NY, USA

Federico Coló, Breast Surgeon, Private Institute of Oncology Alexander Fleming, Buenos Aires, Argentina

Maurício Magalhães Costa, Breast Surgeon, President of Senologic International Society, Breast Center of Americas Integrated Oncology Center, Rio de Janeiro, Brazil and Member of the National Academy of Medicine, Council Member of International Gynecologic Cancer Society, and Head of the Breast Unit of Americas Centro de Oncologia Integrada

Mahmoud Danaei, Breast Surgeon, Marienhospital, Aachen, Germany

Evandro de Azambuja, Medical Oncologist, Bordet Institute, Brussels, Belgium

Geertruida H. de Bock, Epidemiologist, Professor of Epidemiology, University of Groningen, University Medical Center Groningen, The Netherlands

Wim Demey, Medical Oncologist, AZ KLINA, Brasschaat, Belgium

Carmen D. Dirksen, Professor of Health Technology Assessment of Clinical Intervention, Department of Clinical Epidemiology and Medical Technology Assessment, Care and Public Health Research Institute (CAPHRI), Maastricht University Medical Centre+, Maastricht, The Netherlands

Catherine Duggan, Principal Staff Scientist, Public Health Sciences and BHGI, Fred Hutchinson Cancer Research Center, Seattle, WA, USA

François P. Duhoux, Associate Professor Medical Oncology at Cliniques universitaires Saint-Luc and Université catholique de Louvain, Belgium

Nagi S. El Saghir, Professor of Medical Oncology, American University of Beirut, Lebanon

Paul A. El-Tomb, Medical Oncology, American University of Beirut, Lebanon

Alexandru Eniu, Head of the Day Hospital Unit, Cancer Institute 'Ion Chiricuta', Department of Breast Tumors, Cluj-Napoca, Romania

Marc Espié, Associate Professor, Medical Oncology, Hôpital Saint-Louis, Paris, France

Marion Essers, Medical Physicist, Institute Verbeeten, Tilburg, The Netherlands

Carlos A. Garcia-Etienne, Breast Surgeon, Fundazione IRCCS Policlinico San Matteo, Universita degli Studi di Pavia, Italy

Anna Gavin, Director, Northern Ireland Cancer Registry, Queen's University Belfast, North Ireland

Victoria Harmer, Macmillan Consultant (Breast) Nurse, Imperial College Healthcare NHS Trust, London, UK

Rishi Hazarika, Past Vice President, Global Implementation and Courses ICHOM, UK

Teresa Heckel, Project Director, Clinical Programs Sarah Cannon, Colorado Springs, CO, USA

Sylvia Heywang-Köbrunner, Referenzzentrum Mammographie, Munich, Germany

Sandra Hol, Radiation Therapy Technologist, Institute Verbeeten, Tilburg, The Netherlands

Aafke Honkoop, Medical Oncologist, Isala Kliniek Zwolle, The Netherlands

Emilie Hoogland, Local Assistant, European Parliament, Brussels, Belgium

Cathy Hughes, Consultant Nurse Gynaecology/Oncology, Imperial College Healthcare NHS Trust, London, UK

Paul B. Jacobsen, Division of Cancer Control and Population Sciences, National Cancer Institute, Bethesda, MA, USA

Stephen Jan, Professor of Health Economics, The George Institute for Global Health, Sydney, Australia

Manuela Joore, Professor of Health Technology Assessment & Decision Making, Head of the Department of Clinical Epidemiology and Medical Technology Assessment, Care and Public Health Research Institute (CAPHRI), Maastricht University Medical Centre+, Maastricht, The Netherlands

Hans Junkermann, Senior Consultant, Section of Senology, Heidelberg University Hospital, Heidelberg, Germany

Orit Kaidar-Person, Radiation Oncology Unit, Rambam Medical Center, Haifa, Israel

Merel Kimman, Department of Clinical Epidemiology and Medical Technology Assessment, Care and Public Health Research Institute (CAPHRI), Maastricht University Medical Centre+, Maastricht, The Netherlands

Betsy Kohler, Executive Director, North American Association of Central Cancer Registries, Inc. (NAACCR, Inc.) NJ, USA

Nuria Kotecki, Medical Oncologist, Institut Jules Bordet, Brussels, Belgium

Inge Kriel, Primary Care Physician, Johannesburg, South Africa

Christine Langenaeken, Medical Oncology–Palliative Medicine, AZ KLINA, Brasschaat, Belgium

Daniel Leal, Plastic Surgeon, Rio De Janeiro, Brazil

Paulo Roberto Leal, Associate Professor, Plastic Surgery, Uni Rio, Rio De Janeiro, Brazil

Donata Lerda, Health Quality Group Leader, ECIBC, Ispra, Italy

Roma Maguire, Professor of Digital Health and Care, University of Strathclyde, Glasgow, UK

Christos Markopoulos, Professor of Surgery, National & Kapodistrian University of Athens, Athens, Greece

Lawrence B. Marks, Professor and Chair, Department of Radiation Oncology, Lineberger Cancer Center, University of North Carolina, Chapel Hill, NC, USA

Lorenza Marotti, Executive Director EUSOMA, Firenze, Italy

Shahla Masood, Professor and Chair, Department of Pathology and Laboratory Medicine, University of Florida, Jacksonville, FL, USA

Tomohiro Matsuda, National Cancer Center, Registry Section, Tokyo, Japan

Ryan M. McCabe, Senior Manager, National Cancer Data Base, American College of Surgeons, Chicago, IL, USA

Jumana Mensah, Certification Department, German Cancer Society, Berlin, Germany

Michael Michell, Consultant Radiologist, King's College Hospital, London, UK

Alexander Mundinger, Professor of Radiology, Niels-Stensen-Kliniken, Osnabrück, Germany

Liz O'Riordan, Oncoplastic Surgeon, Ipswich Hospital, Ipswich, UK

Groesbeck Parham, Professor of Obstetrics and Gynaecology, University of North Carolina, Chapel Hill, NC, USA; Global Women's Health Fund, Zambia

Johanna Pas, Patient Advocate, Antwerp, Belgium

Rudi Pauwels, Pharmaceutical Scientist, Founder Biocartis, Belgium

Sanne Peters, The George Institute for Global Health, University of Oxford, Oxford, UK

Raghu Ram Pillarisetti, Oncoplastic Breast Surgeon, Director, KIMS-Ushalakshmi Centre for Breast Diseases, Hyderabad, India

Antonio Ponti, Center of Oncology Prevention, CPO Piemonte, Turin; Director, EUSOMA Data Centre, Florence, Italy

Philip Poortmans, Professor of Radiation Oncology, Curie Institute, Paris, France

Xavier Pouwels, Department of Clinical Epidemiology and Medical Technology Assessment, Care and Public Health Research Institute (CAPHRI), Maastricht University Medical Centre+, Maastricht, The Netherlands

Diane M. Radford, Associate Professor of Surgery, Cleveland Clinic Lerner College of Medicine of Case Western Reserve University, Cleveland, OH, USA

Bram Ramaekers, Department of Clinical Epidemiology and Medical Technology Assessment, Care and Public Health Research Institute (CAPHRI), Maastricht University Medical Centre+, Maastricht, The Netherlands

Peter Regitnig, Medical University of Graz, Diagnostic and Research Institute of Pathology, Graz, Austria

Mark E. Robson, Director, Clinical Genetics Service, Memorial Sloan Kettering Cancer Center, New York, NY, USA

Julia H. Rowland, Senior Strategic Advisor, Smith Center for Healing and the Arts, Washington DC, USA

Fernando Suarez, Medical Science Lead, IBM, Watson Health, Toronto, Canada

Roberto Salgado, Department of Pathology, GZA Hospitals, Antwerp, Belgium

Terry Sarantou, Professor of Surgery, Levine Cancer Institute & Department of Surgery, Carolinas HealthCare System, Charlotte, NC, USA

Marjanka K. Schmidt, Professor, Genetic Epidemiology of (Breast) Cancer, Division of Molecular Pathology, Netherlands Cancer Institute, Amsterdam, The Netherlands

Gilberto Schwartsmann, Professor, Medical Oncology, Academic Hospital (HCPA), Federal University (UFRGS), Porto Alegre, Brazil

Gary Schwitzer, Publisher, HealthNewsReview.org, Adjunct Associate Professor, University of Minnesota School of Public Health, Minneapolis, MN, USA

Isabelle Soerjomataram, Medical Epidemiologist, Section of Cancer Surveillance, International Agency for Research on Cancer (IARC), Lyon, France

Luis Teixeira, Medical Oncologist, Associate Professor, Diderot University, Paris, France

Soo Hwang Teo, Genetic Epidemiology, Kuala Lumpur, Malaysia

Francisco Terrier, Breast Surgeon, Breast Clinic, Italian Hospital, La Plata, Argentina

Luzia Travado, Head of Psycho-oncology, Champalimaud Clinical and Research Centre, Champalimaud Foundation, Lisbon, Portugal

Lee F. Tucker, Breast Pathologist, President, Virginia Biomedical Laboratories, Wirtz, VA, USA

Jane Turner, Discipline of Psychiatry, Faculty of Medicine, University of Queensland, Australia

Peter A. van Dam, Professor Gynaecological Oncology, Multidisciplinary Breast Unit, Antwerp University Hospital, and University of Antwerp, Wilrijk, Belgium

Alexandra J. van den Broek, Scientist, Division of Molecular Pathology, Netherlands Cancer Institute, Amsterdam, The Netherlands

Gert G.G.M. Van den Eynden, Department of Pathology, GZA Hospitals, Antwerp, Belgium

Paul van Diest, Pathologist, Head Department of Pathology, University Medical Center Utrecht, The Netherlands; John Hopkins Oncology Center, Baltimore, MA, USA

Xander Verbeek, Information Scientist, Netherlands Comprehensive Cancer Organisation (IKNL) Utrecht, The Netherlands

Adri Voogd, Associate Professor, Clinical Epidemiology, Care and Public Health Research Institute (CAPHRI), Maastricht University Medical Centre+, Maastricht, The Netherlands

Marie-Jeanne Vrancken Peeters, Breast Surgeon, Netherlands Cancer Institute; Antoni van Leeuwenhoek, Amsterdam, The Netherlands

Anna Wagstaff, Freelance Health Journalist, Oxford, UK

Simone Wesselmann, Head of Certification Department, German Cancer Society, Berlin, Germany

Lieve Wierinck, Pharmacist, Member of the European Parliament (MEP), Belgium

Mark Woodward, Professor of Biostatistics, The George Institute for Global Health, University of Oxford, UK; and University of New South Wales, Sydney, Australia

Lynda Wyld, Professor of Surgical Oncology, University of Sheffield, UK

Cheng-Har Yip, Consultant Breast Surgeon, University of Malaya, Kuala Lumpur, Malaysia

Sophia Zackrisson, Associate Professor Diagnostic Radiology, Lund University, Malmö, Sweden

Roberto Zanetti, Director, Piedmont Cancer Registry, Turin, Italy

PART 1

EPIDEMIOLOGY

1

The Global Burden of Breast Cancer in Women

Isabelle Soerjomataram, Claudia Allemani, Adri Voogd, and Sabine Siesling

Introduction

The burden of cancer continues to increase as a result of both population ageing and growth as well as changes in lifestyle and exposure to cancer risk factors (1). Today, breast cancer is the most frequently diagnosed cancer in women, and it is the most common cause of cancer death in women (2). Throughout this chapter, we present the most up-to-date population-based estimates of breast cancer incidence and mortality using data compiled by the International Agency for Research on Cancer (IARC) and the World Health Organization (WHO), and breast cancer survival estimates from the CONCORD programme for global surveillance of cancer survival, led by the London School of Hygiene and Tropical Medicine. We only included primary, invasive breast cancer (International Classification of Diseases, 10th revision: C50), which we refer to as breast cancer. The global estimates for breast cancer incidence, survival and mortality, are dependent on the availability and accuracy of local data sources. Generally, there is a paucity of high-quality cancer registration in low-resource and medium-resource areas, and, hence, interpretation of the estimates from these regions needs to be done with caution.

Data Sources and Methods: Incidence, Survival, Prevalence, and Mortality

Cancer Incidence

Cancer incidence is the frequency of occurrence of new cases of cancer in a defined area, for a specific population, and for a given period of time (3). It can be expressed as the absolute number of cases or as incidence rate per unit time (e.g. 300 cases per 100,000 population per year), where the number of incident cases is divided by the population at risk in a specified period of time. Comparisons of incidence rates can elucidate underlying risk factors help to plan aid and prioritize resources for cancer control, and monitor and evaluate the impact of specific primary prevention interventions (4). Cancer incidence data are collected and classified in population-based cancer registries (PBCR, see Chapter 2), which are either national or regional in their coverage.

Using these data, national cancer incidence is estimated within the GLOBOCAN project for 184 countries world-wide.

Population-Based Survival

Population-based survival is estimated from data provided by PBCRs, and it is a key measure of the overall effectiveness of the health system in managing cancer in a given country or region (5). Population-based survival estimates provide a sharp contrast with survival estimates in randomized clinical trials, which are designed to determine the highest achievable survival in a group of patients selected on age, stage of disease, and lack of comorbidity by comparing short-term outcomes in patients treated either with the best-known treatment to date or with the latest proposed improvement. Trials typically involve <5% of adult cancer patients. By contrast, population-based survival is a measure of the average survival achieved by *all cancer patients*, young and old, rich and poor, with and without comorbidity, and with early or advanced disease at diagnosis. Generally, population-based survival is presented as *net survival*, which is the probability for cancer patients to survive their cancer after controlling for competing causes of death (background mortality), which are higher in the elderly (3).

Cancer Prevalence

Prevalence is the number of persons in a defined population alive at a given time, who have had cancer diagnosed at some time in the past (3). It helps to quantify the medical attention required by individuals who have been affected by cancer. Prevalence is commonly presented as limited duration (partial) prevalence, which is the number of patients diagnosed with cancer within a fixed time in the past (e.g. within the last 5 or 10 years) and is likely to be pertinent in estimating the needs for cancer services according to specific phases of cancer care (4). It can be directly estimated in PBCRs by counting the number of patients still alive, but this method requires long-term registration and follow-up. Alternatively, partial prevalence has been calculated as a product of incidence and time-specific survival (3).

Cancer Mortality

Cancer mortality measures the average risk to the population of dying from a specific cancer and provides a measure of the outcome or impact of cancer (3). Similar to incidence, it is expressed as either the number of deaths occurring or as a mortality rate per unit time. Data are derived from vital registration system, where usually a clinical practitioner certifies the fact and cause of death. The WHO mortality databank contains national cancer mortality data of ~100 countries, and, for many of these, over extended periods of time. Global mortality estimates by country are estimated at IARC and are available for 184 countries worldwide.

Global Burden of Breast Cancer

Incidence, Prevalence, and Mortality by World Region

Breast cancer is the most common cancer in women in 140 of 184 countries (Figure 1.1) and is an important cause of death from cancer. In 2012, breast cancer was responsible for an estimated 1,671,000 new cancer cases (12% of all cancers in women) and 522,000 deaths (6% of all cancer deaths in women); an estimated 6.2 million women were survivors living with a breast cancer diagnosed within the previous 5 years (partial prevalence) (6).

The risk of being diagnosed with breast cancer varies widely by world region (Figure 1.2). In North America, the risk of getting breast cancer before the age of 70 years is 8%, meaning that one out of 12 women in North America will be diagnosed with breast cancer before the age of 70 years. This is followed by 7% and 6% among women in the Oceania region and in Europe, respectively. The risk is lowest for women in Asia and sub-Saharan Africa, ranging from 2.5% to 3%. On the other hand, despite the diverse risks in getting breast cancer, the risk of dying from breast cancer is quite similar across the world region: on average only 1% of all women aged <70 years is expected to die from breast cancer.

Due to differences in population size, and Asia being the most populated region with two-thirds of the total world population, the Asian continent reports the highest number of new cancer cases (36%, including 11% in China and 9% in India) followed by Europe (28%) and North America (16%). By contrast, earlier diagnosis and more effective treatment of breast cancer lead to fewer deaths in these regions, and ultimately a higher number of survivors (prevalence), with Europe and North America showing the highest proportion of prevalent breast cancers (Figure 1.3).

International variation in breast cancer incidence and mortality has been linked to differences in risk factors, early detection practices, and to the effectiveness of cancer treatment (2). Epidemiological studies have identified various modifiable risk factors for breast cancer in the general population. The consumption of alcoholic beverages, overweight, lack of physical activity, and exposure to radiation are all factors that increase one's risk of breast cancer. About 40% of all breast cancers could have been prevented by reducing exposure to these factors, namely, alcohol consumption, adult weight gain, physical inactivity, and current postmenopausal hormone use (7). Breast cancer is also highly related to various reproductive factors, such as family history of breast cancer, personal history of benign breast disease, attained height, age at menarche, age at menopause, age at first birth, and parity. The contribution to the overall risk of breast cancer of these factors, which are generally considered as not modifiable,

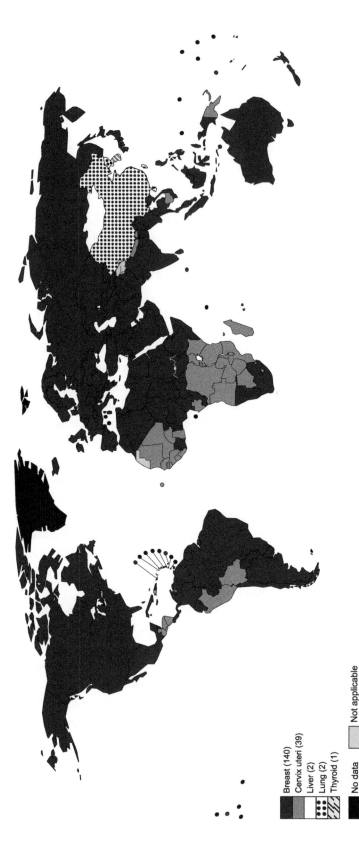

Figure 1.1 Ranking of breast cancer among all cancer diagnosis in 2012 by country. Data source: GLOBOCAN 2012.

Legend:
- Breast (140)
- Cervix uteri (39)
- Liver (2)
- Lung (2)
- Thyroid (1)
- No data
- Not applicable

The boundaries and names shown and the designations used on this map do not imply the expression of any opinion whatsoever on the part of the World Health Organization concerning the legal status of any country, territory, city or area or of its authorities, or concerning the delimitation of its frontiers or boundaries. Dotted and dashed lines on maps represent approximate border lines for which there may not yet be full agreement.

Data source: GLOBOCAN 2012
Map production: IARC
World Health Organization

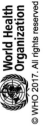
World Health Organization

© WHO 2017. All rights reserved

Reproduced with permission from Ferlay J, Soerjomataram I, Ervik M, Dikshit R, Eser S, Mathers C, Rebelo M, Parkin DM, Forman D, Bray, F. GLOBOCAN 2012 v1.0, Cancer Incidence and Mortality Worldwide: IARC CancerBase No. 11 [Internet]. Lyon, France: International Agency for Research on Cancer; 2013. Available from: http://globocan.iarc.fr

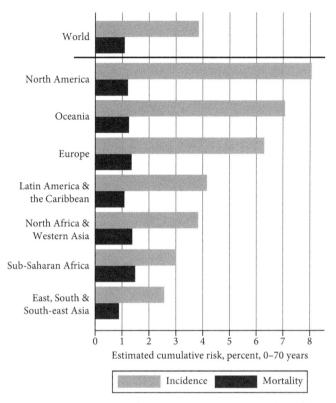

Figure 1.2 Estimated cumulative risk of being diagnosed (grey bar) and dying (dark grey bar) from breast cancer among women before 70 by world region. Data source: GLOBOCAN 2012.

Reproduced with permission from Ferlay J, Soerjomataram I, Ervik M, Dikshit R, Eser S, Mathers C, Rebelo M, Parkin DM, Forman D, Bray, F. GLOBOCAN 2012 v1.0, Cancer Incidence and Mortality Worldwide: IARC CancerBase No. 11 [Internet]. Lyon, France: International Agency for Research on Cancer; 2013. Available from: http://globocan.iarc.fr

depends on their prevalence in a population and may be substantial (8). Nonetheless, a considerable proportion of breast cancers might be avoided by adopting a healthier lifestyle.

Further international differences in breast cancer burden, namely in incidence, survival, and mortality, can be partly linked to variation in early detection programmes or breast cancer screening. In breast cancer screening, the primary target is to detect early invasive cancer, but in-situ carcinomas are also detected with up to one-fifth of the frequency of invasive cancer. Implementation of a breast cancer screening programme causes a temporary increase in incidence because of the detection asymptomatic breast cancers, that would have been diagnosed clinically at some point in the next few years. Further, it has been estimated that biannual mammography screening in females aged 50–69 years improves survival and, consequently, reduces mortality from the cancer by ~20% (7). As such, coverage, quality, and effectiveness of breast cancer screening programmes markedly affect national burden of breast cancer.

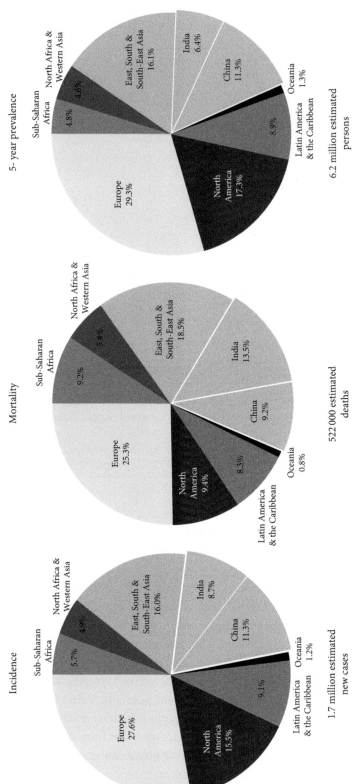

Figure 1.3 Incidence (new cases), mortality (deaths) and 5-year prevalence (survivors) of breast cancer by world region in 2012. Data source: GLOBOCAN 2012.

Reproduced with permission from Ferlay J, Soerjomataram I, Ervik M, Dikshit R, Eser S, Mathers C, Rebelo M, Parkin DM, Forman D, Bray, F. GLOBOCAN 2012 v1.0, Cancer Incidence and Mortality Worldwide: IARC CancerBase No. 11 [Internet]. Lyon, France: International Agency for Research on Cancer; 2013. Available from: http://globocan.iarc.fr

Trends in Breast Cancer Incidence and Mortality

Trends in Breast Cancer Incidence

High-quality cancer registry data provide some salient features for cancer incidence trends over time. Generally, we observed that breast cancer incidence has been increasing in almost all countries and in all age groups. The increases seem to be larger in the older age groups, with an average yearly increase of 2% (>50 years) as compared to 0.8% among the youngest age group (<50 years). In several high-income countries, e.g. the USA, Australia, and Norway, we started to find a stabilization or decline in the rate of breast cancer diagnoses for the older age groups (Figure 1.4).

These rising trends point to the westernization effect in countries, especially those in high- or medium-resource levels, which is likely linked to the increasing adoption of some reproductive, dietary, metabolic, and hormonal risk factors that are akin to those more commonly observed in the west (1). Increasing awareness of breast cancer and early detection (or screening) programmes have also been suggested to play a role in the rising rate of breast cancer, especially the early stages and in ductal carcinoma in situ (a non-invasive type of breast cancer). On the other hand, decreased use of hormonal replacement therapy (HRT) following the announcement of its carcinogenic effects has largely impacted breast cancer incidence rates, particularly in countries such as the USA, where the use of HRT was high, and this may partly explain the observed decrease in incidence rates in such populations (8).

Trends in Breast Cancer Mortality

As for mortality rate, we observed a decreasing trend across countries overall and particularly in higher-income countries in Europe, North America, and Oceania as opposed to many Asian and sub-Saharan countries, where a rising trend of death from breast cancer was still seen (Figure 1.5). The observed declines in mortality rates were largest in the youngest age group (<50 years, on average 2.5% yearly), and smallest in the oldest age group (>70 years, 0% change).

Cancer screening programmes and improvements in treatment are both major contributors to these observed favourable trends in mortality from breast cancer (7). The impact of breast cancer screening on mortality in the general population can best be seen in the age groups targeted by screening (50–69 years) and in countries where screening has been implemented since the late 1980s such as in Sweden, the UK, and the Netherlands (9). Early declines in mortality, before the start of national screening programmes and in age groups outside of the screening coverage (<50 and >70 years), suggest that improved treatment, but also population awareness and hence earlier detection, have had a major impact and explain this pattern.

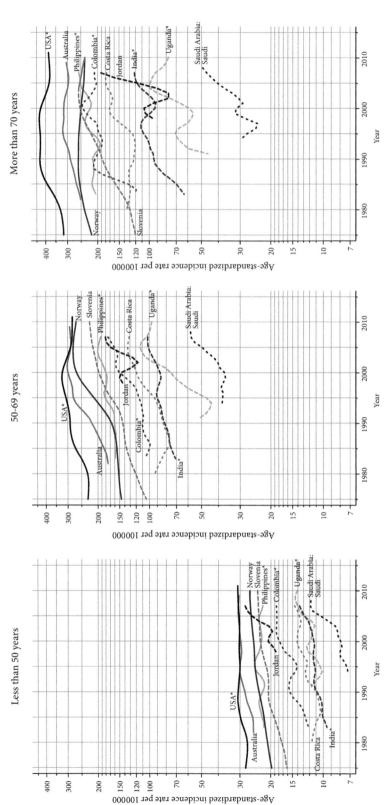

Figure 1.4 Trends in breast cancer incidence rates according to age groups (<50, 50–69, ≥70 years) in a few representative countries. Data source: Cancer Incidence in 5 Continents.

Reproduced with permission from Bray F, Colombet M, Mery L, Piñeros M, Znaor A, Zanetti R and Ferlay J, editors (2017). Cancer Incidence in Five Continents, Vol. XI (electronic version). Lyon: International Agency for Research on Cancer. Available from: http://ci5.iarc.fr

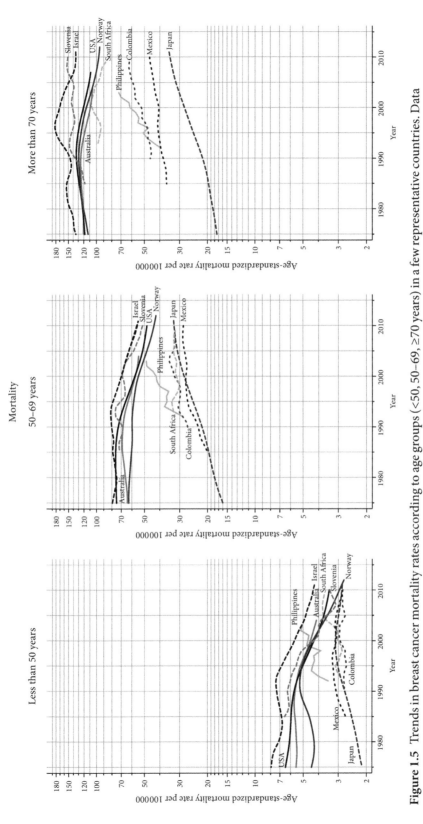

Figure 1.5 Trends in breast cancer mortality rates according to age groups (<50, 50–69, ≥70 years) in a few representative countries. Data source: WHO Mortality Database.

Reproduced with permission from Bray F, Colombet M, Mery L, Piñeros M, Znaor A, Zanetti R, and Ferlay J, editors (2017). Cancer Incidence in Five Continents, Vol. XI (electronic version). Lyon: International Agency for Research on Cancer. Available from: http://ci5.iarc.fr

Yet, without adequate management of the breast cancer, screening would only have a minor benefit, and treatment is also more likely to be effective if cancer is detected, and treated, at earlier stages. High-income countries have made remarkable progress in improving outcomes from breast cancer, whereas, in many low- and medium-resource countries, breast cancer mortality is still rising. Part of this success in high-income countries originates from better adherence to guidelines for surgery and radiotherapy, the introduction of more effective systemic treatment, namely adjuvant chemotherapy especially among patients aged <50 years, and, particularly, hormonal and targeted therapies in those aged >50 years.

Population-Based Breast Cancer Survival

Trends in Breast Cancer Survival

Population-based survival from breast cancer in women has greatly improved over the last few decades. The third cycle of the CONCORD programme analysed data for 6,422,553 women who were diagnosed with breast cancer during 2000–2014, provided by 298 cancer registries in 66 countries (10). Age-standardized 5-year net survival increased steadily in most developed countries up to 2014. For women diagnosed during 2010–2014, age-standardized 5-year net survival was ≥85% in 25 countries. However, worldwide differences in survival remain striking (Figure 1.6).

Continents are displayed from top to bottom in alphabetical order: Africa, Central and South America, North America, Asia, Europe, and Oceania. Survival estimates for each country are ranked from highest to lowest within each continent. To facilitate examination of trends, the ranking for 2010–2014 is also used for 2000–2004 and 2005–2009. Where data were available for more than one registry in a given country, the 5-year survival estimates in Figure 1.6 were derived by pooling the data for that country, excluding data from registries for which the estimates are considered less reliable.

Determinants of Breast Cancer Survival

The stage of disease at diagnosis is a key determinant of long-term survival for almost all malignancies including breast cancer. Differences in cancer survival between population subgroups, i.e. by socioeconomic status or ethnicity within a country, or between countries, may be explained, at least in part, by differences in the stage of disease at diagnosis in the cancer patient populations being compared (11). The survival of all women with breast cancer, for example, may be lower in one country than another because women in that country are generally diagnosed with more advanced disease that is less susceptible to treatment of curative intent. Alternatively, their survival may be poorer at each stage of disease, which may imply that optimal treatment is not available in that country, particularly for early-stage tumours. Thus, both more advanced disease and lower stage-specific survival may play a role in international differences in survival (5).

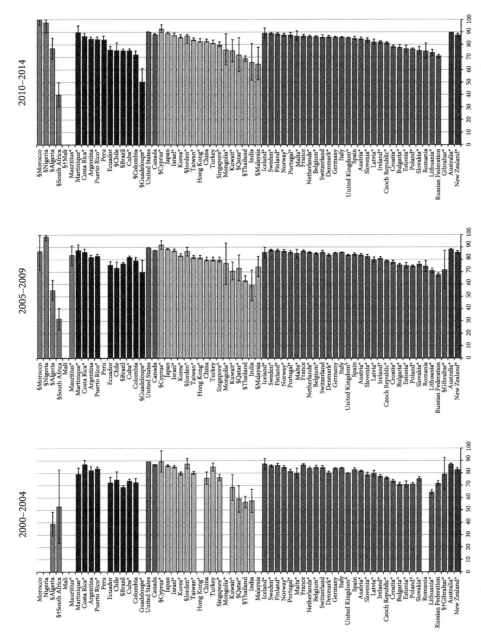

Figure 1.6 Global distribution of age-standardized 5-year net survival (%) from breast cancer in women (aged 15–99 years), by continent, country, and calendar period of diagnosis. *Data with 100% coverage of the national population. †National estimate not age-standardized. §National estimate flagged as less reliable because the only data available were from a registry or registries in this category. Data source: CONCORD programme.

Reproduced with permission from Allemani, Claudia et al. 'Global surveillance of trends in cancer survival 2000–14 (CONCORD-3): analysis of individual records for 37 513 025 patients diagnosed with one of 18 cancers from 322 population-based registries in 71 countries.' *The Lancet*, Volume 391, Issue 10125, pp. 1023–1075. Copyright © Elsevier Ltd. DOI: https://doi.org/10.1016/S0140-6736(17)33326-3.

More in-depth analyses of data on stage collected by the CONCORD programme showed that age-standardized 5-year net survival for women diagnosed during 2004–2009 with a localized tumour was ~90% or higher in most of the 62 countries (12). By contrast, survival for women diagnosed at an advanced stage varied widely between countries. The proportion of women with breast cancer who are diagnosed at an early stage seems to play a key role in the overall levels of net survival for all women combined, both in developed and developing countries.

Analyses of 5-year net survival for women diagnosed in 2005–2009 show a curvilinear relationship with gross domestic product (GDP) (13). This type of curvilinear relationship is well known between life expectancy at birth and GDP. This means that the relationship between 5-year net survival and GDP remains curvilinear, even after controlling for competing causes of death (background mortality, which is closely related to life expectancy). Thus, 5-year net survival from breast cancer increases with GDP, but reaches an asymptote around $30,000/35,000 per capita purchasing power parity (Figure 1.7, left-hand panel). In other words, above a certain level of wealth, it does not matter how rich the country is, because survival remains stable. By contrast, 5-year net survival increases more linearly with total national expenditure on health, when expressed as a proportion of GDP. Similar correlations were found for women diagnosed

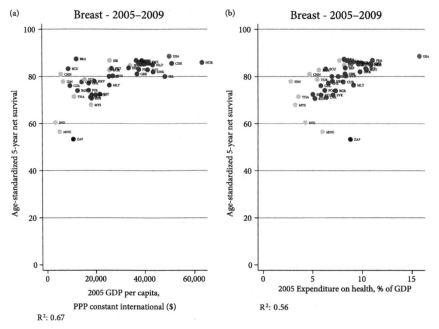

Figure 1.7 Breast cancer, 2005–2009: global distribution of age-standardized 5-year net survival (%) in adult women (aged 15–99 years), by country, gross domestic product (GDP, left-hand panel; PPP, purchasing power parity), and total national expenditure on health (right-hand panel). Data source: CONCORD programme.

Reproduced with permission from Allemani, Claudia et al. 'Global surveillance of trends in cancer survival 2000–14 (CONCORD-3): analysis of individual records for 37 513 025 patients diagnosed with one of 18 cancers from 322 population-based registries in 71 countries.' The Lancet, Volume 391 , Issue 10125, pp. 1023–1075. Copyright © Elsevier Ltd. DOI:https://doi.org/10.1016/S0140-6736(17)33326-3.

in 1995–1999 and 2000–2004 (CONCORD-2 data, not shown). Further analyses of these and more recent data are in progress.

Key Messages

- The risk of being diagnosed with breast cancer varies widely by world region.
- Breast cancer is estimated to be the most common cancer in women in 140 of 184 countries.
- Breast cancer incidence has been increasing in almost all countries and in all age groups, and the number of women diagnosed each year is projected to reach 2.2 million world-wide by 2035.
- Epidemiological studies have identified several recommendations to modify risk factors such as adopting a healthy body weight, reducing alcohol consumption, and increasing physical activity.
- Survival up to 5 years after diagnosis continues to increase, has reached ≥85% in many countries, but global variation remains wide.
- In 2012, an estimated 6.2 million women were survivors living with a breast cancer diagnosed within the previous five years.
- A decreasing trend in mortality in higher-income countries is observed, but there are also striking worldwide differences.
- Early diagnosis and access to effective treatment are crucial in order to achieve further improvements in survival and, over the longer term, reductions in mortality.

References

1. Bray F et al. Global cancer transitions according to the Human Development Index (2008–2030): a population-based study. *Lancet Oncol* 2012;13(8):790–801.
2. Torre LA et al. Global cancer in women: burden and trends. *Cancer Epidemiol Biomarkers Prev* 2017;26(4):444–457.
3. Porta M, editor. *A Dictionary of Epidemiology*, 6th ed. New York: Oxford University Press; 2014.
4. Parkin DM. The role of cancer registries in cancer control. *Int J Clin Oncol* 2008;13(2):102–111.
5. Allemani C. The importance of global surveillance of cancer survival for cancer control: the CONCORD programme. *Cancer Control* 2017:19–22.
6. Ervik M et al. Cancer Today Lyon: International Agency for Research on Cancer. 2016. Available from: http://gco.iarc.fr/today
7. Marmot MG et al., The benefits and harms of breast cancer screening: an independent review. *Br J Cancer* 2013;108(11):2205–2240.
8. Ravdin PM et al. The decrease in breast-cancer incidence in 2003 in the United States. *N Engl J Med* 2007;356(16):1670–1674.
9. Carioli G et al. Trends and predictions to 2020 in breast cancer mortality in Europe. *Breast* 2017;36:89–95.
10. Allemani C et al. Global surveillance of trends in cancer survival 2000–14 (CONCORD-3): analysis of individual records for 37 513 025 patients diagnosed with one of 18 cancers from 322 population-based registries in 71 countries. *Lancet* 2018;391:1023–1075.
11. Allemani C et al. Breast cancer survival in the US and Europe: a CONCORD high-resolution study. *Int J Cancer* 2013;132(5):1170–1181.

12. Allemani C et al., on behalf of the CONCORD Working Group. World-wide variation in breast cancer survival by age, stage, and morphology. North American Association of Central Cancer Registries; Conference proceeding 2016; St. Louis, Missouri, USA.
13. Allemani C et al., on behalf of the CONCORD Working Group. To what extent do national wealth and expenditure on health explain world-wide variation in cancer survival? North American Association of Central Cancer Registries; Conference proceeding 2015; Charlotte, North Carolina, USA.

2

Cancer Registries

Sabine Siesling, Freddie Bray, Roberto Zanetti, Tomohiro Matsuda,
Anna Gavin, Adri Voogd, Betsy Kohler, and Ryan M. McCabe

Introduction

Cancer registry actions date back to the 1900s, when a German committee for cancer research presented the first 'Klinisches Jahrbuch' describing the incidence, survival, prevalence, and mortality in Germany and Leiden, a city in the Netherlands (1). By 1946, cancer registries had been established in Hamburg in Germany, Connecticut and New York in the USA, Denmark, Belgium, Saskatchewan in Canada, England, and in Wales. To obtain comparable data, experts in clinical and experimental oncology, pathology, and cancer statistics met in September 1946 at the Danish cancer registry and decided that a proper system of data collection on cancer was required (2). The international group noted that the information available based on point prevalence data, mortality statistics, and clinical observations was inadequate, and they prepared a formal recommendation to the Interim Commission of the World Health Organization (WHO) in collaboration with the Danish and British governments. This report outlined that (3):

1. great benefit would follow the collection of data about cancer patients from as many different countries as possible;
2. such data should be recorded on an agreed plan so as to be comparable;
3. each nation should have a central registry to arrange for the recording and collection of such data;
4. there should be an international body whose duty it should be to correlate the data and statistics obtained in each country.

The recommendations were implemented by WHO and formed the impetus for building on the work of the pioneer registries to create an international forum. The WHO Subcommittee on the Registration of Cases of Cancer as well as their Statistical Presentation was based on the Copenhagen meeting recommendations, and held its first meeting in Paris in 1950. The Union for International Cancer Control (UICC) set up a Committee on Cancer Incidence in 1964, which produced a Technical Report in 1966, the first volume of *Cancer Incidence in Five Continents* (4). The International Association of Cancer Registries (IACR [http://www.iacr.com.fr/]) was subsequently established with the aim of improving the quality of data on cancer incidence and comparability between registries by standardizing methods of registration, definitions, and coding of a minimal dataset (5). This minimal dataset includes morphology of the tumour and primary site conforming to ICD-O coding and vital status. Moreover, advice on the uniform gathering of supplementary items is given, such as on stage and primary treatment. The IACR is a non-governmental organization and has been in official relations with WHO since January 1979. The IACR is a professional society dedicated to fostering the aims and activities of cancer registries worldwide. It is primarily focused on population-based registries which collect information on the occurrence and outcome of cancer in defined population groups (usually the inhabitants of a city, region, or country). The IACR convenes an annual scientific meeting that rotates through different continents to make participation possible for all members. IACR works in close collaboration with the International Agency for Research on Cancer (IARC, http://www.iarc.fr/en/about/), which is WHO's specialized cancer agency. The objective of the IARC is to promote inter-disciplinary international collaboration in cancer research and bring together skills in epidemiology, laboratory sciences, and biostatistics in order to identify the causes of cancer so that preventive measures may be adopted and the burden of disease and associated suffering reduced. IARC has an important role in describing the burden of cancer worldwide through co-operation with, and assistance to, cancer registries and in monitoring geographical variations and trends over time. Key publications include the Cancer Incidence in Five Continents series, GLOBOCAN (Figure 2.1), and the interactive web-based platform the Global Cancer Observatory (GCO, http://gco.iarc.fr/) presenting global cancer statistics to inform cancer control and cancer research.

IARC developed CanReg5, an open source tool to input, store, check, and analyse cancer registry data. It has modules to do data entry, quality control, consistency checks, and basic analyses of data. The main improvements from the previous version are the new database engine, the addition of multi-user capabilities, and the migration to an open-source platform that permits users to modify source code as needed. Also included is a tool to facilitate the establishment of a new, or modification of an existing, database by customizing fields such as adding new variables, tailoring the data entry forms, etc. More recently, additional analysis functions have been added to generate standard registry reports and allow users to customize graphics.

Cancer Registries in Low- and Middle-Income Countries

Many low- and middle-income countries lack quality data. In response, the Global Initiative for Cancer Registry Development (GICR, http://gicr.iarc.fr/) was launched in 2012. The first worldwide strategy to inform cancer control through better data, the GICR is a partnership based on the commitment of leading cancer organizations to address inequities in underserved countries. Six IARC Regional Hubs for Cancer Registration have been established to provide technical support and training for Africa, Asia, the Caribbean, Latin America, and the Pacific Islands. Each IARC Hub acts as

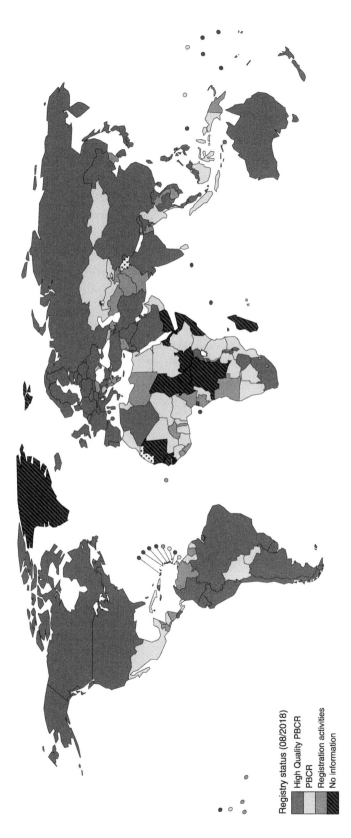

Registry status (08/2018)

- High Quality PBCR
- PBCR
- Registration activities
- No information
- Not applicable

The boundaries and names shown and the designations used on this map do not imply the expression of any opinion whatsoever on the part of the World Health Organization concerning the legal status of any country, territory, city or area or of its authorities, or concerning the delimitation of its frontiers or boundaries. Dotted and dashed lines on maps represent approximate border lines for which there may not yet be full agreement.

Data source: GICR
Map production: IARC
World Health Organization

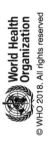

World Health Organization

Figure 2.1 Global overview of established cancer registries (2018). Data source: GICR.

Reproduced with permission from https://gicr.iarc.fr/

the main point of contact for countries within its catchment area to coordinate and deliver regional activities and strengthen capacity building. Recently, some of the Hub/Collaborating Centre countries in Asia, Latin America, and Oceania are running high-quality cancer registries themselves and providing reliable cancer statistics routinely.

Cancer Registries in Europe

The European Network of Cancer Registries (ENCR, http://www.encr.eu/) was established within the framework of the Europe Against Cancer programme of the European Commission on the initiative of IARC, Association of Nordic Cancer Registries (ANCR), IACR, and Latin Language Registry Group (GRELL) and has been in operation since 1990. Besides the minimal dataset, many of the European cancer registries gather supplementary data on stage and treatment, which leads to an increase in use of the data (6). In 2012, the two Directorate-Generals of the European Commission (DG SANTE and the DG JRC) entered a formal collaboration to address actions in support of the ENCR and have paved the way towards further coordination and harmonization of cancer data in Europe. The support has also ensured the continuity of the ENCR secretariat, including the administrative functioning and networking of the ENCR, which is hosted at the European Commission's Joint Research Centre in Ispra, Italy. ENCR is affiliated to the IACR, and by 2016 more than 200 cancer registries are active in Europe.

The Network has the following objectives:

- improve the quality, comparability, and availability of cancer incidence data;
- create a basis for monitoring cancer incidence and mortality in the European Union;
- provide regular information on the burden of cancer in Europe;
- promote the use of cancer registries in cancer control, health-care planning, and research.

Cancer Registries in North America

SEER

The Surveillance, Epidemiology, and End Results (SEER, https://seer.cancer.gov/registries/) Program of the National Cancer Institute (NCI) has been an authoritative source of information on cancer incidence and survival in the USA since 1973. SEER currently collects and publishes cancer incidence and survival data from population-based cancer registries covering approximately 28% of the US population. The SEER Program registries routinely collect data on patient demographics, primary tumour site, tumour morphology and stage at diagnosis, first course of treatment, and follow-up for vital status. The mortality data reported by SEER are provided by the National Center for

Health Statistics. The population data used in calculating cancer rates are obtained periodically from the Census Bureau. Updated annually and provided as a public service in print and electronic formats, SEER data are used by thousands of researchers, clinicians, public health officials, legislators, policymakers, community groups, and the public.

NPCR

The National Program of Cancer Registries (NPCR), administered by the Centers for Disease Control and Prevention (CDC), was established by the US Congress in 1992 through the Cancer Registries Amendment Act. Before NPCR was established, 10 states had no registry, and most states with registries lacked the resources and legislative support they needed to gather complete data. As of 2018, CDC supports central cancer registries in 46 states, the District of Columbia, Puerto Rico, the US Pacific Island Jurisdictions, and the US Virgin Islands. These data represent 97% of the US population. NPCR cancer registries collect and process more than 1.7 million new cancer cases annually. The registries collect data on patient demographics, primary tumour site, tumour morphology, stage at diagnosis, first course of treatment, and outcomes. NPCR registries also link with the National Death Index and/or conduct active patient follow-up to collect survival information. NPCR coordinates with NCI's SEER Program to produce the US Cancer Statistics, which are the official federal cancer statistics. The US Cancer Statistics include information from the entire USA and can be used to identify populations most affected by cancer, investigate potential causes of cancer, and evaluate prevention and screening activities. The data are available online (http://www.cdc.gov/uscs) and in multiple formats, including a public-use database and data visualizations tool.

NCDB

The National Cancer Database (NCDB) was founded in 1989 to capture clinical data from patients being treated in hospitals accredited by the Commission on Cancer. NCDB is jointly sponsored by the American College of Surgeons and the American Cancer Society, collects data from ~1500 accredited hospitals across 50 states, and includes more than 36 million cancer cases covering 78 different diseases. Hospital registrars abstract data on all of their reportable cancer cases and submit more than 250 data variables, including patient demographics, current AJCC staging and tumour characteristics and modalities and dates of treatment, to the NCDB for each patient. These data encompass 72% of all newly diagnosed patients in the USA. The hospital-based registries are also required to provide long-term follow-up mortality data, recurrence data, and an increasing number of organ-specific prognostic data. NCDB is a *hospital-based* registry and provides data-driven insight into the quality of patient at the point of care.

Hospitals are provided real-time data-driven web-based tools regarding individual patient alerts for timing of therapy, quality measure compliance results, and performance comparisons with regional and national benchmarks.

Historical cases diagnosed two or more years ago are used to update trends in quality measures and complex surgeries, local patient migration, and research tools such as stage-based survival statistics and de-identified, organ-based case-level data made available to Commission on Cancer member researchers, and thousands of research articles concerning these updates have been published by clinical investigators over the past several years.

The American Cancer Society Surveillance and Health Services Research division produces dozens of publications each year examining national trends in patient disease and care.

NAACCR

Established in 1987, the North American Association of Central Cancer Registries (NAACCR), Inc., is a collaborative umbrella organization for cancer registries, governmental agencies, professional associations, and private groups in North America interested in enhancing the quality and use of cancer registry data. All central cancer registries in the USA and Canada are members. NAACCR develops and promotes uniform data standards for cancer registration in North America, provides education and training, certifies population-based registries meeting objective criteria for timeliness, accuracy, and completeness of data, aggregates and publishes data from central cancer registries, and promotes the use of cancer surveillance data and systems for cancer control and epidemiologic research, public health programmes, and patient care to reduce the burden of cancer in North America. NAACCR has produced Cancer in North America for more than 20 years and works closely with cancer surveillance standard developers to ensure comparability and consistency of data throughout North America. For more information see https://www.naaccr.org/.

(Future) Use of Cancer Registry Data

In addition to the data gathered for public health indicators on the burden of cancer, aetiology, and monitoring of screening programmes, increasingly cancer registries gather supplementary data on tumour characteristics (molecular profiles), diagnostics, stage, treatment, and outcome (recurrence, and including patient reported outcome) (5). Cancer registries will soon have information on the complete personalized care pathway.

Additional data can be captured manually or by record linkage to other data sources such as clinical audit/hospital-based data, general practitioners, financial sources, and screening programmes. Linkage to screening programmes could support the monitoring of the screening centre by determining the screen-detected cancers, by giving information on stage of these screen-detected cancers, and by identifying the interval cancers. Moreover, breast cancer molecular profiles will be increasingly used to target the treatment as much as possible to patients who benefit from a specific treatment, and preventing unnecessary treatment.

Better data recording in the patient files by caregivers and record linkage offers a great opportunity to registry data for monitoring quality of cancer care and outcomes research. For example, many registries are currently developing technologies that will increase the efficiency of data collection and submission, expand the scope of disease-specific prognostic factor data, and enable the use of patient-reported outcomes and physician-based reporting.

The great advantage of cancer registry data is complete and objective data gathering, which results in comprehensive data on all newly diagnosed patients in a population. It is possible to determine the care given and monitor the implementation of novel treatment modalities in daily practice. This can provide insight into the actual delivered care, implementation of new recommendations, or novel technologies and treatment modalities as well as allow for the monitoring of quality of care and the effect on the outcome. For example, data from cancer registries on breast cancer are being used extensively to support clinical auditing (Chapter 7).

Nevertheless, one must realize that research on outcomes based on cancer registry data can be prone to confounding, since the application of care is not random. Close contact between cancer registry personnel/researchers and the researchers analysing and interpreting the data will improve the quality and ability to understand the significance of the findings. Keeping this in mind when analysing the data and interpreting results on outcomes and comparisons between groups is essential to gain more insight and support hypothesis generation for further research.

Key Messages

- Cancer registries provide insight into the burden of cancer by systematically recording data on new (pre-)malignancies and/or in-situ tumours within a specific region, area, or treatment setting.
- Cancer registries comprise an essential element in the planning and monitoring of cancer control strategies and for identifying priorities in public health.
- By incorporating more data on treatments and outcomes (such as recurrences), cancer registry data can be used for monitoring quality of care, guideline adherence, and outcome research.
- Close contact between the cancer registry, researchers, and caregivers will improve the quality and use of the data and ability to understand the significance of the findings.

References

1. Van Leyden E et al. *Klinisches Jahrbuch*. Komitee für Krebsforschung; 1900.
2. Whelan et al. International Association of Cancer Registries—a history. *Asian Pacific J Cancer Prev* 2010; 10 IACR supplement.
3. Clemmesen J. Statistical studies in the aetiology of malignant neoplasms. *Acta Pathol Microbiol Scand* 1974;Suppl 247:1–266.
4. Doll J et al. *Cancer Incidence in Five Continents: A Technical Report*. New York: Springer-Verlag; 1966.
5. Jensen OM et al. Cancer registration: principles and methods. *IACR Scientific Publication* No. 95, 1991.
6. Siesling S et al. Uses of cancer registries for public health and clinical research in Europe: results of the European Network of Cancer Registries survey among 161 population-based cancer registries during 2010–2012. *Eur J Cancer* 2015;51(9):1039–1049.

PART 2

QUALITY MANAGEMENT OF BREAST CANCER

Accreditation Programmes and Quality Control

3

Opportunities and Pitfalls of Quality Management

Didier Verhoeven, Sabine Siesling, and Lee F. Tucker

Quality Management: 'The Key to Better Care'

Quality of care has been described in several ways (1). Campbell defines two principal dimensions of quality of care for individual patients: access and effectiveness (2). The Institute of Medicine put forth one of the most influential frameworks of quality assessment, which includes the following six aims for the health care system: safe, effective, patient-centred, timely, efficient, and equitable (https://www.ahrq.gov).

Obtaining the best quality of care is a very complex process and can be achieved through good quality management consisting of a combination of tools such as guidelines, protocols, care pathways, registries, evaluation and monitoring, and improvement projects. Quality management follows the principle of the Plan–Do–Check–Act (PDCA) cycle of Deming and is a continuing process in which all phases influence one another, and where all stakeholders of the patient pathway should be closely involved (Figure 3.1). Among these stakeholders are both intra- and extra-mural caregivers, governments, clinical scientific associations, cancer societies, and patient coalitions giving input from the patients' perspective regarding needs and priorities. Health insurers can also play a role.

Five Deming Principles to Improve Health Care
(http://www.deming.org)

- Quality improvement is the science of process management.
- If you cannot measure it, you cannot improve it.
- Managed care means managing the processes of care.
- The right data at the right time in the right hands.
- Engage the smart cogs of healthcare.

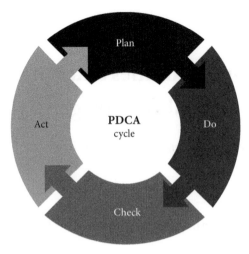

Figure 3.1 Plan–Do–Check–Act cycle of Deming.

Measuring Quality of Care: Quality Indicators

Lord Kelvin wrote: 'To measure is to know. If you cannot measure it, you cannot improve it' (3). Monitoring quality and the implementation of quality management tools can be accomplished with quality indicators, whose aim is to give insight into the quality of the provided care, guarantee a better quality of care and quality of life, and achieve a clinical outcome which approaches the requested standard, or even best practice, as closely as possible. Donabedian divided indicators into three categories: structure, process, and outcome indicators (4).

Structure indicators are related to the organization of the health care system.

Process indicators are related to the way care is given and measure what is done, often in comparison with (local) guidelines. The process indicator is expressed as a percentage based on a specific calculated field.

Outcome indicators measure the results of the given care. They are the most difficult to define and interpret because of the difficulties in tracking down the essential factors influencing the achieved value of the indicator. Moreover, outcome indicators are not easy to register, since the events of interest often take place long after treatment and possibly not in a hospital. Some examples of outcome indicators are recurrence-free survival and overall survival. Their usefulness is debatable, since they may reflect results of actions taken in the past. Treatment modalities might have changed over time, and this renders the results of the outcome indicator less valuable for a current situation.

Recently, more patient-oriented outcome indicators such as patient-reported outcomes (PROMs) and patient-reported experiences (PREMs) were identified. Both indicators assess the quality of received care from the patients' perspective. PROMs measure a patient's health-related quality of life and are collected through self-completed questionnaires (Chapter 6). PREMs focus on experiences with the structure and process and address practical issues such as waiting times, facilities, follow-up, and the experience of shared decision-making conducted mostly by questionnaires.

Criteria for Developing Quality Indicators

Quality indicators should meet specific criteria. They must be defined in such a way that the interpretation and calculation is easy. Moreover, the indicators must be reliable, not sensitive to chance, and valid. They should measure what they are supposed to measure without selection bias, measurement bias, or confounding. Related to this, indicators should also differentiate between hospitals with no influence of possible case-mix factors (differences between hospitals in underlying patient population, i.e. more severe or elderly patients) or random variation. To be able to reveal actual differences between hospitals, the number of underlying patients should be large enough to have small confidence intervals. They should be both acceptable and relevant and address the challenges confronting doctors and patients every day. They must be usable and have a high level of evidence. In order to be useful for internal improvement, they should be available in a timely manner. Moreover, they should be actionable; if the underlying factors cannot be adapted, the indicators are useless. Finally, they must incorporate medical practice, quality of life, and costs.

Indicators with no direct influence on outcomes can be presented to patients in order to help them choose the care that best fits their personal situation. The indicators should always be interpreted cautiously and be seen in light of the complete set, since one indicator can influence the other.

Furthermore, the data needed for the indicator must be easy and reliable to register with a low registration burden, and they should be cost-effective. Preferably, the data are gathered, and the indicator is generated by an independent trusted party in order to assure objectivity and prevent fraudulent reporting (5).

Development of Quality Indicators

Developing and defining quality indicators is a key service the medical community provides to society, and this process requires the participation of stakeholders such as recognized experts in the multidisciplinary breast cancer field as well as patient advocates. Knowledge and experience in the process of care, the existing guidelines, changeability, and the possibility of obtaining data for the indicators are required.

The development of indicators closely linked to the available guidelines is often accomplished using the Delphi method (http://www.thehealthcompass.org). First, an initial list of indicators is defined based on a literature review. After about two or three rounds of questionnaires and review rounds, the indicators are rated by means of pre-defined inclusion criteria resulting in a limited set of indicators describing the quality of care.

Adoption of specific indicator definitions used by other organizations or institutions is important, whenever possible, to prevent unique data collections. By standardizing the definitions of numerator and denominator, it becomes possible to compare performance measures across institutions, regions, and countries.

Quality Management with Indicators in Daily Practice

The aim of quality management is to transform the distribution function of the outcome for number of patients from a curve with a broad and flat distribution to one with a taller and narrower distribution and a better average outcome (Figure 3.2). All of this must be done while taking the financial challenge of cancer care into account, i.e. more expensive care options with a limited budget (6). However, many indicators do not lend themselves to a narrower bell-curve (Gaussian distribution). Examples are the 'wait time for screening mammogram appointment in days' or 'the % of patients biopsied with guided needle biopsy as opposed to open surgical excision'. In these examples, the goal of quality management is to shift, but not narrow, the curve (and its mean or median) towards a benchmark value (along the x-axis).

Performance, as measured by indicators, reflects the given care and is influenced by the available evidence for treatment, the patient's and doctor's preferences (ideally as a shared decision), and the health care system.

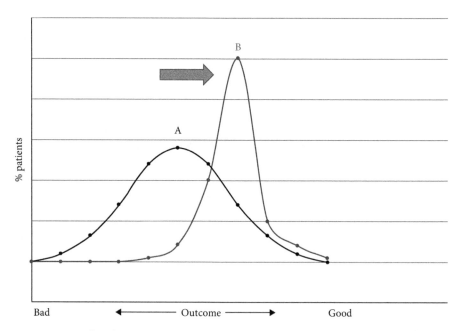

Figure 3.2 Aim of quality management: to transform the distribution function of the outcome for a number of patients from a curve with a broad and flat distribution (A) to one with a taller and narrower distribution and a better average outcome (B).

Indicators can and should be used by the breast care team to monitor the delivered practice and not used in isolation from care delivery. Regular discussion of the results of the indicators within the multidisciplinary team will keep the PDCA cycle in motion and support the continuity of the quality improvement process. Nevertheless, in practice most indicators are often only reviewed when they must be sent to the inspectorate, health insurers, or auditors.

Furthermore, only in cases where the definitions of numerator and denominator are exactly the same and data gathering has been done reliably can indicators be compared between hospitals (the so-called benchmark). Large inter-hospital variations may reflect different patient populations, lack of evidence, lack of consensus regarding scientific evidence or guidelines, or, ultimately, true differences in quality of care. Possible differences in underlying patient populations can be considered with case-mix corrections of the indicators, e.g. age or socioeconomic status.

Variation in cancer care is not wanted in cases where evidence clearly shows poorer outcomes for patients not receiving specific care. In these examples, clear guideline recommendations are preferable. Nevertheless, the correct interpretation and definition of the optimal standard may present difficulties. Quality is much more than numbers. A study conducted in the Netherlands illustrates the use of preoperative diagnostic magnetic resonance imaging (MRI) as a function of the number of breast cancer patients having surgery as their primary treatment, which showed a large variation between hospitals irrespective of patient volume (7). Which hospitals deliver health care in the most cost-effective way? Are they the ones who performed over 70%, or are they the ones with only 10% of preoperative MRI? If case variation reflects a lack of evidence, the variation seen can be used to gain new evidence by comparing outcome between the different treatment groups. In this analysis it should always be kept in mind that the groups were not generated randomly as in a randomized clinical trial, and they might be prone to confounding factors.

Moreover, the development of personalized treatment resulting in smaller patient groups will make evaluation of guidelines and monitoring care with general indicators more difficult in the future.

Variation could also represent the patients' choice of a different treatment from what the guidelines advise, either due to their social situation or to their own beliefs. Although health care outcome is often defined in terms of overall survival, progression-free survival, and quality of life, subjective toxicities and patient satisfaction with care must also be considered. What is the purpose of improving survival by three months or less, when most of that time is then spent in the hospital because of side-effects? In such cases, a 'suboptimal' outcome may be acceptable for some patients.

The process of care surrounding the patient may also have a significant impact on the outcome. Factors such as 'hospital environment' and 'patient characteristics', e.g. education and social situation, also play an important role. Problems with adherence to medication, the therapy proposed by the physician, and the application of alternative therapy are well-known factors. For example, in studying the adherence and compliance of breast cancer patients to hormonal therapy, regular intake of tamoxifen decreased to as low as 50% over a 5-year period, and a similar result was observed with aromatase inhibitors (8).

Another important issue is the patient–doctor interaction. Among UK surgeons, a variation in mastectomy rates of 20% to almost 100% was observed. This huge difference raises the question: 'Who decides the type of surgery for these women?' In addition, the analysis of the Breast Reconstruction Audit in the UK showed a very important network variation. Overall, reconstruction offered after mastectomy rates varied from 23% to 75%, whereas immediate reconstruction rates varied between 8% and 43%. An extended theory of planned behaviour could provide a basis for understanding the choices women make (attitudes, subjective norms, perceived behavioural control, and anticipated regret (9).

Looking at quality indicators from a global perspective, it is clear that guidelines for treatment and technical investigations are not uniform. Attitudes differ regarding various endpoints. Geographic and socioeconomic differences add further complications (10). Moreover, significant differences between countries are observed regarding cancer care outcomes such as mastectomy rate, reconstruction rate, percentage of screening mammographies, radiotherapy, and systemic therapy. Therefore, it is an important task of all governments to stimulate quality improvement and quality research.

Pitfalls: Critical-Confounding Factors of Quality Indicators

Many pitfalls threaten the quality management of our patients. Conflicts of interest, overuse, underuse, and misuse of diagnostic and treatment modalities may harm patients and are difficult to detect. In addition, good leadership, use of accurate data sources, optimal standards, trust, and integrity are extremely important.

The use and coupling of quality indicators to a 'Pay for Performance' system has led to some adverse effects on the quality of care. Physicians are tempted to 'game' the system to maximize their incomes (11). Several scandals have been reported concerning research fraud, fraud with waiting lists as in the Colchester Scandal in the UK, and the mismanagement at the Veterans Affairs Department and its vast network of medical facilities in the USA make us suspicious of inadequate medical care (12).

The many challenges and confounding factors present in developing high-quality indicators are obvious. They must be defined correctly and calculated using accurate data sources. In addition, we are confronted with resistance to change and difficulties with self-assessment. In most cases, organizations are not rewarded for acknowledging deficiencies. The proliferation of measures leads to measurement fatigue without commensurate results. The pitfall of having too many indicators will reflect on the registration burden. Beyond the concern of too many measurements, there is the concern that quality improvement programmes are not using the correct ones. Mostly, we focus on limited areas of care and do not consider coexisting medical conditions nor the complete care pathway outside the hospital. In addition, large parts of the clinical practice cannot be measured (e.g. a 'good' talk).

Advancements in the possibilities of electronic health record systems and third-party applications capable of integrating other outside-the-hospital-data are continuously reducing complexity and offering new modalities. Nevertheless, a balance is required between capturing all valuable information and spending an acceptable amount of time and budget on it.

Key Messages

- Overall quality of care depends on the optimal quality at any stage of the health care process.
- Clear indicators developed by experts in the multidisciplinary breast cancer field and patient advocates are the basis for any effective monitoring and evaluation system.
- Quality measurement must be integrated in daily practice (PDCA cycle) available in the electronic hospital system and not isolated from care delivery.
- Indicators and performances must be registered and monitored by an 'independent' trusted third party.
- Differences in quality indicators lead to benchmarking and better outcome at a lower cost.
- Quality measurements must lead to quality measures.
- Determination of the right standards is key.

References

1. Ayanian J and Markel H. Donabedian's lasting framework for health care quality. *N Engl J Med* 2016;21:205–207.
2. Campbell S et al. Defining quality of care. *Social Sci Med* 2000;51(11):1611–1625.
3. Manary M et al. The patient experience and health outcomes. *N Engl J Med* 2013;368:201–203.
4. Donabedian A. Evaluating the quality of medical care. *Milbank Mem Fund Q* 1966;44:166–206.
5. Verhoeven D et al. Quality management for systemic treatment of breast cancer. *Belg J Med Oncol* 2018;12(1):16–22.
6. Ganz P. Charting a new course for the delivering of high-quality cancer care. *J Clin Oncol* 2013;36:4485–4487.
7. van Bommel AC et al. Clinical audit as an instrument for quality improvement in breast cancer care in the Netherlands: the NABON breast cancer audit. *J Surg Oncol* 2017;115(3):243–249.
8. Niravath P et al. Aromatase inhibitors adverse effects: are we sweeping them under the rug. *J Clin Oncol* 2014;32:3779.
9. Swell S et al. Factors influencing the surgery intentions and choices of women with early breast cancer: the predictive utility of an extended theory of planned behavior. *BMC (Med Inform Decis Mak)* 2013;13:92.

10. Wheeler S et al. Disparities in breast cancer treatment and outcomes: biological, social and health system determinants and opportunities for research. *Oncologist* 2013;1:986–993.
11. Bloche M. Scandal as a sentinel event—recognizing hidden cost-quality trade-offs. *N Engl J Med* 2016;374:1001–1003.
12. Miller S and Wherry L. Health and access to care during the first 2 years of the ACA Medicaid expansions. *N Engl J Med* 2017;376:947–956.

4

EUSOMA

Pioneering Mastology and Breast Centres Networking

Lorenza Marotti, Luigi Cataliotti, and Robert Mansel

EUSOMA

The European Society of Breast Cancer Specialists (EUSOMA) (1) is the only multi-disciplinary society dedicated to breast cancer. EUSOMA aims to harmonize breast cancer care in Europe, foster the set-up of certified Breast Centres, and improve quality control.

Following the first European Breast Cancer Conference, EUSOMA defined the requirements for a specialist Breast Centre in 2000 (2), and these requirements are regularly updated (3).

The basic requirements include the minimum number of new breast cancer cases, i.e. 150 new breast cancers each year, provision of all services necessary from genetics and prevention through the diagnosis and treatment of primary tumour, follow-up, the care of advanced disease, and palliation. The Breast Centre must have a dedicated team of specialists who regularly meet in the multidisciplinary meeting. The Breast Centre must have a database to perform regular data collection and auditing. This is facilitated by a dedicated breast data manager.

Through this publication (2,3), EUSOMA emphasized two basic concepts in breast cancer care: multidisciplinary approach and quality control, which were not consolidated behaviours in the early 2000s.

In 2010, Eusoma published a position paper describing a set of benchmark quality indicators that could be adopted by Breast Centres to allow standardized auditing and quality assurance as well as establish an agreed minimum standard of care (4). This publication was recently updated to include new scientific knowledge in the field (5).

Following the first EUSOMA publication on the requirements for a Breast Centre (2), dedicated health professionals began to evaluate their activity and compliance and to measure themselves with the EUSOMA requirements; this rapidly became the reference document with regard to the requirements for a Breast Centre, not only for the scientific community but also for national governments regulating breast disease management within their own country.

With this in mind, EUSOMA developed a voluntary certification process, (i) to monitor Breast Unit compliance based on annual site visit and yearly data transfer on primary breast cancers, and (i) monitor Breast Unit performance with regard to

EUSOMA requirements and Quality Indicators (QIs) (4). Interest in this process grew at European level, and Breast Units were enthusiastic for such a peer-to-peer process. Therefore, following the pilot phase a dedicated organization was set up to run the process to comply with EU regulation on certification.

In the 2013 Breast Centre Certification, a partnership between a scientific non-profit organization (BCCert) and a certification body (Italcert) was set up in order to run the voluntary European certification process on Eusoma requirements (3), which subsequently gained accreditation by the Italian Accreditation body. As this national body is part of the European Accreditation Multilateral Agreement, the certificates issued have value among the European signatory countries. This recognition is important, because it gives an added value to the certification itself.

In the last few years, not only have dedicated health professionals shown great interest in the process, but also hospital managements now consider this voluntary certification process a constructive way to monitor the performance and activity of their breast centre.

The certification process allows breast centres to improve the quality process in terms of modifying clinical attitudes towards the benefit of increased quality in the standard of care as well as to dedicate sufficient time to regularly monitor and analyse the breast centre organization, activity, and performance.

The certification process lasts three years. Entry requirements are that the Breast Centre treats at least 150 newly diagnosed breast cancer cases annually, has a clinical director, and uses a database validated by EUSOMA, because data monitoring is an important step of the audit process.

A Breast Centre undergoing the process is requested to fill in an online questionnaire based on the EUSOMA requirements. The questionnaire aims to check the availability of data to ensure the feasibility of the audit visit and enables the auditors to have an overview of the Breast Centre before the visit.

In the first year, an initial audit is conducted to evaluate all EUSOMA requirements. The visiting team comprises five experts, i.e. a lead auditor coordinating the visit, a surgeon, a radiologist, a pathologist, and a breast care nurse. During the visit, the experts meet their local colleagues in the different disciplines, visit the breast centre, and, supported by documents of evidence, go through the patient pathway to objectively evaluate compliance with EUSOMA requirements. The visiting team also observes a multidisciplinary meeting (MDM) run by the Breast Centre, because the MDM represents one of the core tasks of the breast centre in terms of deciding the most appropriate treatment modality for each patient. The visiting team does not participate in the MDM decision-making process, but simply observes the conduct of the MDM.

At the end of the visit, the audit team has a private internal meeting and issues a report in which any non-conformity on mandatory requirements, recommendations, and observations are highlighted. The report is presented and discussed with the Breast Centre during the closing meeting.

Following the audit, the Breast Centre is required to send a proposal for corrective actions, which should list actions regarding the recommendations listed in the audit report. Non-conformities must be resolved within four months, and the evidence for changes is reviewed prior to issuing certification. BCCert experts review these documents, and, following a positive evaluation, the Breast Centre can be certified and be listed in the directory of certified Breast Centres.

The Breast Centre certification scheme (6) focuses on real data, essential clinical skills, structure and procedure, and aims to improve the quality process in terms of modifying clinical attitudes to the benefit of increased quality in the standard of care and dedicating sufficient time to a multidisciplinary analysis of the Breast Centre organization, activity, and performance.

In order to monitor Breast Centre adherence to EUSOMA QIs (4,5), EUSOMA has created a data warehouse to which Breast Centres undergoing certification transfer anonymous data on a yearly basis. The EUSOMA data centre then performs an analysis on the data and issues a data report showing Breast Centre performance on the selected QIs (see Table 4.1).

Breast Centres undergoing certification have generally already reached a good level of performance, but continued monitoring, auditing, and benchmarking helps maintain a high standard, improve data collection, and adherence to guidelines.

Because of the availability of this prospectively collected data and analysis, Breast Centres under the umbrella of EUSOMA may collectively publish scientific papers on selected topics. Through these kinds of publications, the impact of EUSOMA certification has been evaluated with respect to the evolution, i.e. before and after certification, of the Breast Centres' performance regarding quality indicators (7). This study showed a great improvement for the following quality indicators: preoperative definitive diagnosis, complete pathological recording for invasive carcinoma, postoperative radiation therapy for invasive cancer following conservative surgery, and ductal carcinoma insitu treatment without axillary clearance. Such an improvement is part of an active process of auditing, analysing, and monitoring performance. This study showed that dedicated Breast Centres are already providing a high level of care when they approach the certification process, but that such a process is pivotal in monitoring, improving, and sharing new challenges in improving care for breast cancer patients.

Data monitoring is also important for monitoring changes in treatment following new information from new trials, is helpful in identifying the need to update recommendations, and is a tool for validating the introduction of new quality indicators.

Key Messages

- EUSOMA has defined the requirements for a specialized Breast Centre and the quality indicators for breast cancer care.
- EUSOMA fosters a multidisciplinary approach to the management of Breast Cancer.
- EUSOMA has developed an active process of auditing, analysing, and monitoring Breast Centre performance.

Table 4.1 List of selected indicators for certification

	Indicator	Minimum standard	Target
1	Proportion of women with breast cancer (invasive or in situ) who had a preoperative histologically or cytologically confirmed malignant diagnosis (B5 or C5).	85%	90%
2	Proportion of invasive cancer cases for which the following prognostic/ predictive parameters have been recorded: histological type (according to WHO Classification of Tumours of the Breast), grading (according to WHO and EU Guidelines: Elston and Ellis modified Bloom and Richardson Grading system), ER, PgR*, HER-2/neu, Proliferation index (Ki67)*. *This marker is recommended but not mandatory, and does not need to be included in the calculation for compliance with the QI For patients receiving primary systemic treatment (PST), characterization on core biopsy prior to therapy is mandatory. For patients receiving primary surgery, characterization may be performed on the surgical specimen only. In addition to the above parameters, the following parameters must be recorded after surgery: pathological stage (pT and pN, or ypT and ypN in case of PST), Size in mm for the invasive component, Peritumoral vascular invasion (L,V), Distance to nearest radial margin	95%	98%
3	Proportion of non-invasive cancer cases for which the following prognostic/predictive parameters have been recorded: Grading (according to WHO Classification of Tumours of the Breast), dominant histologic pattern, size in mm (best pathology or radiology estimate if 2 stage pathology), distance to nearest radial margin, ER.	95%	98%
4	Proportion of patients with invasive breast cancer (M0) who received post-operative radiation therapy (RT) after surgical resection of the primary tumour and appropriate axillary staging/surgery in the framework of BCT.	90%	95%
5	Proportion of patients (BRCA1 and BRCA2 patients excluded) with invasive breast cancer not greater than 3 cm (total size, including DCIS component) who underwent BCT as primary treatment.	70%	85%
6	Proportion of patients with non-invasive breast cancer not greater than 2cm who underwent BCT.	80%	90%
7	Proportion of patients with DCIS only who do not undergo axillary clearance.	97%	99%
8	Proportion of patients with endocrine sensitive invasive cancer who received endocrine therapy.	85%	90%
9	Proportion of patients with ER– (T > 1 cm or Node+) invasive carcinoma who received adjuvant chemotherapy.	85%	95%
10	Proportion of patients (invasive cancer only) who received a single (breast) operation for the primary tumour (excluding reconstruction).	80%	90%
11	Proportion of patients (DCIS only) who received just one operation (excluding reconstruction).	70%	90%
12	Proportion of patients with invasive cancer and clinically negative axilla who underwent sentinel lymph-node biopsy (SLNB) only (excluding patients who received PST).	90%	95%

Table 4.1 Continued

	Indicator	Minimum standard	Target
13	Proportion of patients receiving immediate reconstruction after mastectomy.	40%	NA
14	Proportion of patients with invasive cancer who underwent sentinel lymph-node biopsy with no more than 5 nodes excised.	90%	95%
15	Proportion of patients with HER2 positive (IHC 3+ or fluorescent in-situ hybridization positive) invasive carcinoma (T > 1 cm or N+) treated with chemotherapy who received adjuvant trastuzumab.	85%	95%
16	Proportion of treated patients for which the breast centre collects data on life status and recurrence rate (for at least 5 years).	80%	90%
17	Ratio of benign to malignant diagnoses based on definitive pathology report (surgery only, non-operative biopsies excluded).	1:4	1:5

For the complete description of each of the above indicators, please refer to the Eusoma document "Quality indicators in breast cancer care".

Reproduced with permission from Biganzoli, L. et al. 'Quality indicators in breast cancer care: An update from the EUSOMA working group.' *European Journal of Cancer*. Volume 86, pp. 59–81. Copyright © Elsevier Ltd. DOI: https://doi.org/10.1016/j.ejca.2017.08.017

References

1. EUSOMA [Internet]. Available from: https://www.eusoma.org/
2. Blamey RW and Cataliotti L. The requirements of a specialist breast unit. *Eur J Cancer* 2000;36(18):2288–2293.
3. Wilson AR et al. The requirements of a specialist Breast Centre. *Eur J Cancer* 2013;49(17):3579–87.
4. M. Rosselli Del Turco et al. Quality indicators in breast cancer care. *Eur J Cancer* 2010;46:2344–2356.
5. Biganzoli L et al. Quality indicators in breast cancer care: an update from the EUSOMA working group. *Eur J Cancer* 2017;86:59–81.
6. Breast Centres Certification [Internet]. Available from: https://www.breastcentrescertification.com/
7. van Dam PA, et al. EusomaDB Working Group. The effect of EUSOMA certification on quality of breast cancer care. *Eur J Surg Oncol* 2015;41(10):1423–1429.

5

What Defines a Breast Centre?
An NAPBC Vision

Cary S. Kaufman and Terry Sarantou

Breast Centre Definitions

Since breast cancer is the most common cancer in women over most of the globe, the organized approach to diagnosis and treatment should be easily defined. Breast centres and breast units populate all major cities and countries, yet a unified definition of a breast centre or unit has not been accepted. There are several definitions from major organizations:

- European Society of Breast Cancer Specialists (EUSOMA) definition (1): 'The Breast Centre is made up by a cohesive group of dedicated breast cancer specialists working together as a multidisciplinary team with access to all the facilities required to deliver high quality care throughout the breast cancer pathway ... from genetics and prevention, through the treatment of the primary tumour, to care of advanced disease, palliation and survivorship.'
- National Accreditation Program for Breast Centers (NAPBC) definition (2): 'A breast centre provides comprehensive care that has met or exceeds quality standards established by the National Accreditation Program for Breast Centers.'
- National Quality Measures for Breast Centers (NQMBC) definition (3): 'The definition of a breast center is a physical setting where breast health care services are provided. The management of breast diseases ... requires the interaction of multiple specialists ... surgery, medical oncology, radiation oncology, radiology, pathology, plastic surgery, physical therapy, behavioral medicine and nursing. Quality care means providing the patient with accurate evaluation and appropriate services with compassion in a technically competent and timely manner, with good communication and shared decision making in a culturally sensitive fashion.'

The common threads noted in all these statements define the building blocks of optimal breast care. Breast centres should have the following components which will be clarified throughout this book. The building blocks of breast centres are described in Table 5.1.

Table 5.1 Components of a breast centre

Breast programme leadership with local authority	A small leadership team of the breast centre with authority to direct actions and direction of the breast centre.
Multidisciplinary providers of care	A team of dedicated clinical professionals with specialty expertise with regards to breast disorders.
Regular multidisciplinary breast conferences	Regularly scheduled multidisciplinary meetings of the breast centre clinical team with pretreatment discussion of all patients.
Set of approved treatment guidelines	An agreed upon set of standards, guidelines or treatment schemes that guide the initial approach for each unique clinical situation.
Concurrent database management	Ongoing real-time monitoring of clinical care facilitated by maintaining a database on all patients.
Maintained equipment for diagnosis and treatment	A fully equipped breast centre with up-to-date supplies and functioning equipment within the practical restrictions of the region.
Quality improvement programmes	Regular quality improvement projects initiated and completed by the multidisciplinary team and reported to the breast centre leadership. This may often include clinical research projects.
Clinical research opportunities	Provide patients with opportunities to participate in clinical research.
Community outreach and awareness programmes	Outreach efforts to provide and inform the local community of the need for screening as defined by your region.

The NAPBC in the USA has established a set of standards that embody these principles for breast centres (4). The first three foundation requirements include the leadership team, multidisciplinary care, and a regularly scheduled multidisciplinary meeting to recommend and coordinate care. All breast centres must have these three components to be accredited (5). In the USA, the term 'accredited breast center' is used rather than 'certified breast center' as is common in Europe.

A Leadership Team (Mandatory)

A designated leadership team of the breast centre should have the authority to direct actions and direction of the breast centre. Since breast centres may reside within larger medical facilities, it is important that there is some ability for self-control of the actions of the breast centre. Without the authority to decide on directions, many breast centres fail in their ability to provide the optimal care. Although there may be a single individual identified as the leader, often designated leadership will be a small team of specialists who make strategic decisions for the breast centre to confirm the centre stays on a course of optimal care for their patients (NAPBC Standard 1.1) (4).

Multidisciplinary Care (Mandatory)

The breast centre engages a team of dedicated professionals. For any woman with a breast cancer diagnosis, a team of clinicians is required to provide optimal care. The team has a central core including a breast imager, a pathologist, a breast surgeon, a medical oncologist, a radiation oncologist, a plastic surgeon, a breast care nurse (navigator), and a psycho-oncologist. Beyond that core team are administrators, technologists, mammographers, physical therapists, rehabilitation specialists, psychologists/therapists, and social workers. Even beyond those clinicians are other supportive individuals. The key ingredients require that each individual is dedicated, competent, experienced, and maintains their competence with ongoing education. Current education activities should be monitored. Individual sites and countries may provide their own definitions of these criteria of professional competence based on local or regional standards. Yet, the constant theme must be proficiency and experience in their discipline as it relates to breast cancer diagnosis and treatment. Ideally, common requirements will be applied to all breast centres in each region (NAPBC Standards 2.1, 2.2, 2.8, 2.10, 2.11, 2.12, 2.13, 2.14, 2.15, 2.16, 2.18, 2.19, 5.1) (4).

Multidisciplinary Meetings (Mandatory)

Multidisciplinary meetings of the breast centre team are scheduled at frequent regular intervals. Perhaps the most important aspect of a breast centre is the agreement to approach each patient in a multidisciplinary way. Each patient will receive the benefit of all the breast care specialties by having their case presented on a regular basis to the multidisciplinary conference. At each conference, attendance is taken to document that all specialties and all active breast centre participants attend the meeting to provide a healthy discussion on each new and returning patient. It is essential that discussions take place before any major treatment has occurred. Many centres will have a conference discussion after initial diagnosis (e.g. needle biopsy), and then a second multidisciplinary discussion after initial treatment (e.g. surgery). Further discussion on this topic may be found in Chapter 10 (NAPBC Standard 1.2) (4).

Evidence-Based Guidelines

A set of standards, protocols, guidelines, or treatment schemes that guide initial approach to care for each unique clinical situation are available. Since no single set of guidelines can provide the answers to all situations, the set of documents noted here is used to initiate the discussion and approach to clinical situations. Thereafter, with discussion and the joint experience of the group, decisions of care can be generated from the outlines provided by this set of standard approaches. When the team of professionals is gathered in meetings, a mutually agreed-upon set of guidelines promotes uniformity of care within the breast centre. Ongoing monitoring of results of treatment using a database is a vital part of providing comprehensive breast cancer care. All patients should be entered into the breast centre database for long-term assessment of quality (NAPBC Standard 1.3) (4).

Equipment

Breast centre equipment must be up to date and current within the practical limits of the region. Breast cancer is the first or second most common cancer in women around the globe. Since it affects all areas, regional financial support for breast centres will, to some degree, determine the spectrum of equipment available to each breast centre. With that in mind, there are some pieces of equipment that are vital to the success of any breast centre. Equipment is not limited to mammogram machines or breast magnetic resonance imaging, but also includes the spectrum of surgical and pathology laboratory equipment needed to obtain and examine each patient's findings (NAPBC Standards 2.8, 2.10, 2.11, 2.12) (4).

Clinical Database Management

Ongoing monitoring of clinical care as well as quality assurance with continuous quality-of-care monitoring requires a concurrent clinical database. Changes in breast cancer care occur at a rapid pace, and breast centres must continually assess whether they are providing state-of-the-art quality care. A database should be available to enter clinical data on all patients seen at the breast centre that includes information of their entire breast care journey. The database should be current, searchable, and regularly report outcomes based on database content. In addition, specific quality measures and programmes should be integrated in the care of all breast cancer patients. These quality measures may be sourced from programmes like the NAPBC, NQMBC (3), EUSOMA, SIS, and other regional quality programmes (e.g. the German system (6)) (NAPBC Standards 2.3, 2.4, 2.5, 2.6, 2.7, 2.9, 2.20) (4).

Quality Improvement and Research

Regular quality improvement projects should be initiated and completed by the multidisciplinary team and reported to the breast centre leadership. During administrative meetings or multidisciplinary meetings, areas for quality improvement may become apparent. Resources should be dedicated to investigate those areas and consider options for improvement. The real-time clinical database will be helpful in gathering data on specific quality questions to achieve valid answers. Each year, several quality questions should be initiated, researched and results reported to the breast centre leadership. It is helpful to compare performance with other similar centres. Performance comparisons may be found in programs such as the National Quality Measures for Breast Centres (3). Focused research projects may also highlight quality care. A breast centre should provide patients with information on the availability of applicable clinical trials and offer patients the opportunity to participate in the advancement of evidence-based medicine (NAPBC Standards 3.1, 3.2, 6.1) (4).

Community Outreach

The breast centre's outreach efforts educate the local community of breast health and provide the value of screening as defined by your region. Regardless of the country, some patients arrive too late to benefit from modern treatment. Increasing breast health awareness to the community surrounding the breast centre should be an obligation of each breast centre. A competent and fully equipped breast centre without any patients is an unfortunate situation. Methods of ongoing outreach should be developed and maintained to ensure that those who will benefit from a high-quality breast centre are made aware and seek care (NAPBC Standards 2.17, 4.1) (4).

Summary

Although there are multiple definitions of a breast centre, the list of breast centre components in Table 5.1 helps define the optimal breast centre. This list also helps developing breast centres ensure comprehensive care for their patients by attending to the list of standards and components. Guided by this chapter and bringing together specialists with the goals of providing comprehensive multidisciplinary care will optimize breast cancer care in your community.

Key Messages

- Breast centres require defined leadership with authority over the centre's actions and direction.
- All breast centres should provide multidisciplinary breast cancer clinicians who meet regularly to discuss patients at diagnosis and treatment.
- A current maintained clinical database is essential to assess breast centre performance and quality.
- Breast health education and outreach to their local community is a responsibility of each breast centre.
- The NAPBC maintains a list of quality standards to monitor breast centre performance.

References

1. Cardoso F et al. European Breast Cancer Conference manifesto on breast centres/units. *Eur J Cancer* 2017;72:244–250.
2. National Accreditation Program for Breast Centers. Available from: https://www.facs.org/quality-programs/napbc/accreditation/resources/patient-resources/faq
3. National Consortium of Breast Centers I. Becoming a Certified Quality Breast Center of Excellence. Available from: https://www.nqmbc.org/
4. NAPBC Standards. Available from: https://www.facs.org/quality-programs/napbc/standards
5. Moran M, et al. What currently defines a breast center? Initial data from the national accreditation program for breast centers. *J Oncol Pract* 2013;9(2):e62–e70.
6. Wallwiener M, et al. Multidisciplinary breast centres in Germany: a review and update of quality assurance through benchmarking and certification. *Arch Gynecol Obstet* 2012;285(6):1671–1683.

6

A View on Patient-Reported Outcome Measures

François P. Duhoux and Rishi Hazarika

Patient-Reported Outcome Measures

Breast cancer treatments vary widely across institutions and countries. Nowadays, since different treatments may lead to equivalent survival outcomes, the value each patient places on potential gains and losses associated with each treatment option plays an important role in the treatment choice.

Monitoring symptoms and health-related quality of life (HRQoL) has been shown to improve not only patient satisfaction but also clinical outcomes, to reduce the number of emergency room visits and hospitalizations, to allow longer duration of palliative chemotherapy, and to increase quality-adjusted survival (1). Because health care professionals or relatives give a less accurate estimate of HRQoL than patients themselves, patient-reported outcome measures (PROMs) are being used more frequently to monitor HRQoL. They are captured by asking patients to complete questionnaires about their functioning and wellbeing.

PROM tools such as the European Organisation for Research and Treatment of Cancer (EORTC) Quality of Life Questionnaire C-30 (for cancer) and BR-23 (specifically for breast cancer) have been validated for use in research and routine settings. However, whereas they are widely used in a clinical research setting, their implementation into routine clinical practice is, unfortunately, still very limited. This may be due to the length of the questionnaires themselves or to the lack of enthusiasm of health care professionals to implement these tools more broadly.

The International Consortium for Health Outcomes Measurement (ICHOM) strives to develop standardized health outcome measures for the most frequent diseases. Their mission is to 'unlock the potential of value-based health care by defining global Standard Sets of outcome measures that really matter to patients for the most relevant medical conditions and by driving adoption and reporting of these measures worldwide.' (2). These standard sets have a fourfold aim:

- reduce health care costs by preventing medical errors and unnecessary treatments;
- support informed decision-making and allow patients to choose their physician based on valid data;
- support informed decision-making by enabling physicians to better discuss treatment options with their patients;

- improve health care quality by allowing physicians to compare their health outcomes data to other providers.

The breast cancer standard set (Figure 6.1) was recently published in *JAMA Oncology* following a rigorous process in which patients, health care providers, and health registries prioritized a series of potential health outcomes regarding the relevance of these outcomes for patients (3). Using a predefined methodology initially developed at Harvard Business School, 26 health care providers and patient advocates developed this standard set, which encompasses survival, cancer control, and disutility of care outcomes (e.g. acute treatment complications) to be collected through administrative data and/or clinical records. Selected case-mix factors are to be collected at baseline.

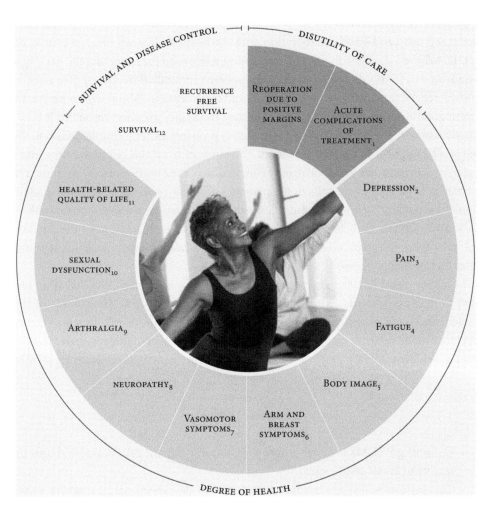

Figure 6.1 The ICHOM Breast Cancer Standard Set comprises items related to degree of health, survival, disease control, and disutility of care.
Reproduced courtesy of Matthew Billingsley
More information can be found at: http://www.ichom.org/medical-conditions/breast-cancer/

Most importantly, the ICHOM standard set relies on a combination of multiple PROM tools to capture long-term degree of health outcomes. The following outcomes are thus captured in all patients: overall wellbeing, physical, emotional, cognitive, social, and sexual functioning, ability to work, anxiety, depression, insomnia, financial impact, pain, fatigue, and body image. In addition, patients treated with surgery and/or radiotherapy are asked to complete questionnaires about satisfaction with breast(s), arm symptoms, and breast symptoms, whereas patients receiving systemic therapy are interrogated on vasomotor symptoms, peripheral neuropathy, vaginal symptoms, and arthralgia.

The ICHOM breast cancer standard set can be used for both the early and the metastatic setting. Some outcomes that are traditionally gathered in the context of breast cancer have been removed, such as progression-free survival, because these were judged non-essential for patients.

Implementing the standard set is both complex and time-consuming. It requires a dedicated team and good collaboration with the hospital IT team. It is, of course, essential to have a database in place, but the parameters used for exporting the data must be adapted to ICHOM's requirements. The patient's individual treatment plan must be considered, because patients receiving different treatment modalities will complete different questionnaires. It is also essential to have the ability to collect these PROMs in a timely manner. The pen-and-paper approach is probably easier to implement initially, but it also requires more staff to encode the answers from the questionnaires into a database. On the other hand, electronic completion of the questionnaires (prompted by e-mails sent at regular intervals to the patients) does not require any additional handling of the data by the site staff, but it has been shown that patients' responses to these e-mails are limited. Only a small number of hospitals currently implement the standard set, but others will join, once they realize the clear advantages that such a system can offer for the quality of care.

In addition to PROMs, patient-reported experience measures (PREMs) were created to measure patients' experience with health care providers. An example of this stakeholder involvement is the Dutch Consumer Quality Index (4). Despite the importance of the patient's experience in metastatic breast cancer, little research has been conducted. Measurements such as PREMs must be easy to complete, requiring ≤5 min.

Key Messages

- Collecting PROMs is key in improving not only patient satisfaction but also the quality of breast cancer care.
- This process will likely become mandatory in developed nations, where value-based health care is becoming increasingly popular.
- The implementation of a standard set, such as that proposed by ICHOM, requires resources and dedicated site personnel, which are not feasible in all countries.
- The greatest added value of PROMs will be the direct feedback in the consulting room to support detection of complaints and need for care.

References

1. van Roij J et al. Measuring health-related quality of life in patients with advanced cancer: a systematic review of self-administered measurement instruments. *Qual Life Res* 2018;27(8):1937–1955.
2. ICHOM (International Consortium for Health Outcomes Measurement). Available from: http://www.ichom.org/
3. Ong WL et al. A standard set of value-based patient-centered outcomes for breast cancer. *JAMA Oncol* 2017;3(5):677 685.
4. Delnoij D et al. The Dutch Consumer Quality Index: an example of stakeholder involvement in indicator development. *BMC Health Services Res* 2010;10:88.

7

Examples of National Programmes on Quality Management

Sabine Siesling, Jumana Mensah, Sara Y. Brucker, Simone Wesselmann,
Marie-Jeanne Vrancken Peeters, Aafke Honkoop, Francisco Terrier,
Federico Coló, and Tomiro Matsuda

The German Perspective

The German Cancer Society (Deutsche Krebsgesellschaft) and the German Society for Breast Diseases (Deutsche Gesellschaft für Senologie) introduced, with strong support from self-help groups, a joint certification system for Breast Cancer Centres in 2003. This initiative was based on the findings of the EUROCARE project, which revealed a 5-year survival of 70% for breast cancer patients diagnosed in Germany between 1978 and 1985 (1). This survival rate placed Germany in an intermediate band among the European member states. In line with the European Parliament motion for a resolution on breast cancer in the European Union, the certification system was designed to permit 'all women suffering from breast cancer ... to be treated by a multidisciplinary team' and 'to establish a network of certified multidisciplinary breast centres which cover the entire population' (2).

Structure of the Certification System

The certification system is geared towards the organization and amelioration of multidisciplinary, cross-sectoral, and multi-professional cooperation in oncologic care. Its starting point was the cooperation of providers of breast cancer care in certified Breast Cancer Centres. According to the German Cancer Plan (http://www.bmg.bund.de/nationaler-krebsplan), a Cancer Centre is a structured (regional) 'network of qualified and jointly certified, multi- and interdisciplinary, trans-sectoral ... facilities ... which ... covers, if possible, the entire chain of care' (3). Hence, all specialist disciplines and professional groups relevant to (breast) cancer care must be integrated into the structure of the centre.

To ensure a maximum level of transparency and reliability, the certification system is subject to a separation of powers.

THE GERMAN PERSPECTIVE 51

1. The legislative powers reside with an independent and multidisciplinary certification commission. The commission assembles nominated representatives from scientific societies of all medical specialties and disciplines involved in breast cancer care (including gynaecologists, radio-oncologists, pathologists, radiologists, etc.) as well as representatives of psychosocial care and cancer registries. Patient perspectives are represented in the system through involvement of self-help group representatives. The certification commission works under the chairmanship of the German Cancer Society, which provides the organizational frame for the certification process.

2. The executive part of the certification system is represented by oncology specialists, who ascertain adherence to all certification requirements. This is achieved by systematic review of the centre's documentation followed by standardized annual audits on site. The auditors are experts in breast cancer care, are guided by the independent certification institute OnkoZert, and participate in specific training on all aspects of the certification process prior to their service. To ensure clear division of all three parts of the certification system, auditors are not permitted to be active panel members in the certification commission.

3. Audit results are summarized in an audit report and include a recommendation by the auditor as to whether the certificate should be awarded. This report, along with the documentation provided by the centre, is submitted to a Certificate Award Committee for final evaluation and decision. This committee consists of three auditors for every certification procedure and constitutes the judicial force in the certification system. Committee members are excluded from active participation in the certification commission to assure sovereignty of all certification bodies.

Quality Indicators

In collaboration with the German Guideline Program in Oncology (GGPO, https://www.leitlinienprogramm-onkologie.de), tumour-specific quality indicators (QIs) are derived from the evidence-based national treatment guideline for breast cancer (3). The certification requirements, as defined by the certification commission, include quality standards that best outline the specific requirements of optimal breast cancer care for every discipline as well as the QIs derived from the national treatment guideline (http://ecc-cert.org/certification-system/organ-cancer-centre). Implementation of these indicators, and therefore of guideline recommendations, is promoted via the certification process. The certification commission regularly updates and adapts the catalogue of certification requirements to ensure timely incorporation of updated guideline recommendations, national legislation, among others.

To ensure standardized documentation, data quality, and analysis of the QIs, an XML-OncoBox (http://www.xml-oncobox.de) uses a defined algorithm for calculating each indicator. The auditors validate the individual results of each centre during the on-site audit process. QI results for all certified Breast Cancer Centres are centrally evaluated and published in an annual benchmarking report, which includes pooled anonymized data and is openly available to the general public. In addition, each centre can request an individual benchmarking report to assess its own performance and quality results for that respective year compared with previous indicator years.

Albeit participation in the certification process is not mandatory for health care providers, 10 years after inauguration, 1,340 sites had already participated in the certification system for different tumour entities. These included 236 Breast Cancer Centres with a total of 281 sites and 14 centres outside of Germany (http://www.oncomap.de). Of the estimated 70,170 new annual breast cancer cases in Germany, ~54,122 are treated within the certified Breast Cancer Centres, which is equivalent to 74.5% of all new breast cancer cases.

In summary, the certification system is a broadly established, transparent, and inclusive instrument for quality assurance in oncologic care. It works independently of political trends or influence by the pharmaceutical industry.

Aim of the Certification System

The certification process aims to accomplish the following.

- **Enhance individual performance of each certified centre.**
  Breast Cancer Centres analyse their treatment quality in a regular and systematic manner in on-site audits and using the annual benchmarking report. This allows an objective comparison of individual results with those of all certified Breast Cancer Centres. Thus, the certification process is an important component in Plan–Do–Check–Act (PDCA) cycles for quality improvement, which is valued by the centres (4).
- **Systematically improve breast cancer care in Germany and beyond.**
- **Provide transparent information on quality of breast cancer care to health policymakers, scientific societies, and the general public.**
  All acquired data from the certified Breast Cancer Centres are made available to the general public in an anonymized fashion.
- **Include the patients' perspectives in the structure of breast cancer care.**
  The certification system, its requirements, and the process are performed in close cooperation and communication with self-help organizations and oncologic patient initiatives. It includes periodic evaluation of patient surveys in the clinical routine (5).
- **Promote research on the structure and quality of cancer care.**
  Research projects on all cancer types and disciplines, funded by different authorities and initiatives, are routinely included in the works of the certification system.

The reporting system, a threefold, cyclical process.

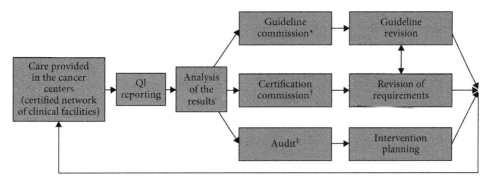

Figure 7.1 The report system, a threefold, cyclical process.

QI, Quality Indicator. (*) Leitlinienprogramm Onkologie. (†) Deutsche Krebsgesellschaft. (‡) Deutsche Krebsgesellschaft and OnkoZert.

Reproduced with permission from Kowalski, C. et al: 'Reporting Program for Cancer Care Quality Indicators'. *Journal of Oncology Practice*. Volume 11, Issue 2, pp. 158–160. Reprinted with permission. © 2015 American Society of Clinical Oncology. All rights reserved DOI:10.1200/JOP.2014.001339 (6)

Future Perspectives

Benchmarking reports were designed to provide comprehensive information for healthcare professionals and serve as tools for quality management and health services research (Figure 7.1) (6). Patient involvement is one focal element of the certification system, thus provision of patient friendly information is essential. Along with the 'translation' of the treatment guidelines into a language easily understandable by patients and their relatives, a conversion of QI results into a patient-friendly version is in process. There are several additional projects with a focus on health services research in oncologic care and intensification of patient involvement, and these are rooted in the certification system. Integration of patient-reported outcomes in quality improvement is piloted in the PCO (Prostate Cancer Outcomes, http://www.epic26.de/info) study, which combines clinical data with patient-reported results. The certification system fosters integration of clinical research into oncologic care through a mandatory requirement for Certified Centres to offer clinical trial participation to their patients.

The Dutch Perspective

In the Netherlands, quality of breast cancer care was enhanced by national organizations such as the National Breast Cancer Organisation Netherlands (NABON) that defined and distributed guidelines containing multidisciplinary criteria for providing good-quality breast cancer care as well as actual treatment guidelines (http://www.oncoline.nl).

After reports in 2003 of variations in care for breast cancer patients in the Netherlands, the Dutch Health Care Inspectorate was the first to introduce QIs to measure the quality of healthcare. They used 39 indicators that should indicate substandard performance of a hospital, and six of these QIs involved oncologic conditions. After this introduction, many others followed, and insurance companies, patient federations, consultancy agencies, and the media all started to use QIs to evaluate hospital performance. In 2008, the Dutch government introduced the 'Healthcare Transparency Program' urging the need for an audit for 80 different conditions including breast cancer care. The NABON started with a working group (the latter NABON Breast Cancer Audit (NBCA) scientific committee) in 2009. This NBCA scientific committee consisted of mandated members of all medical associations involved in breast cancer care in order to constitute a national clinical audit. These included the Dutch Radiological Society, the Dutch Society for Pathology, the Association of Surgeons of the Netherlands, the Netherlands Society for Plastic Surgery, the Dutch Society of Radiotherapy and Oncology, and the Dutch Society of Medical Oncology. The Breast Cancer Patients Association participated to represent the patients' voice. Later, a representative of the Dutch health care insurance companies joined the scientific committee, and in 2015 a mandated member of the Dutch Society for Clinical Genetics joined the working group. The primary goal of the NBCA is the nationwide monitoring of quality of breast cancer care and the provision of feedback to the participating individual hospitals on their results in relation to 'real-time' national benchmark information.

The Comprehensive Cancer Organisation the Netherlands (IKNL; http://www iknl. nl) and the Dutch Institute for Clinical Auditing (DICA; http://www.dica.nl) collaborate within the NBCA. IKNL is a quality institution for oncological and oncological palliative care, which hosts the Netherlands Cancer Registry in which data of all newly diagnosed malignancies in the Netherlands are registered since 1989. Information regarding treatment and outcomes of breast cancer is extracted from the medical records by specially trained data-managers in each hospital in the Netherlands. The DICA, currently facilitating 22 different audits, was founded in 2011 with the objective to facilitate the start-up of new nationwide clinical audits following the successful initiation of the DICA in 2009. Participation in the NBCA is one of the core indicators of the Health Inspectorate, and all hospitals in the Netherlands participate.

NBCA in Practice

Participating hospitals can either register the data themselves (facilitated by the web-based data-collection system of DICA) or have the data registered by IKNL data managers. A manual is available to secure uniform data acquisition. When data are registered by IKNL, which is in practice in about 75% of the 79 hospitals, hospitals can check the indicators and data at the patient level for possible inconsistencies before the data are transferred to the DICA system, in which data from all participating hospitals are gathered. Patient information is anonymized before transfer of the data to the national database. Each year, hospital-specific outcomes on all QIs become publicly available.

Individual hospitals have continuous insight into their own performance on the QIs along with other baseline information such as patient-, tumour-, and treatment characteristics; these are regularly updated on their secured MijnNBCA website. The QIs are nationally benchmarked against the other (anonymously presented) hospitals using funnel plots showing the 95% confidence interval in conjunction with the benchmark results. The NABON will set up the audit visits to the hospitals together with the scientific societies of the specialists.

Results

All surgically treated patients diagnosed with primary invasive breast cancer or ductal carcinoma in situ (DCIS) in the Netherlands are included in the NBCA. Patients diagnosed with lobular carcinoma in situ, phyllodes tumours, sarcomas, and lymphomas are not included. Patients are included based on the date of the histologically confirmed diagnosis. Information regarding diagnostic procedures, surgery, reconstructive surgery, radiotherapy, neo-adjuvant, and adjuvant systemic treatment are collected.

From the data set, the first set of indicators was established by the NBCA scientific committee in 2011, and these cover different aspects of the multidisciplinary care path for breast cancer patients from diagnostic work-up to the different treatment options. Evaluation of the results of four-year NBCA showed an overall high quality of breast cancer care in all hospitals in the Netherlands. For most QIs, improvement was seen over time, whereas some indicators showed unexplained variation (7). In 2015, 32 QIs measuring structure, processes, and outcomes of breast cancer care were available for benchmarked feedback. All these indicators were transparent to the public. For 10 indicators, a professional standardized norm was available, i.e. a generally accepted cut-off value, implying that a hospital should perform above (e.g. in case of preoperative multidisciplinary team (MDT) meeting) or below (e.g. in case of tumour-positive margins) a predefined standard. Other indicators were merely defined to explore institutional variation in treatment patterns. Standardized cut-off values denominating a level of quality are not (yet) available for these indicators. By 2017, more than 100,000 breast cancer patients had been registered in the NBCA. The NBCA QIs are evaluated annually by the scientific committee on their validity, and indicators may be adapted or removed when considered appropriate. During the seven years in which the NBCA has been active, and considering 2011 as the start-up year, improvement in the proportion of patients discussed in an MDT (from 91% in 2012 to 98% in 2017) and the decrease in variation between the hospitals reveals quality improvement (Figure 7.2). Moreover, it also showed that this indicator is redundant and will be removed from the list.

Future Perspectives

To decrease the registration burden, the Health Inspectorate urged limiting the number of indicators, and this led to a list of ten indicators in 2018. More effort will be made to include additional patient-reported outcomes such as quality of life of

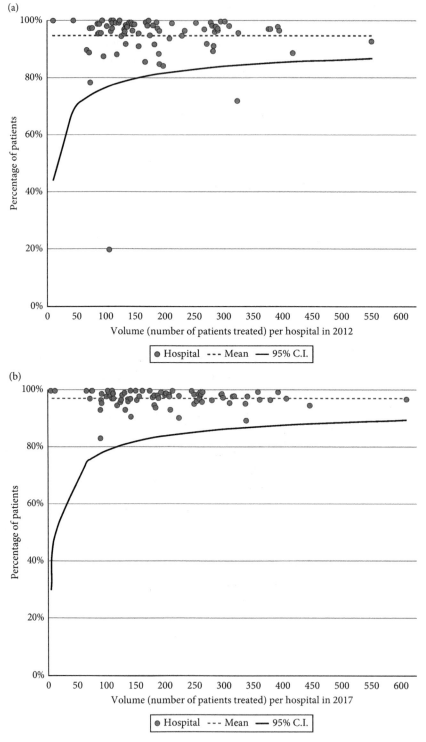

Figure 7.2 The increasing proportion of patients that has been discussed in an MDT (both pre- and postoperative) in 2012 (a) and 2017 (b): variation between hospitals is decreased.

With courtesy of Dutch Institute for Clinical Auditing (DICA), year report 2017, https://dica.nl/nbca/home'.

patient experiences of their received care. This will align with the ICHOM initiative (Chapter 6).

The Argentine Perspective

In Argentina, the Argentine Society of Mastology (Sociedad Argentina de Mastología, or SAM; http://www.samas.org.ar) is the entity that brings together, nationwide, the various specialists devoted to breast disease and plays a pivotal role in education. Based on the conviction that breast cancer units or mastology units are today the most appropriate structures to deal with breast disease, especially breast cancer, SAM, through the Sub-Committee on Standards for Mastology Units (created in 2012), urges the various institutions to start an interdisciplinary approach in their services in order to build the MUs. SAM launched their official Accreditation Program in 2014–2015.

Mastology Units

Mastology units (MUs), breast cancer units, or breast centres are defined as organizations within a hospital or clinic with various general care services, institutions purely devoted to breast disease, or several institutions collaborating in 'centres without walls'. In these MUs, a multidisciplinary group of sub-specialists in charge of the diagnosis and treatment of breast disease combine efforts to coordinate and streamline procedures. At the core of all MUs, and as a result of their integration, lies the periodic multidisciplinary meeting (MDM), where the various steps to be taken are agreed. If a facility does not hold periodic MDMs, it is not a MU, it is a medical centre with different services, but with a fragmented approach to health care. An essential aspect is the team head, the mastologist, who supervises and coordinates the different stages of treatment. According to SAM a well-functioning MU must treat at least 150 breast cancer cases per year.

All MUs must have a Board of Directors, Steering Committee, or Director. The role of this office is to coordinate the operation of the individual parties, to ensure implementation of the MDMs, and to fulfil and update the protocols to be followed. The specialists within the MU must be dedicated to breast cancer and demonstrate this through their education and experience. Moreover, it is crucial that the MU participate in training activities related to the sub-specialties it includes, covering key areas such as mastology, breast radiology, oncology, and any others present in a fully developed MU. This will ensure the best training for specialists, with the aim of already starting their career in the MU environment and its guiding principle of multidisciplinary team work. SAM recommends that the institution and its members are actively involved and participate in educational and prevention activities at the community level. These activities should take place not only within the institution, but also move to other areas in the region where the MU stands in order to reach the different educational, economic, and social levels of the community.

The MU must have some key components and deliver specific services such as sentinel node biopsies, oncoplastic and reconstructive surgery, appropriate imaging equipment, close contact to a radiotherapy facility, and an updated database, where patient information is stored. SAM suggests using one's own database (SAM-RCM). The database must meet all legal requirements and contain the required fields for the breast centre to regularly audit its results and keep track of its performance. To complete the service of the MU, close contact with other specialists and facilities, i.e. medical genetics, nuclear medicine service, rehabilitation, and social work service, is preferred.

Criteria

The MU must fulfil performance criteria (indicators) such as at least 50% conservative surgery at early stage breast cancer (0–II) and the performance of a sentinel node biopsy with acceptable quality. The histopathology report should include all the prognostic and predictive factors necessary for the treatment of breast cancer (at least): tumour size in millimetres, distance to nearest margin in millimetres, histological type, histological grade, vascular and lymphatic invasion, determination of oestrogen and progesterone receptors, Her-2 determination, conventional study of resected lymph nodes, and, if necessary, immunohistochemistry studies.

Moreover, the core of the MU, the MDT, should also fulfil a set of criteria. It must meet the basic condition of being in full contact with the rest of its components, cases of breast cancer (or any other breast disease) should be presented prospectively for multidisciplinary discussion and consensus, representatives of all specialties considered as essential components of the MU must attend (irrespective of their location/building), and clinical practice guidelines should be available. MDMs must be recorded in a common database. The MDM must be held regularly according to the number of cases treated annually; the frequency should not be lower than fortnightly. The MDT does not involve active participation or presence of patients.

Certification and Accreditation Programme

The certification and accreditation of MUs are two different instances with different objectives, needs, and implications. Certification might be the beginning of the process that could finish with accreditation, but this is not scheduled to be the final outcome.

Certification
Certification involves the recognition by the SAM, that a certain MU has at its disposal the key components to begin the process of interdisciplinary unification. Furthermore, certification involves the members' intention to pursue this process until it reaches its

full certification. The certification process means SAM committing itself to provide direct and active counselling through the Subcommittee on Mastology Units. The application must be made by a SAM member (Active Member or Associated Member). After completing the necessary documents, the Board of Directors shall evaluate the application and, if approved, allocate two members of the corresponding Sub-Commission to visit the MU and formally begin the certification process. For the certification process, some of the key components might be as described above, but to achieve accreditation, they must be part of the MU. A diploma will be issued and signed by the chairman of the SAM granting certification to the MU concerned, and this certification is valid for three years. The certification granted by the SAM might be renewed only once and for a period of three years, after which the MU must proceed to the Accreditation Program. For the MU to have access to a new certification, its directors must apply to the Board of SAM. In turn, two auditor doctors shall be appointed to visit the MU and with the same agenda as planned for the first certification process.

Accreditation

After completing its initial period (no less than three years in service) and having fulfilled the first certification by SAM, the MU can proceed to the Accreditation Program. MUs that have not been submitted to the initial certification and which deem themselves eligible for accreditation can formally start the application process by submitting the relevant documents through the centre's managers. Having analysed and approved the application, the Board of SAM will refer it to the MU Sub-Committee in order to assess the data and quality standards required in the programme. Subsequently, the Board of Directors will allocate two or three auditor doctors who will visit the MU in order to survey the facilities and verify all previously submitted data. Once the audit is complete, SAM will have a period of 30 days to issue the final report; said report shall contain the observations carried out by the auditor physicians and shall be submitted to the Board of Directors with a recommendation on whether to award the accreditation. The certificate issued by SAM to an accredited MU implies that it complies with the necessary requirements in order to provide comprehensive health care at the highest international standards. MU accreditation by SAM is valid for five years, after which there will be access to its renewal. In such a case, MU directors will submit a formal application to the Board of SAM together with the relevant documents. The Board of SAM will then appoint two or three auditor doctors and will make arrangements for a visit. The following process is similar to that described in the initial accreditation.

Current Status of the Programme

The certification/accreditation program was presented in September 2015. Updated 1 January 2019, seventeen centres were accredited, one received certification, and two centres were rejected. A subcommittee is currently analysing the information sent by other additional centres.

The Australasian Perspective (derived from the website)

The Royal Australasian College of Surgeons (RACS; https://www.surgeons.org/about/), formed in 1927, is a non-profit organization training surgeons and maintaining surgical standards in Australia and New Zealand. The college represents nine regions: the eight states and territories of Australia, plus New Zealand. The aim of the RACS is to lead surgical performance, professionalism, and improve patient care by advocating surgical standards and education. Values are: service, integrity, respect, compassion, and collaboration. The RACS has a specific RACS Section of Breast Surgery. They developed the National Breast Cancer Audit.

BreastSurgANZ Quality Audit (BQA)

The Breast Surgeons of Australia and New Zealand (BreastSurgANZ) Quality Audit (BQA) (https://bqa.org.au) of the RACS was started in 1998 as the pilot study National Breast Cancer Audit (NBCA) and has been run by the BreastSurgANZ since 2010 (8). It has been collecting information from surgeons on the treatment of their patients who were diagnosed with breast cancer. This data is used to assess surgeon performance, as well as for research into early breast cancer treatment in Australia and New Zealand. The BQA aims to improve the quality of care by surgeons for patients with early and locally advanced breast cancer in Australia and New Zealand. Participants can self-assess their clinical performance against set key performance indicators. Research into breast cancer treatment and outcomes using de-identified audit data also forms an important part of the audit's value. BreastSurgANZ, directors of the audit, require Full members to submit data on all cases of early and locally advanced breast cancer. The BQA Subcommittee is responsible for providing direction, oversight, and clinical advice to the operation of the audit.

The key set of indicators are all evidence-based and determined through extensive examination and discussion by audit governance as well as by consultation with other experts and stakeholders in the field. They all have a defined threshold. In November 2017 high-quality performance indicators were added to the BQA system. This is a set of six indicators which are in a pilot phase and are being tested on their practical value on patients diagnosed since October 2017.

The BQA applies the full cycle of clinical auditing and disseminates the audit results. Surgeons can review and benchmark their practice.

Furthermore, the RACS Section of Breast surgeons, having 262 members, describes the involvement of surgeons in the multidisciplinary care teams breast surgeon [8]. The recommendation of the national Breast Cancer Centre to include six core disciplines was well represented in all teams.

As the data does not include information on how many patients survive, researchers decided to link the audit database to the central database of deaths at the Australian Institute of Health and Welfare, the National Death Index. The NBCA data only uses the first three letters of the patient's name and the date of birth, to protect privacy. A recent study showed that the data of the NBCA and the National Death Index can be linked successfully. The NBCA data can now be used to consider how factors such as age, screening, and differences in treatment affect the survival of Australian breast cancer patients.

The Japanese Perspective

The quality of medical care is evaluated in Japan by the Ministry of Health, Labour and Welfare. The measurement of quality of cancer care is not implemented on a national level in Japan. Since 2010 QIs are selected and clinical data of cooperating hospitals are collected and analysed. The National Hospital Organisation is one of the outsourcing organizations of the project, which sets outcome indicators and process indicators of 87 items, called 'clinical quality indicators'. Some clinical quality indicators selected for breast cancer are: (i) sentinel lymph node biopsy implementation rate for invasive breast cancer patients (stage I); (ii) implementation rate of breast-conserving surgery for breast cancer (stage I) patients; (iii) implementation rate of hormone receptor and HER-2 test against breast cancer patients; (iv) administration rate of combination of 5-HT3 receptor antagonistic antiemetic drugs and steroid during chemotherapy with high risk of nausea. These indicators were updated in 2016.

Japanese Breast Cancer Society (JBCS)

Since the publication of the Medication Therapy Guidelines in 2004, JBCS has published guidelines for five fields: surgery, radiation therapy, screening, diagnosis, and prevention/ epidemiology, every three years. Since recent advances in medical technology and drug therapy are remarkable, and in order to respond quickly to the changes, the JBCS prepared an online guideline that integrates all fields and opened it publicly in September 2011. In accordance with the online version, books are issued concurrently and revised every two years. The database of the cancer registry for breast cancer organized by JBCS has now been combined with the National Clinical Database, which has made it possible to examine clinical prognostic data. A QI subcommittee within the clinical practice guidelines committee developed eight QI items, such as 'Tamoxifen administration rate as postoperative endocrine therapy for premenopausal hormone receptor positive stage I–III invasive breast cancer patients', based on clinical practice guidelines.

Research Group of the National Cancer Centre

The research group of the National Cancer Centre has launched a project to establish QIs for clinical practice of cancer care in 2007. It states that it is the responsibility of the government to promote 'equalization of cancer treatment' by allowing equal and appropriate cancer treatment to the entire public through the establishment and enforcement of the Cancer Control Act (2006). In order to evaluate the progress of 'equalization of cancer treatment', it was necessary to develop a standard method to measure quality of cancer care, grasp the current state of cancer medical quality, and to understand to what extent the disparity has been resolved. Five major cancers (breast, liver, stomach, colon, and lung) and palliative care were the target. The QI of medical treatment is roughly divided into 'structure' indicators such as improvement of equipment and human resources, 'process' indicators represented by standard medical practice implementation rate, and 'outcome' indicators such as survival rate and length of hospitalization. For regular monitoring, the research group has identified the standard procedures based on clinical practice guidelines and created QI using the RAND/UCLA Appropriateness Method. As examples, two indicators concerning radiation therapy were selected: (i) radiation therapy after breast-conserving surgery aged <70 years (within 180 days after surgery); (ii) radiation therapy to patients with high risk of recurrence after mastectomy T4 or four or more lymph node metastases.

In 2016, studies were done to measure the adherence rate of breast cancer QIs of 308 hospitals. One study used administrative claims date (9), and another used a retrospective record review of hospital data (10) representing nearly half of all Japanese breast cancer patients. In the retrospective study, the quality data of 15,227 patients with breast cancer were analysed. Drug adherence had a low score (52.8%). A great variation was observed across facilities for HER-2 testing and for radiation therapy after breast-conserving surgery.

Quality Evaluation

Quality management of breast cancer is not conducted in a standardized way in Japan. Efforts are planned to widen the implementation of indicators and to evaluate and publish more efficiently and reliably the quality of breast cancer care nationwide.

Key Messages

- National programmes on quality management focus on the multidisciplinary approach with the MDT as key element.
- The programmes should encourage regular quality monitoring and improvement within the hospitals/MU.
- Reliable data on the delivered care and information (indicators) generated out of (already available) data are key to limiting registration burden.
- Audits, certification, and accreditation are all different levels of quality management.

- All hospitals should monitor and benchmark their own quality of care on a regular basis.
- A single set of QIs must be defined per country, answering the need of all involved parties (including the government).

References

1. Sant M et al. Survival of women with breast cancer in Europe: variation with age, year of diagnosis and country. The EUROCARE Working Group. *Int J Cancer* 1998;77(5):679–683.
2. European Parliament, Committee on Women's Rights and Equal Opportunities: Report on breast cancer in the European Union (2002/2279(INI)), A5-0159/2003 2003.
3. Kreienberg R et al. Leitlinienprogramm Onkologie (Deutsche Krebsgesellschaft; Deutsche Krebshilfe; AWMF): Interdisziplinäre S3-Leitlinie für die Diagnostik, Therapie und Nachsorge des Mammakarzinoms, Langversion 3.0, 2012, AWMF-Registernummer: 032/045OL. 2012.
4. Kowalski C et al. Quality of care in breast cancer centers: results of benchmarking by the German Cancer Society and German Society for Breast Diseases. *The Breast* 2015;24(2):118–123.
5. Kowalski C et al. The patients' view on accredited breast cancer centers: strengths and potential for improvement. *Geburtshilfe Frauenheilkd* 2012;72(2):137–143.
6. Kowalski C et al. Reporting program for cancer care quality indicators. *J Oncol Pract* 2015;11(2):158–161.
7. Van Bommel AC et al. Clinical auditing as an instrument for quality improvement in breast cancer care in the Netherlands: the national NABON Breast Cancer Audit. *J Surg Oncol* 2017;115(3):243–249.
8. Marsh CJ et al. National Breast Cancer Audit: the use of multidisciplinary care teams by breast surgeons in Australia and New Zealand. *Med J Aust* 2008;188:385–388.
9. Iwamoto M et al. Monitoring and evaluating the quality of cancer care in Japan using administrative claim data. *Cancer Sci* 2016;107(1):68–75.
10. Mukai H et al. Quality evaluation of medical care for breast cancer in Japan. *Int J Quality Health Care* 2016;28(1):110–113.

8

Educational and Training Harmonization in Breast Care

Lynda Wyld and Christos Markopoulos

Introduction

Training and education in breast care across all disciplines (surgery, medical and radiation oncology, oncology nursing, palliative care, radiology, pathology, etc.) are critical to the quality of care delivered and are highly variable among European countries and beyond. Undoubtedly, much of the variation observed in practice is due to differential funding and access to health care, which, in turn, restrict access to screening and early diagnostic services, more advanced types of surgery, and systemic therapies. However, training limitations are also restricting, and improving the quality of training would help to improve care.

Fellowships to refine specialist training are not mandatory but are much more likely to occur in high-income countries. Low-income countries lack access to high-level training locally and surgeons and other medical staff often seek this specialized training abroad, which limits its availability due to costs. Thus, there will be widely varying standards of breast cancer care due to this limited access to training in some countries. Efforts have been made to develop training curricula that would have global applicability (1). The delivery of, and access to, the required training are also major limiting factors. Many developed countries do facilitate training opportunities for graduates of low-income countries, although the relevance of this training may be limited when trainees return to their own health system, which may be unable to afford application of their new skills, and where disease and patient factors may preclude their use. For example, in high-income countries some 90% of all breast cancers are stages 1 and 2 at diagnosis, whereas in low-income countries this falls to 40% or less. Therefore techniques such as sentinel node biopsy and breast reconstruction surgery are inappropriate for the majority of women, even if they were able to afford them.

European Breast Training

Training in Europe has some degree of harmonization. Since 1996, European Law mandates that all European member states (plus European Economic Area (EEA) states) mutually recognize each other's primary medical qualifications. In theory, therefore, at the start of specialist training the standard of knowledge and practice should be similar. The situation is similar at the completion of specialist training, where European Law again mandates mutual recognition of specialist training certification or licensing (European Specialist Medical Qualifications Order 1995). Therefore, a surgeon who has completed training in one member state should be able to apply for a consultant post in any other member state (subject to ability to speak the host language). In most states there is a regulatory body (competent authority) that oversees the process of confirming eligibility (based on certification and experience) and linguistic competency. In theory, at least, there should be parity of skills, knowledge, and practice across Europe. However, national guidelines vary widely across Europe, and national funding models have different priorities and thresholds.

A recent review of the length of training in cancer surgery across Europe found that total training time (from medical school to completion of training) varied between 9 and 18 years, and the duration of surgical specialist training varied between 4 and 7 years just within Europe (see Figure 8.1) and there is an even wider global variation (2). Even within a single specialist area (breast surgery, for example) the host specialty may vary (breast surgery is part of general surgery in some countries, in others it is part of gynaecology). Again, in breast surgery, some countries include breast reconstruction as integral to breast surgery training (the UK or Germany for example), whereas in others reconstructive surgery is part of plastic surgery training (The Netherlands, Sweden). In many countries standard training is not felt to provide adequate training in all the complexities of breast surgery, especially in oncoplastic and reconstructive surgery. Many trainees seek formal fellowships as part or after completion of their training (3) to ensure that they have the necessary, non-mandatory, competencies.

There have been efforts to develop a training curriculum for breast surgery to support the Union of European Medical Specialists (UEMS) Breast Examination, but this has no national or pan European mandate, and taking the exam is voluntary. In most countries surgical training is regulated at the national level with varying degrees of rigor. Some countries have very detailed systems with curricula, multiple objective assessments, log books, and annual progress reviews with examinations (the UK Joint Committee for Higher Specialist Training and Royal Colleges, for example). Other countries have very informal arrangements with simple, local peer review.

The European Society for Therapeutic Radiotherapy and Oncology (ESTRO) has published a curriculum for radiotherapy training which has led to improved standardization of training in Europe for radiation oncologists (4). This curriculum now includes quite detailed objective assessments and log book review to enhance reliability and reproducibility (5). Similarly, the European Society of Medical Oncology (ESMO) developed a European training curriculum in collaboration with the American Society for Clinical Oncology (ASCO) (6). None of these curricula, however, are specific for breast cancer.

As can be seen from the above, heterogeneity of training is an ongoing issue across the European Union (EU), and harmonization of training would help to improve and standardize outcomes. In an effort to address this issue the UEMS was established in

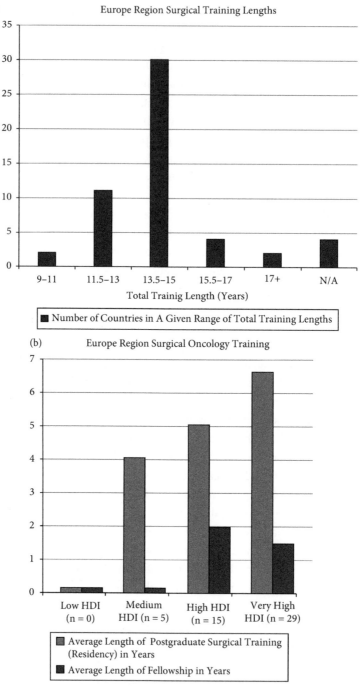

Figure 8.1 Length of surgical training and cancer surgery residency and fellowships in European countries.

Reproduced with permission from Are, C. et al. 'Variations in training of surgical oncologists: Proposal for a global curriculum'. *European Journal of Surgical Oncology*. Volume 42, Issue 6. pp. 767–778. Copyright © 2016 Elsevier Ltd. DOI: 10.1016/j.ejso.2016.04.004

1958 and now comprises 43 specialist sections, each representing an independently recognized discipline. Breast surgery is a specialist division within the section of surgery, and breast care is formally represented as a pan-European multidisciplinary joint committee (MJC) at the UEMS in recognition of the highly multidisciplinary nature of its management (7). In addition, there are sections for medical and radiation oncology and for plastic and reconstructive surgery which include aspects of breast care.

Many of the sections have examination boards and run pan-European exams, of which the European Breast Exam is one. The exam was established in 2010 as a joint endeavour between the UEMS, European Society of Breast Cancer Specialists (EUSOMA), and European Society of Surgical Oncology (ESSO), and the number of applicants is growing steadily. A curriculum for training has been established, and eligibility criteria for the exam map to this. The exam assesses candidates against the standard of a newly qualified European consultant surgeon who has just completed training. It comprises a written exam and a rigorous oral exam with complex case management discussions and academic critique of the recent scientific literature. Knowledge of oncoplastic and reconstructive techniques is embedded in the syllabus, as is awareness of the latest evidence-based guidelines and research interpretation. Whereas the exam is not yet officially recognized by any national regulatory body, it is gaining in popularity and is widely recognized as a marker of high-quality practice.

In a similar way, the UEMS section of plastic and reconstructive surgery has a training syllabus and exam which cover aspects of breast care from a plastic surgery perspective.

Another issue is the ongoing education of specialist licensed surgeons. Once again, the UEMS offers pan-European accreditation to ensure that high-quality standards are met for Continuing Medical Education (CME) via its EACCME (European Accreditation Council for CME) Council. There is a huge number of accredited high-quality courses in various aspects of breast care. However, there is no formally agreed and recognized breast syllabus upon which content can be standardized. There are also several formal university degrees in postgraduate breast cancer management including the University of Ulm (Germany)/In cooperation with European School of Oncology Certificate of Competence in Breast Care, and the University of East Anglia (UK) Master's Degree in Oncoplastic Breast Surgery.

The last issue concerns the quality of the centre where breast training is provided. High-quality training posts should have access to a high throughput of complex cases, a properly constituted multidisciplinary team, good quality training, good imaging and pathology input, research and academic support, and excellent technical equipment (magnetic resonance imaging, digital mammography, reconstruction resources, and training). The quality standards for such posts are not standardized across Europe (and indeed absent in some states), which adds a further source of variability to the quality of training. Trainers themselves must be trained and their skills and knowledge assessed regularly.

In an attempt to harmonize care, EUSOMA published in 2016 an updated version of 'The requirements of a specialist Breast Centre' to define the minimum requirements and quality indicators that are essential to improve organization, performance, and outcome in breast care. Such organized Breast Units can provide the optimal environment for training of breast specialists.

Breast Surgery Training in the USA

By comparison with Europe, breast surgical training in the USA is tightly regulated with formal residency programmes in general breast surgery or plastic surgery, professional exam certification at the end of residency programmes, and mandatory re-certification at intervals. Specialist training fellowships approved by the American Society of Breast Surgeons, American Society of Breast Diseases, and the US Society of Surgical Oncology are also offered by many large US centres. Breast Surgery fellowships offered by some universities are usually of 12 months in length and include training for the management of breast diseases and cancer, participation in the multidisciplinary aspects of patient care (including radiation, imaging, plastic surgery, and pathology), and engagement of fellows in clinical research activities. The length of training in the USA, from the start of medical school to completion of training, is also one of the longest, and specialist fellowships are more common.

Key Messages

- Harmonization of training in breast care is not widely recognized by national certification bodies.
- Integrated standardized high-quality international curricula for training in breast care that cover surgery, radiology, pathology, medical oncology, radiation oncology, and genetics are required.
- Standardized certification in breast care disciplines, either via professional examinations (e.g. UEMS), degrees, or diplomas should be mandatory before a specialist may be appointed.
- A standard curriculum to which the content of EACCME accredited courses may be mapped.
- Formal recognition of certified training centres regulated nationally in accordance to high international standards.

References

1. Are C et al. Global curriculum in surgical oncology. *Ann Surg Oncol* 2016;23(6):1782–1795.
2. Are C et al. Variations in training of surgical oncologists: proposal for a global curriculum. *Eur J Surg Oncol* 2016;42(6):767–778.
3. Fitzgerald JE et al. Clinical fellowships in surgical training: analysis of a national pan-specialty workforce survey. *World J Surg* 2013;37(5):945–952.

4. European Society for Radiotherapy & Oncology. Recommended ESTRO core curriculum for radiation oncologists/radiotherapists, 3rd ed.; April 2010. Available from: https://www.estro.org/binaries/content/assets/estro/school/european-curricula/cc_finalapprovedestro_ccapril2010.pdf

5. Eriksen JG et al. The updated ESTRO core curricula 2011 for clinicians, medical physicists and RTTs in radiotherapy/radiation oncology. *Radiother Oncol* 2012;103(1):103–108.

6. Dittrich C et al. ESMO/ASCO Recommendations for a Global Curriculum in Medical Oncology, Edition 2016. *ESMO Open* 2016;1:e000097.

7. European Union of Medical Specialists, Section of Surgery & European Board of Surgery. Available from: https://www.uemssurg.org/divisions/breast-surgery

PART 3
THE GUIDELINES

9

The Role of Guidelines in Breast Cancer Management in Different Resource Settings

Catherine Duggan, Alexandru Eniu, and Benjamin O. Anderson

Introduction

Cancer care in any country is a costly, complex, and multi-step endeavour, especially for breast cancer, a heterogeneous disease, where effective treatment depends on early detection and diagnosis. Efforts to provide the best evidence-based care for breast cancer patients, ensure optimal use of resources, reduce variation in practice, assist practitioner and patient decision-making, and standardize appropriate health care across institutions and/or countries have resulted in the development of many clinical practice guidelines (CPG) which translate evidence-based research into methodological standards. Guidelines, defined by the Institute of Medicine as 'Statements that include recommendations intended to optimize patient care that are informed by a systematic review of evidence and an assessment of the benefits and harms of alternative care options' (1), address specific clinical situations (disease-oriented) or use of approved medical products, procedures, or tests (modality-oriented). Curated websites such as the Guideline International Network and the US-based National Guideline Clearinghouse list 167 and 151 breast cancer related guidelines, respectively (see https://www.guideline.gov/ and http://www.g-i-n.net/home). However, these represent only a fraction of the available international guidelines on the management of breast cancer.

An ideal CPG follows a stepwise development process that includes specification of topic and methodology, review of the literature, synthesis of evidence, incorporation of expert opinion, consideration of public policy, drafting of a document, and circulation for peer review (2). A quality guideline should also be continuously reviewed and updated. Bodies such as the World Health Organization (see WHO Handbook for Guideline Development, http://www.who.int/publications/guidelines/handbook_2nd_ed.pdf) and the Institute of Medicine (1) have published guidelines and standards for CPG development including directives on establishing transparency, guideline development group composition, performing systematic reviews, determining quality of evidence, and updating recommendations, among others.

In 1999, Woolf and colleagues published a paper on the potential benefits, limitations, and harms of clinical guidelines (3). The authors stated that benefit from guidelines might encompass improvements in health outcomes by promoting effective interventions and discouraging ineffective ones, reducing morbidity and mortality, improving consistency of care, and supporting quality improvement activities. The latter can improve efficiency (often by standardizing care) and optimizing value for money. The authors also considered a series of harms such as the development of flawed recommendations due to lacking, misleading, or misinterpreted scientific evidence-based recommendations, excessively influential opinions of individual members of the development group, subjective judgements of benefits versus harms, and bias for cost-savings versus optimal care for patients (3).

In response to these concerns, a series of evaluation tools were developed such as the Appraisal of Guidelines for Research and Evaluation (AGREE II) framework, which is used to evaluate and validate existing practice guidelines (4). An analysis of breast-cancer treatment guidelines revealed a large degree of conformity in seven widely used national breast cancer guidelines published between 2001 and 2011 that satisfied inter-nationally recognized methodological criteria (e.g. validity, reproducibility, reliability, representative development, clinical applicability, clinical flexibility, clarity, meticu-lous documentation, and scheduled review) (5). Despite describing an overall high level of conformity among guidelines, the AGREE II study found a minor degree of discordance, especially among recommendations for endocrine therapy. Underlying factors explaining these discrepancies included different dates of publication leading to shifting evidence bases, inconsistency in evidence among trials which causes re-commendations to be less precise, and different interpretations of sufficient evidence. The AGREE II authors suggested that, given the high level of overall concordance, the current practice of developing guidelines at national level, as opposed to international collaborations such as the St Gallen Consensus Conference, should be discussed (5). A 2012 study compared clinical breast cancer guidelines from the American Society for Clinical Oncology (ASCO) (nine guidelines), Cancer Care Ontario (19 guidelines), and the National Institute for Health and Clinical Excellence (NICE, 22 guidelines). The study used the AGREE framework to determine the quality and consistency of content across international organizations and found that recommendations were broadly con-sistent. However, the study found variability both between and within organizations in the quality of guidelines in the domains of stakeholder involvement, applicability, and editorial independence (6).

While review of all breast cancer guidelines is outside the scope of this chapter, we briefly provide an overview of a selection of the most well-known international guide-lines in Table 9.1.

Guideline Compliance and Patient Outcomes

Effectiveness of guidelines relies not only on their quality but also on their level of dis-semination, ease of implementation, and acceptance by both clinicians and the public. Despite the proliferation of CPGs, there are relatively few assessments of the penetra-tion of the CPGs into routine practice, adherence and compliance to CPGs, or differ-ences in approaches taken by institutions in interpreting and implementing CPGs.

Table 9.1 A selection of Clinical Practice Guidelines (CPGs) from high-income countries (HICs)

Guideline	Development process	Grading of recommendations	Review cycle	Setting/ target
ASCO	• Evidence-based consensus approach based on the modified Delphi technique. • Based on a CPG guideline-development protocol worksheet. • Systematic review of selected databases (PubMed/Embase/ Cochrane Library) by ASCO staff and the expert panel using criteria specified in the worksheet. • Specific procedure to be followed when insufficient evidence exists in the literature. • **Consensus development:** iterative process based on panellists rating their agreement with each consensus recommendation on a 5- or 7- point Likert scale. • **See** https://www. instituteforquality.org/ guideline-development-process	**Strong Consensus/ Consensus/No Consensus** based on compiled ratings reaching a minimum threshold for each recommendation to be adopted. Criteria used: study quality, the strength of the evidence and the strength of the recommendations.	**Varies:** ASCO solicits and reviews guideline topic proposals from ASCO members annually.	USA

Cancer Care Ontario	• Follows the Program in Evidence-Based Care (PEBC).
	• Based on developing an evidence base from:
	  • systematic review of PubMed/ Embase/Cochrane Library;
	  • adaption of existing guidelines;
	  • environmental/horizon scanning;
	  • assessment, analysis and reporting of evidence.
	• **Consensus development:** group and methods to achieve formal consensus defined for each guideline (including Delphi rounds).
	• External review process and peer reviewed publication of the document.
	• **See** https://www. cancercareontario.ca/en/cancer-care-ontario/programs/data-research/evidence-based-care
		Grading:
		No formal grading of recommendations, the justification for each recommendation is provided in the document (for example, direct evidence, evidence plus expert opinion, or formal consensus).
			Varies: stakeholders identify a need for a new or revised guideline.	Canada

(continued)

Table 9.1 Continued

Guideline	Development process	Grading of recommendations	Review cycle	Setting/ target
ESMO–ESO Guidelines for Advanced Breast Cancer (ABC)	• Systematic review of current evidence selected by expert authors. • Levels of Evidence and Grades of Recommendation are used for each statement (See http://www.esmo.org/Guidelines/ESMO-Guidelines-Methodology). • ESO-ESMO Consensus Conferences on advanced breast cancer held every two years. • **Consensus development:** modified Delphi method that develops statements by gathering opinion from the consensus panellists; during the conference the statements are voted by the panellists. http://www.esmo.org/content/download/77792/1426729/file/ESMO-Consensus-Conferences-Standard-Operating-Procedures-Jan2017.pdf	**Levels of Evidence** describes the quality of existing evidence. I: Evidence from at least one large randomized, controlled trial of good methodological quality (low potential for bias) or meta-analyses of well-conducted randomized trials without heterogeneity. II: Small randomized trials or large randomized trials with a suspicion of bias (lower methodological quality) or meta-analyses of such trials or of trials with demonstrated heterogeneity. III: Prospective cohort studies. IV: Retrospective cohort studies or case–control studies. V: Studies without control group, case reports, experts' opinions. **Grades of Recommendation** A: Strong evidence for efficacy with a substantial clinical benefit, strongly recommended. B: Strong or moderate evidence for efficacy but with a limited clinical benefit, generally recommended. C: Insufficient evidence for efficacy or benefit does not outweigh the risk or the disadvantages (adverse events, costs), optional. D: Moderate evidence against efficacy or for adverse outcome, generally not recommended. E: Strong evidence against efficacy or for adverse outcome, never recommended.	Varies: updated when the GLC determines that there is a need	Europe

Table 9.1 Continued

Guideline	Development process	Grading of recommendations	Review cycle	Setting/ target
NICE guidelines	• Systematic reviews of best available evidence in answer to the review questions of interest (usually a new drug or intervention) including cost effectiveness analysis to decide reimbursement by the UK National Health System (NHS). • Involves stakeholders in a transparent and collaborative manner. • Primary methodological research and evaluation undertaken by the NICE teams using the Guideline Implementability Appraisal tool. • Processes and methods are based the AGREE II instrument. See https://www.nice.org.uk/process/pmg20/chapter/introduction-and-overview	NICE guidance interprets evidence to formulate recommendations in favour or against reimbursement (Yes/No).	**Varies:** Topics are referred to NICE as stakeholders identify need.	UK
NCI–PDQ Cancer Information Summaries	• Comprehensive, evidence-based summaries covering breast cancer treatment, screening, prevention, genetics, special situations (male breast cancer, pregnancy and cancer), and integrative, alternative, and complementary therapies. • Reviewed regularly and updated as necessary by the PDQ Adult Treatment Editorial Board. • Board members review recently published articles each month to determine whether an article should be discussed, be cited with text, or replace or update an existing article. • **Consensus process:** Board members evaluate the strength of the evidence in the published articles and determine how the article should be included in the summary. See https://www.cancer.gov/types/breast/hp/breast-treatment-pdq#section/_AboutThis_1	Some of the reference citations in this summary are accompanied by a level-of-evidence designation. **Strength of Study Design** 1. Randomized, controlled, clinical trials: i. Double-blinded; ii. Non-blinded treatment delivery. 2. Nonrandomized, controlled, clinical trials. 3. Case series or other observational study designs: i. Population-based, consecutive series; ii. Consecutive cases (not population-based); iii. Non-consecutive cases or other observational study designs (e.g. cohort or case–control studies).	Monthly/as necessary	US/ global

(continued)

Table 9.1 Continued

Guideline	Development process	Grading of recommendations	Review cycle	Setting/target

		Strength of evidence
		A. Total mortality (or overall survival from a defined time).
		B. Cause-specific mortality (or cause-specific mortality from a defined time).
		C. Carefully assessed quality of life.
		D. Indirect surrogates:
		  i. Event-free survival;
		  ii. Disease-free survival;
		  iii. Progression-free survival;
		  iv. Tumour response rate.		

NCCN	• **Annual institutional review** of guidelines by clinical cancer experts at NCCN member institutions of new data/evidence.
	• NCCN Headquarters Guidelines team identify important clinical issues/topics for deliberation at the annual Panel meetings.
	• **Literature Review:** Prior to the annual update of the Guidelines, an electronic search of the PubMed Database, provided by the US National Library of Medicine, is performed to obtain key literature published since the previous Guidelines update.
	• See https://www.nccn.org/professionals/development.aspx
		• **Evidence weighting:**
		  • **Category I**, high level of evidence with uniform consensus;
		  • **Category IIA**, lower level of evidence with uniform consensus;
		  • **Category IIB**, lower level of evidence without a uniform consensus but with no major disagreement;
		  • **Category III**, any level of evidence but with major disagreement.
			Annual	US/global

St. Gallen International Expert Consensus Conference	• Biannual Conference Based Consensus Panel Review of Evidence. • Systematic review of current published evidence (past 2 years) selected by global experts. • Discussion on whether new diagnostic or therapeutic findings are ready for incorporation into routine everyday practice with a focus on controversies in the management of early stage breast cancer.	**Grading:** No formal grading of recommendations. Panellists asked to cast vote (yes/no/abstain) in response to questions posed at panel discussions. After each vote, answers are summarized in percentages.	Biannual	International

Table 9.1 Continued

Guideline	Development process	Grading of recommendations	Review cycle	Setting/ target
	• **Consensus development** modified Delphi method that develops statements by gathering opinion from the consensus panellists; during the conference the statements are voted by the panellists.			

All guideline committees review working groups and guideline development groups for conflict of interest.

AGREE II, Appraisal of Guidelines for Research and Evaluation II; ASCO, American Society for Clinical Oncology; CPG, Clinical Practice Guidelines; ESMO, European Society for Medical Oncology; ESO, European School of Oncology; NCCN, National Comprehensive Cancer Network; NICE, National Institute for Health and Care Excellence; PDQ, Physician Data Query; PEBC, Program in Evidence-Based Care.

A retrospective study of 3976 patients with primary breast cancer reported a significant association between adherence to the German national treatment guidelines and statistically significant improved recurrence-free and overall survival rates. At the same time, they observed a linear association between increasing number of violations in guideline adherence and decreased overall survival (7). A second study examined the association between guideline-adherent adjuvant treatment and survival outcome in 371 patients with triple-negative breast cancer (TNBC) nested within Breast Cancer Care under Evidence-Based Guidelines (BRENDA), an observational, retrospective, multi-centre, cohort study. 66.8% of patients with TNBC were found to have one or more guideline violations, which was also associated with worsened survival outcomes (8). A further evaluation of this cohort demonstrated that rates of guideline adherence were lower in TNBC versus non-TNBC subtypes, especially among TNBC patients aged over 65 years. However, there were no differences in survival between any TNBC age subgroup among patients who experienced 100% guideline adherent treatment (9). By contrast, a large retrospective study of early stage breast cancer identified from the Netherlands Cancer Registry reported that while adherence to treatment guidelines was affected by age, and noting that breast cancer patients aged ≥75 years are less likely to receive guideline-concordant treatment, adherence to guidelines was not associated with overall survival in any patient subgroup (10).

Another review examined compliance with National Comprehensive Cancer Network (NCCN) guidelines during the treatment of 395 breast cancer patients at a single institution. Guideline compliance averaged 94% for initial staging evaluation, 97% for surgery, 91% for chemotherapy, 89% for hormone therapy, 91% for radiation therapy, 85% for follow-up, and 100% for determination of oestrogen receptor/progesterone receptor and HER2 status. Age, comorbidities, and stage influenced guideline compliance, and the main reasons for non-compliance were patient refusal, patient choice after shared decision-making, and overuse of testing (11). By contrast, a large-scale study conducted from July 2006 to May 2011 examined inter-institutional variation for management decisions in a variety of cancers. This study included a breast cancer cohort of 11,293 women derived from NCCN Outcomes Database who presented with incident cancer at 17 NCCN institutions from July 2008 to June 2010. Here, inter-institutional variation was high (median absolute deviation >10%) for 16 out of 76 (21%) breast cancer management decisions. Forty-six percent of high-variance decisions involved imaging or diagnostic procedures, and 37% involved choice of chemotherapy regimen (12). The authors concluded that the substantial degree of variation in institutional practice revealed a lack of consensus concerning optimal management for common clinical scenarios, which, they proposed, should prompt comparative effectiveness research, patient–provider education, or standardized pathway development.

Thirty-five Italian oncology centres participated in an Italian Association of Medical Oncology (AIOM) study to evaluate the concordance between the 2005 AIOM Breast Cancer Guidelines and clinical practice in patients diagnosed with stages I and II invasive breast cancer from 2005 to 2006. Whereas >90% adherence to guidelines for diagnostic and therapy indicators was observed, poor adherence to patient follow-up reduced overall compliance to 64% (13). A Dutch retrospective study from the Eindhoven Cancer Registry documented increases in the use of adjuvant systemic treatment in 8,261 patients with early stage breast cancer, from 37% in 1990–1997 to 53% in 2002–2006, reflecting significant changes in Dutch treatment guidelines for breast cancer. However, the authors noted that despite overall increases in guideline compliance, there were marked differences among hospitals in the adoption of adjuvant treatment for node-negative patients, <2% of patients aged >70 years received any chemotherapy, and there was significant variation in timing of adoption of treatment guidelines between hospitals (14).

A US study examined guideline compliance in the treatment of women with early stage breast cancer in 18 Massachusetts and 30 Minnesota hospitals. Whereas overall compliance with four indicators of quality of care (radiation therapy after breast-conserving surgery, axillary lymph node dissection, chemotherapy for premenopausal women with positive lymph nodes, and hormonal therapy for postmenopausal women with positive lymph nodes and oestrogen receptor-positive tumours) was >80% for three of the four standards, compliance for hormonal therapy for postmenopausal women was 'low' at <64% (15). A Canadian study (British Columbia) reported that, among 939 patients identified from a cancer registry with invasive node-negative breast cancer, compliance to practice guidelines for treatment with adjuvant radiotherapy, chemotherapy, and tamoxifen was 97%, 96%, and 89%, respectively (16).

Several studies examined adherence to more specialized guidelines. An early US-based study from 1992 found that compliance with treatment adherence to standards for appropriately selecting and managing patients who receive breast-conserving therapy was 80% or higher for 16 of the 22 standards across 842 community hospitals treating 7097 patients (17). However, poor compliance was documented for six standards, and there were significant variations in guideline adherence across the type of hospital cancer programme as well as by geographic region (18). The College of

American Pathologists developed guidelines to standardize pathology reporting for breast-conserving surgery, and a study found that patients with non-compliant margin reporting were 1.7 times more likely to undergo re-excision and/or mastectomy than those with maximally compliant reporting (19).

From the studies cited above, it is clear that whereas there is relatively little variation between the guidelines themselves, uptake and compliance vary widely between, and in some cases within, institutions. There are various reasons underlying lack of compliance with CPGs. Barriers to compliance with CPGs for breast cancer care include patient age (10), patient refusal, patient choice after shared decision-making, and overuse of testing (11). At an institutional level, lack of consensus about optimal management for common clinical scenarios (12) was a barrier. More general studies have also examined barriers to guideline compliance. A study of Dutch general practitioners found that while 89% believed that guideline adherence improved patient care, 35% reported difficulties in changing practices to comply with guidelines. Perceived barriers included patient behaviours, preferences, as well as lack of applicability of recommendations both in general and to individual patients (20). An earlier systematic review of barriers to physician adherence to CPGs reported common barriers such as lack of awareness, familiarity or agreement, lack of outcome expectancy, low self-efficacy, ability to 'overcome the inertia of previous practice', and external barriers which might include a lack of equipment, space, educational materials, time, staff, and financial resources (21).

Guidelines in Limited-Resource Settings

One factor concerning the potential harms of guidelines that was not considered in the above-cited studies, perhaps understandably, is their unsuitability in low-resource settings. Before 2005, the only published breast-cancer guidelines available in low-resource settings were those developed in and for high-income countries (HICs). HIC guidelines implicitly or explicitly assume treatment availability and a healthcare infrastructure including high proportions of screen-detected cancers, strong referral systems, and unconstrained health spending levels. In reality, the implementation of HIC guidelines is beyond the reach of most low- and middle-income countries (LMICs), where significant disparities exist in health infrastructure, capacity, and health spending compared to HICs. Attempting to implement 'high-resource' guidelines in low-resource settings can be harmful, because these add excessive burdens on underfunded health care systems that are juggling competing burdens of infectious diseases, maternal, and child mortality with increased incidence of non-communicable diseases including cancer. Woolf et al. commented on the potential benefits and harms of CPG in terms of high resources, and their comments are especially pertinent to LMIC: 'Healthcare systems . . . may be harmed by guidelines, if following them escalates utilization, compromises operating efficiency, or wastes limited resources. Some clinical guidelines . . . may advocate costly interventions that are unaffordable or that cut into resources needed for more effective services' (3).

Historically, breast cancer incidence rates have been significantly higher in HICs than in LMICs, a difference which is due in part to the use of mammographic screening in HICs. However, breast cancer incidence and mortality rates have stabilized or are decreasing in the USA and Western Europe. Meanwhile, incidence rates are steadily increasing in LMICs, and globally 75% of breast cancer deaths are expected to occur in LMICs (22). Bray et al. stratified the Human Development Index, a composite indicator of gross domestic product, life expectancy, and education, to highlight global disparities in cancer incidence and mortality and to predict future burdens of breast cancer in limited-resource settings (23). LMICs share a set of specific challenges that make it impractical, if not unrealistic, to integrate HIC-based guidelines into routine care. These differences include shortage of trained personnel and drugs, lack of infrastructure, and low levels of health spending. Despite the high cancer incidence and mortality in LMICs, a disproportionately low fraction of development assistance for health is allocated to cancer care: of the $37.9 billion allocated in 2016, only 1.7% ($643.8 million) was allocated to all major non-communicable diseases; in 2012, only an estimated 5% of spending on non-communicable diseases was specifically allocated for cancer (24).

Because most HIC practice guidelines generally assume the availability of costly diagnostic and treatment resources applied within a mature and organized health care infrastructure, they make no recommendations concerning how resource expenditures should be prioritized to achieve the greatest clinical benefit and outcome. This makes the applicability of existing practice guidelines of limited use in LMICs. In response to the increasing burden of cancer in LMICs, WHO published an executive summary of their National Cancer Control Programmes, Policies and Managerial Guidelines in 2002 (see http://www.who.int/cancer/media/en/408.pdf). Here, WHO described three country resource scenarios (low, medium, and high) and suggested that actions by national cancer control programmes for cancer early detection, diagnosis, treatment, and palliation should be prioritized based upon available resources. Strategic deployment of scarce health care resources in LMICs may help ensure that the highest proportion of the target population can access and benefit from breast health care in the timeliest fashion. However, at that time there were no guidelines to aid evidence-based decisions in breast cancer care that were appropriate for available resources in LMICs.

From 2002 to 2013, the Breast Health Global Initiative (BHGI), via a series of collaborative Global Summits held from 2002 to 2013, developed a resource-stratified framework to guide all aspects of breast cancer control across all resource settings (25). They used a well-defined and evidence-organized approach (primary literature review, evidence examination, structured multidisciplinary consensus development, team authorship, external peer review, and final publication) and presented their resource stratification methodology in 2005. This comprised a four-tier resource stratification framework—basic, limited, enhanced, and maximal—and resulted in resource-stratified guidelines for breast cancer early detection, diagnosis and pathology, treatment, and healthcare systems. The 2007 summit created a series of implementation metrics linked to the resource stratification tables and addressed resource-allocation monographs on early detection, diagnosis, treatment, and healthcare systems. That summit also developed guidelines on specific implementation issues in breast pathology, breast radiation therapy, and management of locally advanced breast cancer. In 2017, the BHGI, in collaboration with the Union for International Cancer Control and the National Cancer Institute (NCI) Center for Global Health, published 14 Knowledge Summaries for Comprehensive Breast Cancer Control. These summarized content from the guidelines to facilitate decision-making by policymakers, health care administrators, and advocates engaged in implementing breast-cancer control programmes at various resource levels. Each summary contains relevant clinical content, evidence-based approaches to guide breast cancer control, and policy and advocacy considerations to aid in the development and implementation of programmes and implementation of selected strategies. They emphasize coordinated, incremental programme improvements across the continuum of care to achieve the best possible outcomes at each resource level (see http://www.fredhutch.org/en/labs/phs/projects/breast-cancer-initiative_2-5/knowledge-summaries.html).

Complementing this work, at least four other groups have adapted BHGI's framework in resource-stratified guideline development for breast and other cancers including the Asian Oncology Summit guidelines (2009), the World Bank (2015), and ASCO. Finally, in 2017 the 70th World Health Assembly requested the Director-General 'to develop or adapt … resource-stratified guidance and tool kits … to establish and implement comprehensive cancer prevention and control programmes' (26). NCCN has now created its own resource-stratified framework for breast and other cancers which are also based on the BHGI methods and approach (27,28). This framework outlines a rational approach for 'building cancer management systems to provide the highest achievable level of cancer care by applying available and affordable services in a logical sequence.' Each resource level builds on the previous one and provides a framework for improving cancer care with incremental changes to the availability and allocation of resources (see https://www.nccn.org/framework/). Further work, in collaboration with the African Cancer Coalition, led to the NCCN Harmonized Guidelines for Sub-Saharan Africa based on the NCCN Guidelines launched in November 2017. The guidelines are targeted recommendations on treating breast and other cancers, they address cancer pain in adults, and they cover palliative care (see https://www.nccn.org/harmonized/default.aspx).

At present, it is unknown how LMICs will integrate resource-stratified guidelines into routine care. A systematic review of the literature assessed implementation of BHGI guidelines from the creation of knowledge in guideline development through guideline dissemination in the global health published work, and organizational adoption and implementation of the guidelines from 2003 to 2012. They found 552 articles that cited BHGI guidelines, and the majority, 68%, cited them as a method related to disease management and noted that the guidelines could develop a course of action. However, there was low specific implementation of the guidelines in comprehensive cancer control plans in various LMIC. The small number of publications referencing the guidelines as part of a comprehensive plan suggests that implementation remains a significant challenge for most LMICs (29). As discussed earlier, there are many reasons underlying a lack of compliance with CPGs (21), many of which are exacerbated in low-resource settings, where financial constraints are more likely to present significant barriers. Certainly, the existence of guidelines, however appropriate, does not determine or facilitate their use.

Key Messages

- The development and use of guidelines for the management of breast cancer in HICs has led to extensive evidence to support their widespread use.
- Adherence to evidence-based guidelines is associated with improved patient outcomes.
- In resource-rich environments, there is relatively little variation between CPGs themselves, although uptake and compliance vary widely between, and in some cases between and within, institutions.
- As CPGs appropriate for use in LMICs are developed, attention to barriers that may prevent or reduce their implementation efficacy should be assessed.
- Resource-stratified guidelines provide an approach, whereby evidence-based treatment approaches can be adapted to existing practice environments in LMICs.
- Since the implementation of resource-stratified guidelines has not yet been shown to improve cancer outcomes in LMICs, implementation research methodology will need to be developed to assess how improved guideline adherence in LMIC correlates, or fails to correlate, with improved breast cancer outcomes.

References

1. Institute of Medicine (US) Committee on Standards for Developing Trustworthy Clinical Practice Guidelines; Graham R, Mancher M, Miller Wolman D, Greenfield S, Steinberg E, editors. Clinical Practice Guidelines We Can Trust. Washington DC: National Academies Press; 2011. Available from http://www.ncbi.nlm.nih.gov/pubmed/24983061
2. Poonacha TK, Go RS. Level of scientific evidence underlying recommendations arising from the National Comprehensive Cancer Network Clinical Practice Guidelines. *J Clin Oncol* 2011;29:186–191.
3. Woolf SH et al. Potential benefits, limitations, and harms of clinical guidelines. *BMJ* 1999;318:527–530.
4. Brouwers MC et al. AGREE II: advancing guideline development, reporting, and evaluation in health care. *Prev Med* 2010;51:421–424.
5. Wolters R et al. A comparison of international breast cancer guidelines—do the national guidelines differ in treatment recommendations? Eur J Cancer 2012;48:1–11.
6. Hogeveen SE et al. Comparison of international breast cancer guidelines: are we globally consistent? Cancer Guideline AGREEment. *Curr Oncol* 2012;19:e184–e190.
7. Wockel A et al. Effects of guideline adherence in primary breast cancer—a 5-year multi-center cohort study of 3976 patients. *Breast* 2010;19:120–127.
8. Schwentner L et al. Triple-negative breast cancer: the impact of guideline-adherent adjuvant treatment on survival—a retrospective multi-centre cohort study. *Breast Cancer Res Treat* 2012;132:1073–1080.

9. Schwentner L et al. Adherence to treatment guidelines and survival in triple-negative breast cancer: a retrospective multi-center cohort study with 9,156 patients. *BMC Cancer* 2013;13:487.

10. van de Water W et al. Adherence to treatment guidelines and survival in patients with early-stage breast cancer by age at diagnosis. *Br J Surg* 2012;99:813–820.

11. Adegboyega TO et al. Institutional review of compliance with NCCN guidelines for breast cancer: lessons learned from real-time multidimensional synoptic reporting. *J Natl Compr Canc Netw* 2015;13:177–183.

12. Weeks JC et al. Interinstitutional variation in management decisions for treatment of 4 common types of cancer: a multi-institutional cohort study. *Ann Intern Med* 2014;161:20–30.

13. Barni S et al. Importance of adherence to guidelines in breast cancer clinical practice. The Italian experience (AIOM). *Tumori* 2011;97:559–563.

14. Sukel MP et al. Substantial increase in the use of adjuvant systemic treatment for early stage breast cancer reflects changes in guidelines in the period 1990–2006 in the southeastern Netherlands. *Eur J Cancer* 2008;44:1846–1854.

15. Guadagnoli E et al. The quality of care for treatment of early stage breast carcinoma: is it consistent with national guidelines? *Cancer* 1998;83:302–309.

16. Olivotto A et al: Compliance with practice guidelines for node-negative breast cancer. *J Clin Oncol* 1997;15:216–222.

17. Winchester DP, Cox JD. Standards for breast-conservation treatment. *CA Cancer J Clin* 1992;42:134–162.

18. White J et al. Compliance with breast-conservation standards for patients with early-stage breast carcinoma. *Cancer* 2003;97:893–904.

19. Persing S et al. Surgical margin reporting in breast conserving surgery: does compliance with guidelines affect re-excision and mastectomy rates? *Breast* 2015;24:618–622.

20. Lugtenberg M et al. Perceived barriers to guideline adherence: a survey among general practitioners. *BMC Fam Pract* 2011;12:98.

21. Cabana MD et al. Why don't physicians follow clinical practice guidelines? A framework for improvement. *JAMA* 1999;282:1458–1465.

22. DeSantis CE et al. International variation in female breast cancer incidence and mortality rates. *Cancer Epidemiol Biomarkers Prev* 2015;24(10):1495–1506.

23. Bray F et al. Global cancer transitions according to the Human Development Index (2008–2030): a population-based study. *Lancet Oncol* 2012;13:790–801.

24. Institute for Health Metrics and Evaluation (IHME). Financing Global Health 2016: Development Assistance, Public and Private Health Spending for the Pursuit of Universal Health Coverage. Seattle, WA: IHME; 2017.

25. Anderson BO, Duggan C. Resource-stratified guidelines for cancer management: correction and commentary. *J Glob Oncol* 2017;3:84–88.

26. World Health Organization: The Seventieth World Health Assembly. Cancer prevention and control in the context of an integrated approach, in The Seventieth World Health Assembly: A70/A/CONF./9. Geneva: WHO; 2017.

27. Carlson RW et al. NCCN Framework for resource stratification: A framework for providing and improving global quality oncology care. *J Natl Compr Canc Netw* 2016;14(8):961–969.

28. Gradishar WJ et al. NCCN Guidelines Insights: Breast Cancer, Version 1.2017. *J Natl Compr Canc Netw* 2017;15:433–451.

29. Echavarria MI et al. Global uptake of BHGI guidelines for breast cancer. *Lancet Oncol* 2014;15:1421–1423.

PART 4

THE MULTIDISCIPLINARY MEETING

10

The Multidisciplinary Meeting

Hallmark of Multidisciplinary Care

Terry Sarantou, Cary S. Kaufman, Alexandru Eniu, Sabine Siesling, Marc Espié, Xander Verbeek, and Roberto Salgado

Introduction

Over the past 100 years, the care of patients with breast cancer has changed from radical surgical intervention with mastectomy to less aggressive surgical intervention and includes systemic therapy and radiation therapy. New developments in medical oncology, radiation oncology, and reconstruction have become integral to breast cancer treatment. Management of many patients may be straightforward; however, some patients present with diagnostic and treatment dilemmas associated with their age, family history, genetics, presentation, or tumour biology. In the progression towards more personalized medicine as well as patients presenting with unique problems, international guidelines, such as the National Comprehensive Cancer Network (NCCN) and European Society of Medical Oncology (ESMO), or consensus guidelines, such as the St Gallen, may be difficult to interpret in some instances (1–3) (see Chapter 9). Many breast programmes are developing their own breast care guidelines based on consensus and evidence-based data. This promotes teamwork, a sense of ownership, and leads to better participation. Consequently, a more robust multidisciplinary approach with the cooperative efforts of those providers treating patients with breast disease has become increasingly important. Prospective presentation of breast cancer cases at a multidisciplinary breast conference (MBC) or tumour board promotes effective evidence-based care.

Structure of the Multidisciplinary Breast Conference and Multidisciplinary Tumour Decision Teams

The multidisciplinary breast conference (MBC) has evolved from general 'tumour boards', where a variety of cancer cases were presented at regular intervals to review complex treatment regimens and plans for patients, to 'specialized' tumours boards for specific cancers including breast disease. Tumour boards allow experts to review a complex case and work together to develop and refine therapeutic strategy. In the USA, the cancer tumour board is a required component for achieving accreditation through the Commission on Cancer, a quality programme using evidence-based standards and organized through the American College of Surgeons with input from multiple provider organizations. A formal accreditation programme for breast centres also exists, the National Accreditation Program for Breast Centers (NAPBC), which accredits breast centres in the USA and internationally (3–5). The Commission on Cancer and NAPBC accredit cancer programmes through compliance with evidence-based standards for cancer care. The NAPBC requires a formal breast cancer conference with specific guidelines for presenting patients and provider attendance thresholds as part of its accreditation process (see Chapter 5).

Multidisciplinary breast cancer clinics (MDCs) also exist, where patients are seen by multiple providers in one setting, including review of pathology and imaging. MDCs are required in Europe, but not in the USA, and they can represent best practice. MDCs are often seen in academic settings and require resources that may not be available to all providers and/or breast centres.

In Europe, multidisciplinary tumour decision teams (MDTs) are required by accreditation services for breast units in several countries and are mandatory by law in the UK. The MDT is defined as 'A group of people of different health care disciplines which meets together at a given time (whether physically in one place or by video or teleconferencing) to discuss a given patient and who are each able to contribute independently to the diagnostic and treatment decisions about the patient'. The UK Department of Health Manual for Cancer Services (London, Department of Health, 2004) establishes that for breast cancer care, core membership of the MDT includes two designated breast surgeons, a radiation oncologist, medical oncologist, two imaging specialists, two pathologists, two breast cancer nurse specialists, and an MDT coordinator/secretary. Extended team members include a reconstructive/plastic surgeon, physiotherapist/lymphoedema specialist, psychiatrist or clinical psychologist, and a social worker.

The European Society of Breast Cancer Specialists (EUSOMA) has developed requirements for specialist breast units and quality indicators in breast cancer care (6,7) (see Chapter 4). EUSOMA's recommendations aim at improving the quality of breast cancer care and specify that 'The Breast Centre must hold at least weekly a multidisciplinary case management meeting (MDM) to discuss diagnostic, preoperative and postoperative cases, as well as any other issues related to breast cancer patients, which requires multidisciplinary discussion'. At least 90% of all breast cancer cases should be discussed prospectively. To ensure that the best multidisciplinary evaluation is made for each case, several core members of the breast team need to be present: radiologist, pathologist, medical oncologist, surgeon/oncoplastic surgeon, breast care nurse, and radiation oncologist. Additional members are encouraged to participate and should be available for consultation. These include a nuclear medicine specialist, clinical geneticist, psychologist/psychiatrist, physiotherapist/lymphatic drainage specialist, breast care worker, and palliative care specialist. General practitioners are encouraged to participate. A breast centre is required to care for a minimum 150 breast cancer cases for accreditation (8).

Why Do We Need MDTs?

Multidisciplinary breast care should be the goal of all breast programmes. The MBC serves as an organizational structure of a breast programme which facilitates collaborative care between physicians and ancillary staff. Breast conference presentation encourages patient review and provides opportunities for physician and staff education so that patients receive the most up-to-date and relevant treatment. Breast conference presentation also serves as an opportunity to review clinical trial participation, participation in research, complementary/alternative therapies, and the need for psychosocial support.

With increasing knowledge and technological advances, breast health care has become more complex. Patients see multiple specialists for their care, and at times communication between providers and patient is not ideal. Cancer care 'office shuttling' may lead to delays and gaps in patient care treatment. Multidisciplinary breast care 'tumor board clinics' were described in the USA in the 1980s and provided second opinions for care (8). Although multidisciplinary breast clinics were popular in the 1990s and still are today, they face challenges due to cost, required resources, time commitment of physician and ancillary staff, and overload of information on the patient from seeing multiple providers in one setting. MBCs as outlined in the USA and MDTs as outlined in Europe and other settings, as opposed to breast multidisciplinary clinics, provide a practical method for case presentation with review. The observed outcome has been an ongoing blending of MBC and decision team presentation, leading to enhanced patient care plans.

MBC presentation allows for reviewing selected cases that benefit most from collaborative review. MBC and MDT review also provides an opportunity to identify patients for clinical trial and research participation.

Tables 10.1 and 10.2 illustrate some key components of the multidisciplinary breast clinic (MDC) with benefits and challenges (9).

Observational studies have shown the benefits of receiving cancer treatment at a specialist centre, and evidence continues to accrue from comparative studies of clinical benefits of an MDT approach, including improved survival (10). A Scottish study reviewed 13,722 patients undergoing cancer care between 1990 and 2000 in western Scotland (11). Prior to the introduction of multidisciplinary care (September 1995), mortality was 11% higher in the intervention area than in the non-intervention area (hazard ratio: 1.11). The authors concluded that with the introduction of MDTs, mortality was 18% lower in the area where MDTs had been introduced (hazard ratio = 0.82) than in other areas in the region.

Murthy et al. (9) reported that patients presented at MBCs experienced improvement in patient management and treatment: 42% of patients had modified changes in management after presentation at MBCs; 38% of treatment changes were for surgery, 33% for medical oncology (chemotherapy and endocrine therapy), 17% for radiation oncology, 6% for both medical and radiation oncology, and 6% for imaging

Table 10.1 Multidisciplinary clinic (MDC): clinical care

Benefits	Pitfalls
Single site of care	Incompatible space/personnel needs
Decreased cost (volume)	Increased cost (volume)
Enhanced communication	Increased complexity of staff function/training
Coordinated treatment plan	Turf wars, politics
Broad-based patient education	
Coordinated follow-up	

(see Figures 10.1 and 10.2). Most of the changes were made to AJCC Stage IA (27%) followed by AJCC Stage 0 (21%).

Newman et al. showed changes in recommendations for surgical management resulting from review of patients presented at MDCs, with 45% of cases with changes in interpretation from imaging review (12). This resulted in a change in surgical management in 11% of patients. Review of pathology resulted in changes in interpretation in 29% of patients with a 9% change in surgical management; 34% of patients had a change in surgical management after discussion with surgeons, medical oncologists, and radiation oncologists not based on reinterpretation of radiology or pathology. Overall, second evaluation of patients reviewed at MDCs led to changes in recommendation of treatment in 52% of patients.

Table 10.2 Multidisciplinary clinic (MDC): research efforts

Benefits	Pitfalls
Pooled resources	Increased complexities and incompatibilities
Correlations and input across specialties	Scientific disagreements
Enhanced development of evidence	Different 'cultures' and educational backgrounds
Cross training/education across disciplines	Politics of different departments and research units
Ability to train beyond primary discipline	

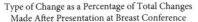

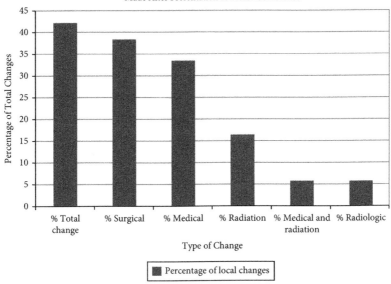

Figure 10.1 Type of treatment modification as a percentage of total change made following discussion at MBC. A total 42% of all cases presented received changes to treatment following discussion at MBC (38.2% surgical, 33.3% medical, 16.6% radiation, 6.8% both medical and radiation, and 4.9% radiologic).

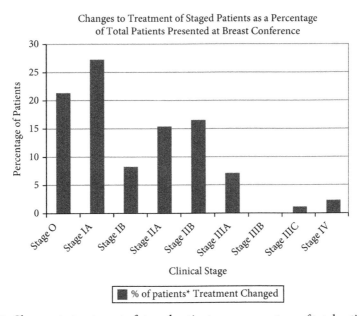

Figure 10.2 Changes to treatment of staged patients as a percentage of total patients presented at MBC. Changes in Stage 0 patient treatment total 21% of total changes. Stage IA: 27%; Stage 1B: 8%; Stage IIA: 15%; Stage IIB: 17%; Stage IIIA: 7%; Stage IIIB: 0%; Stage IIIC: 1%; Stage IV: 2%.

How to Organize a Successful MBC/MDT?

A breast programme leadership committee should be formed to organize the MBC/MDT, ensure multidisciplinary representation, monitor and evaluate meeting frequency unique to individual disciplines and practices, establish attendance thresholds, review prospective and annual case presentation, and include staging and discussion of pertinent treatment guidelines. Support and input from hospital administration is important.

Physicians who wish to be identified as members of a breast programme may formulate a 'contract', where breast programme participants (mainly physicians) agree to present a minimum number of breast cases. The agreement to present cases at breast MBCs/MDTs provides recognition to members of a multidisciplinary breast programme. Good leadership is essential to ensure positive team dynamics, adequate administrative support, recording of the data, and sufficient staff time and funding for the MBC/MDT.

The MBC/MDT should be held at regular intervals (at least biweekly) and, ideally, with most cases presented in a prospective fashion. An MBC/MDT coordinator should be responsible for reaching out to the physicians or staff who wish to present a case, organizing the case presentations with relevant necessary materials, and collaborating with pathology, radiology, and pertinent ancillary staff (Table 10.3).

As defined by the NAPBC, MBC/MDT presentations should include:

- a presentation of relevant history and physical elements, including family history;
- a discussion of stage, risk profile, surgical options/pre-surgical options;
- visual display of pathology slides and radiology imaging, and a discussion regarding radiology–pathology correlation;
- discussion regarding clinical trials, genetics risk, and reconstructive options;
- consideration of nationally recognized guidelines at the conference;
- an open discussion among all conference participants.

Table 10.3 Multidisciplinary breast conference (MBC)/multidisciplinary team (MDT): conference attendees and outcomes

Who should attend?	Conference discussion
Breast and reconstructive surgeons	Different clinicopathologic aspects of disease
Pathology	Up-to-date treatments
Radiology	Sound, unique treatment plan for each patient
Medical and radiation oncology	Clinical trials and data metrics review
Other medical professionals	Provider relevancy

The NAPBC defines prospective case review as:

- newly diagnosed breast cancer and treatment not yet initiated;
- newly diagnosed breast cancer and treatment initiated, but discussion and additional treatment is needed;
- previously diagnosed, initial treatment completed, but discussion of adjuvant treatment or treatment recurrence or progression is needed;
- consideration for clinical trials;
- previously diagnosed and discussion of supportive or palliative care is needed.

Programme circumstances will determine the timing and frequency of case presentation. If there will be a delay in care while waiting for the breast MBC/MDT presentation, physicians can also initiate multidisciplinary communication via electronic methods, e-mail, electronic health record, telephone, or conference call.

Physicians and ancillary staff may face challenges regarding the scheduling and timing of the MBC/MDT conference. They may feel that there might be competing priorities with the time required to attend multiple meetings and conferences. The breast programme must specifically create a dialogue with physicians and ancillary members and emphasize and reinforce the importance of MBC participation. The breast MBC/MDT is often identified as the 'central piece' of a breast programme, and robust participation is vital to the success of the breast centre. Physicians and staff must realize that their lack of MBC participation may be viewed by those in their communities as jeopardizing their relevance as breast centre participants.

Ideally, providers should commit to a prescribed time to attend MBC as part of their patient care routine. Providers may find themselves housed in different locations at the time of MBC. Fortunately, technology now allows for MBC/MDT presentation via different electronic avenues. Advances in video technology allow providers to access conference presentation and review patient information, radiology, and pathology. Providers can also access MDTs from their smartphones or tablets. These technologies are efficient and give providers a sense of active conference participation.

A breast programme should determine the number of cases to be presented at the tumour board. This number can be obtained from reviewing the analytic case load of a breast programme. Depending on resources available, centres may choose to present all cases (ideal) or to select cases that may ideally benefit from multidisciplinary presentation. Other methods of case review exist, including a 'working conference' held on a regular basis, where most breast patients who will be seen at a centre will have their relevant history (including pathology report) and images reviewed and an initial treatment plan formulated. These working conferences allow for more rapid review of many cases and allow time for a more thorough didactic presentation for those cases presented at formal breast MBC/MDTs. The core group of physicians caring for the patients presented at MBC/MDT should be available and participate in the discussion of the patients presented.

A conference organizer can record the recommendations and treatment plan discussed at the MBC. Ideally, a sound, complete, and unique treatment plan should be completed for each patient presented. Options include creating a conference 'tracking sheet', where the conference recommendations can be recorded. In addition to a patient identifier, the tracking sheet should record the stage of breast cancer, brief description of treatment recommendations including relevant surgical, medical, and radiation oncology therapies. Additional topics to be listed in the tracking sheet include discussion of national and breast centre treatment guidelines, genetics, psychosocial support, rehabilitation, and relevant clinical trials (Figure 10.3). Other information can be recorded at the discretion of the breast programme. The breast centre should discuss how this information will be used. The information can be forwarded to the relevant medical providers to be placed into the medical record. The breast programme can audit the information to assess compliance with MBC/MDT recommendations as a quality measure. The confidentiality of all patient information disclosed at MBCs must be maintained by all participants.

Example MDT in the Netherlands

In the Netherlands, MBC/MDT presentation serves as a quality metric for multidisciplinary care (13).

Improved technologies and medicines demand further specialization on the part of professionals and set higher requirements for professional collaboration. At the same time, there is a growing demand for transparency regarding the effectiveness and efficiency of treatments such as the responsible use of new medicines.

The Netherlands Comprehensive Cancer Organisation (IKNL, http://www.iknl.nl) responds to these changes by supporting the MDT in several ways.

- They developed the MDT toolkit, a quality instrument describing quality criteria to achieve an effective MDT. The MDT toolkit contains a regulation code/protocol in which agreements are described with the participating disciplines, participating institutions, responsibilities, preparation and presentation, workflow and decision-making, reporting and availability of relevant information for care partners or a consultant (information standard), documentation/archiving of the outcome of the MDT with a treatment plan.
- They support MDT meetings by hiring consultants or tumour-specific experts, who give their advice through teleconferences if necessary. Previously, consultants

LCI Breast Health Conference
Wednesday, August 1, 2018
****

CASE#	MR#	NAME	DOB	DIAGNOSIS/TITLE	PRESENTING PHYSICIAN
1					

Clinical or Path AJCC Stage   T____N____M____Group_   No AJCC scheme for this histology____

National Guidelines Discussed ☐ NCCN ☐_____ <u>No</u> NCCN Guidelines for this histology ☐

Prognostic Indicators Discussed ☐

Clinical Trials Discussed ☐

Genetic Testing Discussed ☐

Nutrition Referral ☐

Rehabilitation Referral ☐

Reconstruction Referral ☐

Psychosocial Referral ☐

ECOG Performance Status:	ASA Classification:
☐0 - Unrestricted in physical activity	☐1 normal
☐1 - Strenuous activity restricted, able to do light work	☐2 mild sys disease
☐2 - Up and about > 50% waking hrs	☐3 severe sys disease
☐3 - Confined to bed or chair > 50% waking hrs	☐4 severe sys disease w/ constant threat to life
☐4 - Completely disabled.	☐5 imminent risk of death
☐5 - Dead	☐6 brain dead

Surgical Recommendations:_____
_____
_____
_____

Medical Oncology Recommendations:_____
_____
_____
_____

Radiation Oncology Recommendations:_____
_____
_____

Figure 10.3 Conference tracking sheet.

were required to attend the conference, but their attendance was less frequent. Introducing teleconferences required persuasiveness, because clinicians were concerned that a perceived lack of live face-to-face interaction would diminish the effectives of the conference. Video consultation was gradually implemented by continuing with a live bimonthly meeting. Initially, reviewing pathology and radiology correlation was constricted by technology, and there was a perceived awareness of less optimal presenter preparation when using a video format. As technology improved, these obstacles were overcome. Around 2009, all hospitals were able to do video consultation.

- They supported the creation of networks such as the Comprehensive Cancer Networks, in which MDT discussions are not restricted to the knowhow of one hospital/team but can profit from the knowledge of an entire region. Hospitals and cancer programmes are combining into networks, and this is leading to changes in the delivery of breast cancer care. Lower-volume hospitals are increasingly relying on video consultation and development of treatment algorithms to optimize patient care.
- Guidelines (http://www.oncoline.nl) presented in data-driven decision trees are available interactively in 'Oncoguide for tumour board decision support' (http://www.oncoguide.nl). By projecting patient information discussed in the Tumour Board on the decision tree, Oncoguide generates a path through the tree towards a patient-specific guideline-based clinical advice. In addition to guideline-based decision trees, Oncoguide includes prediction models (nomograms) such as PREDICT and the Nottingham Prognostic Index to support clinical decision-making based on risk prediction (14,15).

Does Presentation of Patients and Participation in MBC/MDT Lead to Increased Quality?

Efforts have been made to investigate the role and efficiency of tumour boards in medical systems. The endpoints evaluated in these studies have included patient satisfaction, clinical outcomes, team dynamics, and communication (16). A major goal of MBC/MDT participation is to reduce delays in patient treatment and improve patient satisfaction. Unfortunately, measuring the efficacy of a tumour board is complex and multifactorial, and this creates challenges to objectively quantify endpoints (17). Participation in tumour boards can lead to increased clinical trial participation (18).

MBC/MDT should serve as a mechanism to review specific quality metrics of a breast programme. Attending and presenting at MBC/MDT facilitates discussion regarding the direction of breast programme care for patients. Decisions regarding review of treatment decision pathways and quality metrics can be outlined at MBC/MDT. Treatment pathways can be updated with review of the recent literature. Reviews of metrics and pathways should be performed at least annually.

Review of breast programme metrics, either group or individually based, encourages provider engagement in the breast programme and identifies the MBC as the centrepiece of a breast programme. Some physicians will participate in specialty society or individual data collection. The MBC is an ideal forum for presentation and self-review of breast centre and individual physician metrics. As the electronic medical record matures, it is expected that more of the quality metrics will be incorporated.

Metrics include:

- frequency of the conference (weekly or bimonthly?);
- specialty and individual attendance;
- documentation of conference discussion and recommendations for patient care;
- number of patients discussed;
- presentation: prospective, prior to medical and/or surgical treatment, ongoing care, and survivorship;
- specialty and individual physician quality metrics (determined by breast programme leadership).

Future Perspectives

The contemporary treatment of breast cancer has increased in complexity, and combined modality therapy is the standard of care. An MBC recognizes the need for multimodality treatment in a collaborative setting. Incorporating genomics into patient care is becoming increasingly important.

Multidisciplinary molecular tumour boards are emerging as a post-analytical tool for patient care. Due to the increasing use of high-throughput genomic technologies, clinicians are increasingly faced, in daily practice, with the question of how best to deal with this enormous amount of genomic information. A classical test cycle is defined as having three main components:

- the pre-analytical phase, defined as the phase before testing, when it is important that all conditions of sample handling, e.g. fixation, are adequately controlled;
- the analytical phase, defined as that part of the cycle that concerns performing the assay, when it is important to rigorously validate the assay in terms of sensitivity, specificity, etc.;
- the post-analytical phase, defined as that part of the cycle concerned with, e.g. data-analysis.

It has become apparent that at the pre-analytical and analytical levels, there may not be sufficient constraints to impede an adequate implementation of genomic-driven clinical practice. However, the interpretation of genomic data is still a major hurdle for a substantial number of clinicians (19). In a recent study by Johnson and colleagues, only a minority of clinicians felt comfortable in interpreting, using, and discussing somatic as well as germline test results (20). The authors reasonably conclude that 'To optimise the integration of genomic sequencing into cancer care, methods must be developed to improve basic competencies around cancer-based genomic testing. Given the complexities surrounding variant interpretation and genotype–phenotype relationships, interdisciplinary collaborations are warranted.'

Enter the concept of an MTB, which is defined as a multidisciplinary board comprised mostly of oncologists, pathologists, research scientists, bioinformaticians, and genetic counsellors. This board reviews a patient's chart including pathological, radiological, and molecular information. The goal of an MTB is to advise on the optimal use of the genomic variants encountered. This advice may range from concluding that the obtained genomic information does not lead to a clinical intervention, which is unfortunately still mostly the case, to identifying clinical trial options and/or investigational/off-label use.

It is becoming apparent that the added value of the use of high-throughput genomic technologies in a daily health care setting will depend on the optimal interpretation and subsequent use of identified variants. This necessitates the development of MTB infrastructure, not only at a local level, namely in the hospital where these high-throughput technologies are being used, but also at a regional and even national level, since patients are highly mobile and may visit different centres. The further development and integration of genomic-driven daily practice will not only be impeded by the under-use of the encountered genomic variants due to inexperienced and suboptimally trained clinicians in genomic medicine, but also by the discrepant use of the variants of an individual patient in different hospital settings by different clinicians specifically due to the lack of training and/or harmonization of the use of these variants across different hospital settings. The latter is also of legal importance, since patients are increasingly better informed on the use of this information, and they may not accept that important treatment options are withheld.

Therefore, van der Velden and colleagues have defined a set of recommendations for optimal MTB functioning which ranges from minimal member and operational requirements and includes the need for the development of a policy for unsolicited findings (21).

All the above illustrate that the post-analytical phase is becoming an increasingly important element to consider and develop within this ever-evolving context of genomic-driven medicine.

- Incorporate the results of the MDT in the electronic patient files with different prediction models and supporting data.
- Include the pitfalls of commercial organizations and the advantage of fair data (http://www.navify.com); oncology 360 (Varian); intellispace (Philips).

Presentation and participation in MBC/MDT will also become more important within the current evolving landscape of reimbursement models. It is conceivable that organ-based tumour boards will review patient treatment plans with evidence-based consensus of care with costs including imaging, surgery, systemic therapy, radiation therapy, palliative care, and other key components of care, while also educating patients on the costs of testing.

The interdisciplinary setting promoted by MBC/MDT leads to an environment to produce an organized evidence-based approach to cancer care (Figure 10.4). The knowledge and experience of MBC/MDT participants enhances education among participants and leads to enhanced individual participation in MBC/MDT. Nevertheless, remarkable differences are noted in the mandatory aspects of MDT in different geographic regions in the world (22).

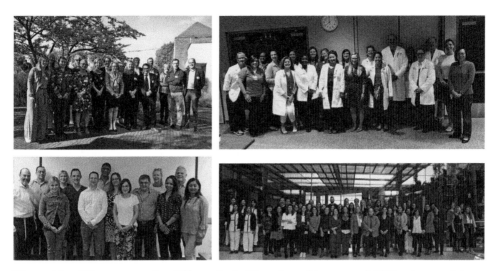

Figure 10.4 'The same goal, a different look. There is nothing more fulfilling in your job than working with the best team in the world.' Teams from Belgium, USA, South Africa, and Portugal.

Key Messages

- Multidisciplinary team work for breast cancer ensures the best options and treatment.
- Although the optimal management of breast cancer requires expertise of different disciplines and multidisciplinary meetings, it is not mandatory in many countries.
- Many patients presented at the MDT discussion had modified changes in management.
- Teleconferences can be helpful, but they require efficient technologies and optimal presenter preparation.
- Multidisciplinary molecular tumour boards will become more important with increasing use of genomic technologies.

References

1. Curigliano G et al. De-escalating and escalating treatments for early-stage breast cancer: the St. Gallen International Expert Consensus Conference on the Primary Therapy of Early Breast Cancer 2017. *Ann Oncol* 2017;28(8):1700–1712.
2. Cardoso F et al. 4th ESO–ESMO International Consensus Guidelines for Advanced Breast Cancer. *Ann Oncol* 2018;(July):1634–1657.
3. National Comprehensive Cancer Network. About the NCCN Clinical Practice Guidelines in Oncology (NCCN Guidelines®). Available from: https://www.nccn.org/professionals/default.aspx
4. Cancer Program Standards (2016 ed.). Available from: https://www.facs.org/quality-programs/cancer/coc/standards

5. National Accreditation Program for Breast Centers Standards Manual. Available from: https://accreditation.facs.org/accreditationdocuments/NAPBC/Portal Resources/ 2018NAPBCStandardsManual.pdf

6. Wilson ARM et al. The requirements of a specialist breast centre. *Eur J Cancer* 2013;49(17):3579–3587.

7. Biganzoli L et al. Quality indicators in breast cancer care: an update from EUSOMA Working Group. *Eur J Cancer* 2017;86:59–81.

8. La Fargue MM, Harness JK. Administrative and leadership challenges in building a new era of breast centers. *Semin Breast Dis* 2008;11(1):38–42.

9. Murthy V et al. Multidisciplinary breast conference improves patient management and treatment. *Surg Sci* 2014;5:214–319.

10. Vrijens et al. Effect of hospital volume on processes of care and 5-year survival after breast cancer: a population-based study on 25 000 women. *Breast* 2012;21:261–266.

11. Kesson M et al. Effects of multidisciplinary team working on breast cancer survival: retrospective, comparative, interventional cohort study of 13722 women. *BMJ* 2012;344:e2718.

12. Newman EA et al. Changes in surgical management resulting from case review at multidisciplinary tumor board. *Cancer* 2006;107(10):2346–2351.

13. Siesling S et al. Impact of hospital volume on breast cancer outcome: a population-based study in the Netherlands. *Breast Cancer Res Treat* 2014;147(1):177–184.

14. Wishart GC et al. PREDICT Plus: development and validation of a prognostic model for early breast cancer that includes HER2. *Br J Cancer* 2012;107(5):800–807.

15. Rakha EA et al. Nottingham Prognostic Index Plus (NPI+): a modern clinical decision making tool in breast cancer. *Br J Cancer* 2014;110(7):1688–1697.

16. El Saghir NS et al. Tumor boards: optimizing the structure and improving efficiency of multidisciplinary management of patients with cancer worldwide. *Am Soc Clin Oncol Educ Book* 2014:e461–e466.

17. Keating NL et al. Tumor boards and the quality of cancer care. *J Natl Cancer Inst* 2013;105(2):113–121.

18. Kehl KL et al. Tumor board participation among physicians caring for patients with lung or colorectal cancer. *J Oncol Pract* 2015;11(3):e267–e278.

19. Gray SW et al. Physicians' attitudes about multiplex tumor genomic testing. *J Clin Oncol* 2014;32(13):1317–1323.

20. Johnson LM et al. Integrating next-generation sequencing into pediatric oncology practice: an assessment of physician confidence and understanding of clinical genomics. *Cancer* 2017;123(12):2352–2359.

21. van der Velden et al. Molecular Tumor Boards: current practice and future needs. *Ann Oncol* 2017;28(12):3070–3075.

22. Saini K et al. Role of the multidisciplinary team in breast cancer management: results from a large international survey involving 39 countries. *Ann Oncol* 2011;23(4):853–859.

PART 5

QUALITY CONTROL OF BREAST CANCER DIAGNOSIS AND TREATMENT

11

Radiology

Hans Junkermann, Wolfgang Buchberger, Sylvia Heywang-Köbrunner,
Michael Michell, Alexander Mundinger, Carol Benn, and Sophia Zackrisson

Methods for Assessment of Breast Symptoms and Screening

Mammography

Imaging Principle

Mammography is an X-ray examination of the breast for screening (early detection) and diagnostic purposes. The image results from the differential absorption of low energy X-rays by the components of breast tissue. Calcifications are the strongest absorbing structures in the breast and are, therefore, easily detectable in all types of breast tissue. Microcalcifications (below 1 mm) often are the first sign of malignancy. The absorption of the other components in the breast is mainly determined by their water content. Thus, malignant tumours, cysts, benign tumours, and fibrous tissue all have a higher absorption than fatty tissue. Therefore, the presence of X-ray-absorbing benign or normal structures may obscure signs of malignancy or simulate the presence of a lesion.

During the second half of the 20th century there was a tremendous development of the mammography technique leading up to the now commonly used digital mammography systems. Today, there are still several types of system in use, including both analogue and digital systems. In analogue systems, also called screen-film mammography, the X-ray beams are collected on a film cassette, the films are developed, and then reviewed on a light-box by the radiologist. Along with the development of digital imaging during the last two decades, so-called flat panel detectors have come into use, which are designed to digitally capture the X-rays (instead of film) and convert the information to a digital image: full-field digital mammography. The digital images are viewed on digital high-resolution monitors and can be digitally stored just like computer files. Both types of system are still in use worldwide. The advantage with digital mammography is that the separate processes of image acquisition, display, and storage enable optimization of each. However, CR systems, in which the information is stored on a special imaging plate that replaces the film cassette and is read out on a separate reader that converts the latent image into a digital image, do not provide the full advantage of full-field digital mammography regarding image quality, radiation dose, and workflow.

The newest development in digital mammography that is now being introduced into clinical practice is tomosynthesis. This method is being used as a complement to, or even as a replacement for, conventional digital mammography at a fast pace (especially in the USA). Tomosynthesis is often described as 'pseudo three-dimensional mammography', since conventional mammography is a two-dimensional imaging technique, whereas tomosynthesis generates a three-dimensional image volume. With the development of the digital detectors and more powerful computers in the late 1990s, the first landmark paper on a digital breast tomosynthesis technique was published. Basically, the X-ray tube moves in a limited arch (typically 11–50°) over the breast, acquiring multiple low-dose projection images, which are mathematically reconstructed into an image volume with around 50–70 slices, usually 1 mm thick, that can be viewed individually, scrolled through, or shown as a cine loop on a computer screen. The major advantage of tomosynthesis is that it reduces the effect of overlapping tissue (especially in dense breasts) making suspicious lesions more visible and detectable compared with two-dimensional mammography while simultaneously reducing the simulation of malignant lesions by superimposition of benign structures.

Most vendors have combined units capable of both mammography and tomosynthesis. Further, to avoid the need for double acquisition of mammography and tomosynthesis, the generation of so-called synthetic mammograms from the tomosynthesis volume is of help for detecting asymmetries and comparing with prior mammograms.

Quality Assurance

Quality assurance (QA) programmes for mammography are highly developed and exist in many national adaptations. A driving force for their development and for their incorporation into national regulations was the importance of radiation protection in the use of a method applied to large numbers of healthy women. Typical examples for QA programmes are the European Guidelines of Quality Assurance in Mammography Screening and Diagnosis and the ACR Manual for QA. These programmes usually encompass assessment of the technical function of the mammography machine in the acquisition, processing, and display of the images. Daily, weekly, and monthly assessments are usually performed by the radiographers working on site, whereas semiannual or annual or assessments must be conducted by trained medical physicists or service technicians. Whereas QA of the digital mammography is by now fairly standardized with moderate differences between individual national programs, the programmes for tomosynthesis are still in development.

Demands on the Surroundings

The mammography machine must be installed in a temperature-controlled environment (digital detectors are temperature sensitive). The room must have adequate protection to prevent radiation from escaping into surrounding environment where non-involved persons sojourn. Most mammography machines are operated in stationary units; however, especially for screening, they are also operated in mobile units (e.g. trucks or busses). This helps in reaching out to less densely populated regions, but mobile units are costlier.

Investment and Running Cost

Mammography machines cost upwards of €60,000. If mammography is used for the assessment of screen-detected lesions and special views in cases of symptomatic women, then magnification and stereotactic-guided vacuum-assisted biopsy must be available. For reading mammograms, monitors with higher resolution (two 4K monitors) than usually used in radiology are necessary. A workstation for reading mammograms costs around €30,000. Whereas the films were a significant financial contribution to the service in analogue film screen mammography, the running costs for digital mammography are only minor. Principally, the cost for running and maintaining a PACS (picture archiving and communication system) to store and distribute the images need to be considered.

Demands on Personnel

For the acquisition of mammograms, well-trained radiographers are needed who also have sufficient regular practice. The positioning and compression of the breast has been described as an art (Figures 11.1 and 11.2). Existing guidelines should be considered in the performance of mammography. All efforts must be made to visualize as much of the breast tissue as possible while also avoiding unnecessary pain during the procedure. The performance of the radiographers should be regularly and systematically

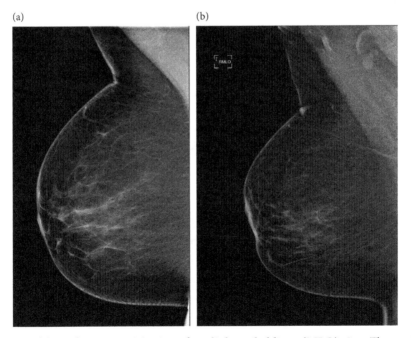

(a)   (b)

Figure 11.1 (a) Inadequate positioning of mediolateral oblique (MLO) view. The pectoral muscle is only marginally visible on the image, indicating that peripheral parts of the breast tissue are not be imaged. (b) Adequate positioning of MLO view. The pectoral muscle is seen down to the nipple line. Peripheral parts of the breast are covered as demonstrated by the imaging of (benign) axillary lymph nodes.

(a)   (b)

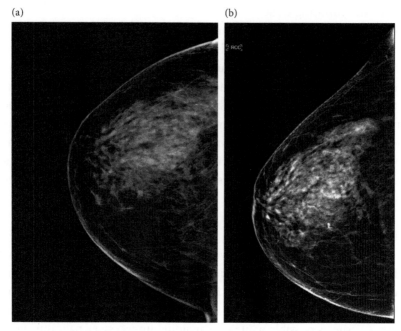

Figure 11.2 (a) Inadequate positioning of the craniocaudal (CC) view. The mammilla is deviating laterally and the lateral part of the breast is not imaged. (b) Adequate positioning of the CC view. The mammilla is pointing centrally and the lateral part of the breast is included, containing some benign microcalcifications.

monitored as part of the QA programme. The examination time for the woman is about the same for a mammography as a tomosynthesis. One technician can perform up to 10 mammographic examinations per hour.

Reading of the mammograms should only be done by specially trained physicians (usually radiologists) with sufficient regular practice. The European Guidelines as well as the ACR guidelines define minimum requirements for the reader (980–1000 cases per year) (1). The European Guidelines also suggest double reading for radiologists reading fewer than 3000 cases per year in symptomatic disease, and a minimum of 5000 cases per year together with double reading of all cases in screening. Reading time is an issue, especially in screening. Using batch reading in screening, one reader needs about 60 s per case. A reading session usually should not last longer than an hour, since it is not possible to maintain concentration continuously for a longer time. The time for reading tomosynthesis (including synthetic two-dimensional images) is about 50–100% longer. Data on the incremental value of double reading with tomosynthesis are not yet conclusive.

Medical Physicists
The technical quality control needs specially trained physicists or regular maintenance by qualified service personnel from the vendor of the equipment.

Ultrasonography

Imaging Principle

Since its introduction in the 1950s, breast ultrasound has evolved significantly and is now an indispensable tool for the detection and staging of breast cancer and for guiding breast interventions.

The technical principle is the transmission of high-frequency sound waves into the tissue, which are absorbed, scattered, partially reflected, and received by the ultrasound probe. From the position of the reflecting interface and the propagation time and amplitude of the reflected sound wave, a two-dimensional greyscale image is calculated (B-mode, brightness mode). High contrast and spatial resolution are achieved by using high-frequency linear array broad bandwidth transducers, usually with a frequency range of 5–12 MHz. Lower transducer frequencies are used for deeper lesions, and higher transducer frequencies are used for more superficial lesions.

Three-dimensional imaging can be achieved either by manually pivoting a two-dimensional linear transducer over a certain volume of the breast or by using matrix array transducers that electronically scan a three-dimensional volume. With a single pass of the ultrasound beam, a three-dimensional volumetric image and three perpendicular reconstructed planar sections—sagittal, transverse, and coronal—are displayed.

Relative Value for Screening and Assessment of Symptoms

Sonography was initially used only for the distinction between cysts and solid lesions. Simple cysts are correctly identified with an accuracy of nearly 100%. Complex cysts and clustered microcysts have a low probability of malignancy (0.8%) and require short-term imaging follow-up or occasionally ultrasound-guided fine-needle aspiration.

With more advanced ultrasound technique and increased experience, distinction between benign and malignant lesions became sufficiently reliable to avoid immediate histological clarification of solid lesions with a very low probability of malignancy. Ultrasound is frequently used for the assessment of palpable breast abnormalities. Approximately 10–15% of palpable carcinomas are occult on mammography but are detectable sonographically. On the other hand, negative mammography and ultrasound in a palpable lesion exclude malignancy with 97–100% confidence. In symptomatic women of average cancer risk aged <30 years in whom the risk of malignancy is less than 1%, assessment can be done with ultrasound alone, provided it demonstrates a benign cause of the symptoms. Otherwise, further imaging with mammography, magnetic resonance imaging (MRI) (especially in high-risk women), and/or needle biopsy is recommended.

Another common indication for breast ultrasound is evaluation of abnormal findings on mammography, including masses, architectural distortions, or asymmetries. Ultrasound is also used for the assessment of MRI-detected abnormalities. These lesions are frequently occult on mammography and can be identified, in part, with second-look targeted ultrasound. A systematic overview demonstrated a wide variation between 22.6% and 82.1% (pooled average 57.5%) in the effectiveness of this procedure. Besides further lesion characterization, ultrasound can be used to guide core needle biopsy. Although mammographically occult multifocal or multicentric disease can be detected sonographically, ultrasound is inferior to MRI in preoperative local staging of breast cancer. However, it can be used to identify abnormal axillary, supraclavicular, and internal mammary lymph nodes.

Ultrasound has also been used as a supplementary screening method in addition to mammography. Due to the expected significant increase in recall rates, biopsy rates, and absent data concerning its effect on mortality reduction or survival, additional ultrasound is currently not recommended in routine screening of women at normal risk for breast cancer. In high-risk women who receive both annual mammography and MRI, screening ultrasound at the time of MRI does not add value or incremental cancer detection.

Because of its easy availability and real-time capacity, ultrasound is the primary technique for guiding interventional procedures. Most palpable lesions, as well as many lesions detected with mammography or MRI, can be biopsied under sonographic guidance. With a false-negative rate of 1.5–3% and a complication rate of less than 1%, automated 14-gauge core needle biopsy is a safe and accurate diagnostic procedure and is adequate for most ultrasound-guided biopsies. Although vacuum-assisted biopsy has lower underestimation rates in high-risk lesions such as atypical hyperplasia, it is a much more expensive and invasive procedure and should only be considered for very small masses (below 5 mm), intraductal or intracystic lesions, or for microcalcifications.

Qualitative Demands and Quality Management

Specifications on the technical equipment and QA, the required qualification of the examiner, and adequate documentation of the examination are summarized in various guidelines, e.g. in the ACR practice guidelines or the EFSUMB guidelines (2). Minimal technical requirements are linear-array and broad-bandwidth transducers operating a centre frequency of at least 12 MHz. Gain settings, focal zone selections, and field of view should be optimized to obtain high-quality images. Equipment performance should be monitored regularly in accordance with existing guidelines. Conspicuous findings should be documented and measured in two perpendicular planes, and the clock position and distance to the nipple should be indicated. The report should be written according to the BI-RADS classification scheme.

Budgetary Impacts: Investment in Machinery, Running Costs, Expert Time Needed

The price for a real-time handheld ultrasound unit suitable for breast ultrasound begins at around €35,000. The annual maintenance costs are 5–10% of the acquisition costs. The time required for hand-guided sonography of both breasts performed by specially trained physicians or technologists is 15–20 min, which significantly adds to the cost of the method.

Magnetic Resonance Imaging

Imaging Principle

MRI uses the magnetic properties of hydrogen nuclei to image tissues based on their differing hydrogen content.

Even though some tissue information is possible without contrast agent, for detection or exclusion of malignancy breast MRI is internationally considered to require the use of MRI contrast agent, i.e. gadolinium chelates, which are administered intravenously. The imaging is thus based on the perfusion and diffusion properties of the contrast agent in diseased tissue compared to healthy tissue. Ongoing research projects are investigating possible new technologies for MRI without contrast media, and these are mainly based on diffusion-weighted imaging sequences, but, so far, equivalence with contrast-enhanced MRI is unproven.

With standard contrast-enhanced MRI, the complete breast is imaged at 2 mm slices using pixel sizes of approximately 1×1 mm. The complete volume (usually both breasts) is imaged once before contrast agent and three to five times after contrast medium every 1–2 min covering about 7–10 min after intravenous injection.

Relative Value for Screening and Assessment

Overall, contrast-enhanced MRI is the imaging modality with the highest sensitivity for the detection of invasive malignancy with sensitivity ranges around 95–99%. For malignancies detected by microcalcifications, the sensitivity is lower. Today, for clinical applications, sensitivities of 99% and specificities of 89% have been reported for MR differentiation of non-calcified mammographic masses, and sensitivities of 87% and specificities of 81% have been reported for MR differentiation of mammographic microcalcifications.

Considering the high sensitivity and negative predictive value in case of non-calcified lesions, the use of MRI for exclusion of malignancy may be justifiable to avoid biopsy for some non-calcified lesions. Appropriate cases might include those with multiple lesions, extensive scarring, and lesions which are difficult to target by percutaneous breast biopsy. However, in the cases where MRI (due to contrast enhancement irrespective of its type) cannot exclude malignancy, biopsy remains necessary.

In summary, data on the use and accuracy of MRI for lesion assessment have increased. Considering the excellent sensitivity of quality-assured percutaneous breast biopsy and its higher specificity compared to MRI, MRI is not currently considered part of the standard diagnostic work-up. For appropriate diagnostic questions, however, the use of MRI for differentiation appears justified.

Even though data concerning mortality reduction are lacking, and this is mostly due to the single-armed study designs, systematic reviews have shown a significant and convincing gain of sensitivity by the added use of MRI in women at high risk with and without gene mutation. High false-positive biopsy rates and the lack of mortality data are accepted in these women in view of expected advantages of earlier detection. For intermediate- and average-risk women, MRI screening is not recommended. However, some larger prospective studies are now investigating the value of screening MRI for certain groups of women at intermediate risk.

Qualitative Demands and Quality Management

Both national and international quality recommendations exist for breast MRI. As previously mentioned, breast MRI can be adequately performed on breast MRI units operating at 1.5–3 T. In addition, a special purpose breast coil is mandatory, and dedicated software is needed for image evaluation. The use of contrast agent is considered mandatory for cancer detection or exclusion.

Most guidelines require sufficient experience with, and availability of, mammography, breast ultrasound, and breast interventional techniques (ACR Practice Parameters 2013). Furthermore, the availability of MRI-guided interventions is considered requisite for anyone performing breast MRI. For MRI-guided breast biopsy, an additional dedicated breast biopsy coil with a corresponding targeting unit is needed. For state-of-the-art MRI-guided percutaneous breast biopsy, an MRI-compatible vacuum pump is necessary. For most institutions, the issue of availability of MRI-guided intervention is, however, solved by cooperation with specialized institutions possessing the equipment and expertise needed for this procedure.

Whereas technical prerequisites are fulfilled in most countries, remaining quality deficits most often concern patient motion, correct identification and interpretation of motion artefacts, and the diagnostic capabilities of the interpreting radiologist. Benchmarks for assessing the quality of MRI performance and results are highly desirable, but these may need to vary depending on the indication. Initial attempts are under way, and these demonstrate the existing limits of 'screening MRI' concerning both sensitivity, interval cancer rate, and positive predictive value of biopsy indications. Even though QA is most important for any screening procedure, an effective QA programme (including controlled training and systematic prospective data collection that would allow systematic evaluation and improvement by continuous feed-back) is, to our knowledge, not yet installed in any health system.

Budgetary Impacts: Investment in Machinery, Running Costs, Expert Time Needed

Costs per breast MRI study include costs for approximately 20 min MRI scanner time, costs of MRI contrast agent and blood tests (to assess kidney function before application of contrast agent), as well as additional costs for the dedicated breast coil, special pulse sequences (if applied), and dedicated evaluation software (for quantitative measurements and possibly motion compensation). Overall, these costs exceed the costs of most other MRI studies, and in most countries amount to three to five times the costs of a mammogram. Abbreviated protocols may allow reducing MRI scanner time. However, adequate testing and decision based on proven advantages and disadvantages remains necessary. If these protocols prove successful, moderate cost reduction may be possible.

Best Practice: Minimum and Ideal Requirements in (Developed) Countries

For Assessment of Symptoms

Introduction

The aim of the diagnostic assessment clinic for a patient presenting with breast symptoms is to provide a definite diagnosis of malignant or benign breast disease or normal physiological breast change (3). This is achieved by use of the multidisciplinary triple diagnostic method: (a) clinical examination; (b) imaging: ultrasound ± mammography; (c) needle biopsy where indicated. The tests used in an individual patient will be determined by the presenting symptoms, the clinical findings, and the age of the patient. The use of the triple diagnostic method enables a diagnosis to be established in the majority of patients, and diagnostic excision is rarely required. The published rate of delayed diagnosis of breast cancer in symptomatic women following triple assessment is 0.2%. The diagnostic clinic should be arranged so that radiological facilities are integrated with or very close to the clinic and organized so that all necessary tests are carried out during the same clinical visit.

(a) Clinical assessment

The clinical assessment should be carried out before imaging and should document the nature, site, and duration of symptoms and record the level of suspicion for malignancy on a scale P1–P5 (P1 = normal, P5 = malignant). The clinical assessment should be carried out by a suitably trained member of the multidisciplinary team. This may be a specialist breast care nurse, radiologist, breast clinician, or breast surgeon. The clinical information should be available to the staff conducting the imaging assessment.

(b) Imaging assessment (ultrasound and mammography)

Requirements:

- High-frequency ultrasound (≥12 MHz);
- Full-field digital mammography with facilities for additional views (spot compression, fine focus, magnification), tomosynthesis, and X-ray-guided biopsy;
- Equipment for image-guided biopsy including core biopsy, vacuum-assisted core biopsy, and fine-needle aspiration cytology (if sufficient expertise for the interpretation of breast disease is available);
- Breast MRI is not required for the initial diagnostic assessment of patients with symptoms (limited data indicate that MRI may add valuable additional information in a small group of selected patients with indeterminate assessment results).

(c) Needle biopsy

The clinical and imaging work-up should be completed prior to needle biopsy, and biopsy procedures should be carried out under imaging guidance in order to achieve optimum accuracy. The most commonly performed procedure in the symptomatic clinic is ultrasound-guided 14G core biopsy. Fine-needle cytology may also be helpful in assessing axillary lymph nodes. A clear local protocol for needle biopsy of breast lesions should be available based on clinical and imaging features and age. For example, a localized lump in a woman aged <25 years with benign clinical features and ultrasound appearances of a fibroadenoma may not require biopsy.

Referral

Patients presenting with breast symptoms are most commonly referred to the diagnostic clinic by the primary care doctor, general practitioner, or in some countries by other disciplines, e.g. gynaecology. Patients with the following symptoms should be referred:

(d) lump, lumpiness, change in texture;
(e) progressive change in breast size with signs of oedema;
(f) skin distortion, dimpling;
(g) nipple symptoms:
   • unilateral blood-stained or serous nipple discharge;
   • nipple eczema, nipple change, retraction/distortion;
(h) breast pain: one-sided, persistent following initial treatment;
(i) axillary lump.

The referring doctor should ensure that all relevant clinical information is provided to the clinic including the site and duration of symptoms and signs. This is best achieved using a standard referral proforma.

Use of Imaging

Ultrasound should be performed for all patients with a lump or localized change of texture found on examination and should be the sole imaging required for most women aged <40 years as well as women who are pregnant or lactating. The ultrasound examination should be targeted to the area of the patient's symptoms or signs and should cover the whole breast and axillary lymph nodes in patients with suspected malignancy.

Mammography should consist of mediolateral oblique and craniocaudal views of each breast and is used in the primary investigation of women aged ≥40 years (unless pregnant or lactating). Mammography should also be used in younger women with suspicious clinical findings (P4 and P5) and should be considered in women with indeterminate (P3) lesions in whom ultrasound is normal as well as after malignancy has been confirmed. The level of suspicion for malignancy on imaging should be recorded on a standard scale (e.g. British Society of Breast Radiology imaging classification, BI-RADS lexicon). Further specialized mammography views including spot compression and magnification views or tomosynthesis are carried out following standard views for the further mammographic assessment of equivocal and suspicious mammographic features and for all cases of malignancy. Tomosynthesis provides a more accurate measurement of local extent of malignant lesions compared to standard two-dimensional mammography.

MRI is only occasionally required in the initial assessment, for example, in suspicious discharge from the mammilla if the underlying abnormality cannot be located with mammography/ultrasound, or with diffuse changes in mammography/ultrasound where guided biopsy is not feasible because no defined target can be delineated.

It is more useful as an adjunct pretherapeutic assessment if malignancy is established but mammography/ultrasound are inconclusive considering the full extent of the infestation of the breast, and, for example, if nodal or distant metastasis suggests a primary in the breast that cannot be found by conventional methods (cancer of unknown primary (CUP) syndrome).

Also, it has advantages in the evaluation of the treatment response, especially in hormone receptor-negative tumours. The frequency of the use of pretherapeutic MRI varies from about 10% to nearly 100% in expert institutions, and this points to the scarce evidence relating the performance of pretherapeutic MRI to the outcome of the treatment.

Outcome and Quality Reporting of Diagnostic Assessment

Following assessment, patients should be clearly informed of the findings. Patients with normal, benign, or physiological changes are reassured. Patients who have undergone needle biopsy are provided with support and an appointment to discuss results. The assessment findings and results of all women who undergo needle biopsy should be discussed in a multidisciplinary meeting attended by radiologist, pathologist, surgeon, and breast care nurse in order to decide on further management.

The report on the results of imaging studies must be clear, exact, and understandable not only for the experts in imaging. In order to facilitate communication, standardized scales have been developed. Of these, the BI-RADS categories of the ACR have gained worldwide acceptance (4). Each imaging result is assigned to a category directly relating to further action that should be taken. The signs leading to each category are based on evidence and described in the BI-RADS lexicon. The BI-RADS reporting system for mammography has seven categories:

- BI-RADS 0: Incomplete—need additional imaging evaluation and/or prior mammograms
  Management: recall for additional imaging and/or comparison with prior examination(s).
  Comment: mostly used in screening
- BI-RADS 1: Negative
  Management: routine mammography screening.
  Comment: completely normal, no notable abnormalities.
- BI-RADS 2: Benign
  Management: routine mammography screening.
  Comment: a notable but clearly benign lesion.

- BI-RADS 3: Probably benign
  Management: short-interval (6-month) follow-up or continued surveillance mammography.
  Comment: a most probably benign lesion (estimated risk of malignancy below 2%). This category should only be assigned after a full diagnostic work-up. Short-term follow-up until malignancy is excluded is advisable. Biopsy is not recommended.
- BI-RADS 4: Suspicious
  Management: tissue diagnosis.
  Comment: intermediate risk of malignancy. Appropriate action to be taken (usually percutaneous biopsy).
- BI-RADS 5: Highly suggestive of malignancy
  Management: tissue diagnosis.
  Comment: almost certainly malignant (above 95%). Immediate action should be taken (histological confirmation and therapy).
- BIRADS 6: Known biopsy-proven malignancy
  Management: Surgical excision when clinically appropriate.
  Comment: this category has been introduced to facilitate QA statistics.

Reproduced with permission from Junkermann, H. et al. 'Breast Imaging Reporting and Data System'. ACR BI-RADS® Atlas, 5th edition. Copyright © 2013 American College of Radiology.

Assessment categories and management instructions are reproduced with permission from Sickles, EA, D'Orsi CJ, Bassett LW, et al. ACR BI-RADS® Mammography. In: ACR BI-RADS® Atlas, Breast Imaging Reporting and Data System. Reston, VA, American College of Radiology; 2013.

Definitions and management specifications for ultrasound and MRI are slightly divergent.

Achieving High-Quality Service
Key requirements are:

(a) effective multidisciplinary working;
(b) high-quality diagnostic equipment;
(c) specialist training for all disciplines;
(d) audit of practice against key standards, e.g.
   - all patients with breast symptoms seen in the clinic within two weeks of referral (standard 93%);
   - all patients requiring triple assessment have all tests performed during first visit (standard 95%);
   - preoperative diagnosis rate—proportion of cancers having a non-operative pathological diagnosis (standard 95%).

Imaging in Low- and Middle-Income Countries
In these countries, the major problem is often not the availability of mammography and ultrasound, but the accessibility of services for the symptomatic women for monetary and geographical reasons as well as cultural beliefs preventing them from seeking

medical assistance. Under these circumstances, it seems reasonable to deviate from the principle of complete imaging at the first visit and provide an accessible, perhaps a mobile, service using ultrasound together with core biopsy in an outreach clinic. More expensive and less mobile mammography is then only secondarily applied in the treatment centre after malignancy has been established.

For Screening

Despite some pronounced critical discussion of the harm:benefit ratio, the majority of international experts judge that mammography screening for breast cancer fulfils the criteria formulated by Wilson and Jungner in their World Health Organization report (1968) for an effective screening programme (International Agency for Research on Cancer, 2015). Mammography is the method of choice for women of average breast cancer risk. The age group that benefits most is women aged 50–70 years. In view of the rising age at death, especially in high-income countries, the extension of mammography screening to 75 years is considered appropriate by many experts and governmental bodies. The extension to the lower age range between 40 and 50 years of age is more equivocal (5).

Since screening addresses apparently healthy subjects of whom only a fraction will develop the disease (lifetime risk in western developed countries is around 10 per 100 women), not only the question of sensitivity but also the question of specificity is of utmost importance. Breast cancer is a heterogeneous disease with large variations in aggressiveness and disease progression. Therefore, the issue of overdiagnosis—i.e. the diagnosis of a breast cancer that, without screening, would never have been detected, caused symptoms, or caused death during a person's lifetime—is an important consideration, especially with respect to screening older age groups. In contrast to the assessment of symptomatic disease, in screening a multimodal approach is usually not appropriate not only for economic reasons, but also because the application of multiple methods adversely affects the balance between sensitivity and specificity.

In order to maintain a positive balance between the harm and benefit of a screening programme, the screening examination should be performed in a strictly quality-assured surrounding. Descriptions of all aspects of QA of an organized screening programme are contained in the 'European Guidelines for Quality Assurance in Breast Cancer Screening and Diagnosis' which are available in their 4th edition (2006), whereas the ACR Best Practice Guidelines address QA in a more open system (6).

In order to make such a programme effective, the aspects detailed in the following sections need to be considered.

Reach the Target Group as Completely as Possible
In general, an invitation model allows the best coverage of the target group irrespective of social factors. This requires registers comprising the whole target group.

Maximize the Early Detection Potential of the Method Used for Screening
Screening for early cancers demands that the methods used are brought to their highest level of performance in order to detect as many cancers in a stage, where effective

treatment can be applied without maximum treatment intensity. In mammography screening, independent double reading of the images improves the sensitivity of the method by about 10% and is recommended in the European Guidelines.

Minimize Inherent Negative Consequences of the Screening Programme

Any screening programme has adverse effects, since no method of detection has complete sensitivity and, especially important in the screening situation, specificity. This leads to additional work-up for ambiguous (false-positive) lesions, which puts emotional and physical strain on healthy participants. To reduce the false positives, the decision to assess a lesion should be made by readers with a high level of experience (the European Guidelines demand 5000 readings per year), and regular feedback on the achieved sensitivity and specificity is necessary in order to allow each reader to adjust his individual working point. In order to reduce the emotional strain until clarification of suspicious lesions, their assessment should be offered in a fast, but not overly rushed, structured process by experienced personnel.

The most serious adverse effect of any screening programme is that disease is detected and treated that may never have surfaced and may never have become a health problem if it had not been detected in the screening programme. In mammography screening, this may not only refer to some of the in-situ cancers that would be treated with local measures (surgery and irradiation) alone, but also to some invasive carcinomas that would be treated with aggressive or longstanding systemic treatment, because we are not able to determine which individual tumour will progress to endanger health during the remaining lifetime of the patient. Reliable estimates of the amount of overdiagnosis are extremely difficult to obtain outside of randomized studies with long-term follow-up and no screening of the control groups, which is the case in only two trials (Malmö and Canada). All other estimates are based on modelling, and are, therefore, less reliable. Comparable amounts of overdiagnosis, however, must be expected for all methods allowing earlier detection effectively.

Foster Participation of the Target Group, While Respecting an Individual's Right to Informed Decision-Making

A screening programme will only be implemented if there is broad consensus in society that it is justified considering the harm:benefit ratio. An individual woman, however, may judge harms and benefits differently. It is a challenge, only recently recognized and tackled, to inform women, in a balanced way, about harms and benefits, so that they can make their individual informed decision about participation.

Provide Adequate Resources not only for the Screening Process but also for the Consequential Assessment of Screen-Detected Lesions and the Treatment of the Detected Tumours

When a screening programme starts, a considerable proportion of women (between 5% and 7% of participating women according to the European Guidelines) will have a suspicious mammogram. The majority of these will be benign after additional assessment.

A large number of prevalent cases will be detected in the first round. The European Guidelines expect a threefold detection of cancers over background. Since about half of all breast cancers are detected in the 50–69-year age group, and half of this target population will be invited every other year, between 12.5% (at 50% participation) and 19% (at 75% participation) of additional cancer treatments must be provided for in the introductory phase. This will level out in the following years, but additional treatments will be required for a long time, since the compensatory decrease will only appear after the women reach the upper age limit of the programme. In addition, some overdiagnosis must be reasonably expected.

The effect of a breast cancer screening programme cannot be evaluated at an individual level, since the heterogeneity of breast cancer biology does not allow assessing the effect of an early detection in an individual case. Therefore, the effectiveness of a screening programme can only be evaluated epidemiologically with a view of the whole targeted group of persons. The effectiveness in the whole target group is the only way to ensure maximal effect for the individual participant. Since the balance between positive and adverse effects of a screening programme is always delicate, the highest reasonably possible level of evidence should be sought before introducing changes into an established effective screening programme.

Cost-Effectiveness

For developed high-income countries, mammography screening can be considered cost-effective according to the amount of money to be invested per year of life saved. Experience shows that such a programme also promotes the quality of the diagnostic process for women who present with or without symptoms outside of the programme.

Screening in Low- and Middle-Income Countries

For lower- and middle-income countries other health problems may be of greater importance. With growing income, however, and adoption of a more western lifestyle, the importance of breast carcinoma is rising. Generally breast cancer screening, however, is not considered cost-effective in low-income countries, since the relation between the number of breast cancer cases that can be saved per capita income is much more unfavourable than in the developed high-income countries. In addition, in many of these countries, economic and social inequalities as well as health care access put the usefulness of a screening programme in question.

In such contexts, the recommendations are to improve awareness of the importance of early detection and strengthen and scale up treatment for clinically detectable cancer combined with open access to health care services for any women with breast symptoms.

In many of these countries, not only economic matters but also cultural beliefs and traditions hinder early presentation and treatment of clinical breast disease. An attempt to improve breast health by early detection must be embedded in a holistic approach considering these societal aspects as well as the attitude of the medical profession.

Ultrasound and MRI as Additional Methods in Dense Breasts

The sensitivity of mammography is highly dependent on the density of the breast tissue. Data from various studies suggest that the addition of handheld ultrasound screening to mammography in women with dense breast increases cancer detection rates by 2.3–4.6 per 1000 (depending on the basic breast cancer risk) at the expense of higher recall rates and lower positive predictive values. The positive predictive value of a biopsy recommendation after full diagnostic work-up has been shown to be 22.6% for mammography, 8.9% for ultrasound, and 11.2% for combined mammography and ultrasound. Screening ultrasound with automated whole breast units yielded similar results to screening with handheld ultrasound. Because of the increased recall rates, and especially the biopsy rates as well as the multifold expert time, additional ultrasound is currently not recommended in routine screening of women at normal risk for breast cancer. Based on the study designs, none of the existing studies can provide sufficient evidence for assessing the effect of additional ultrasound on breast cancer mortality. So far, one single trial exists which promises to answer these essential questions in the future: the randomized J-START trial is being conducted in Japanese women aged 40–49 years. It will remain, however, questionable whether data from Japanese women (with mostly small breasts and dense tissue) can be transferred to the European or US populations.

Whereas MRI surveillance (including MRI and mammography) is internationally accepted as the recommended method of early detection for women at high risk, insufficient data exist supporting MRI screening of women (at intermediate or low risk) with dense breast. None of the available studies has an appropriate design that would enable assessing the effect of MRI screening on breast cancer mortality. Based on the existing studies, the positive predictive value of the biopsy recommendation reported after MRI for dense tissue, ranging from 3% to 33%, is (like the positive predictive value reported for additional ultrasound) considered too low to justify a recommendation for MRI screening. To date, there is only one study ongoing which could, in the future, answer questions concerning the use of MRI for screening dense breasts. This is a randomized controlled trial being run in the Netherlands. As long as there is no clear evidence how the effectiveness of screening may be enhanced by taking the density of the breast tissue into account, it remains questionable whether women should be informed about their breast density and its effect on the sensitivity of mammography.

Risk-Adapted Screening

For special groups of high (usually genetic) risk, MRI can be considered as the method of choice and eventually offered in a multimodal programme (including mammography, where appropriate).

The strongest increase of sensitivity has been observed for mutation carriers, from 38.1% (mammography: MX) to 94.1% (MRI + MX) on average. In spite of the larger contribution from MRI in these (mostly non-blinded) studies, MRI and MX proved complementary, since MX, too, increased the sensitivity from 84.4% (MRI only) to 94.1% (MRI + MX). This contribution by MX was statistically significant for women aged >50 years. Whereas MX contributed significantly to the detection of malignancy in BRCA2 mutation carriers aged <40 years (with 30% only-MX-detected cancers), no additional cancers were detected by mammography in BRCA1 mutation carriers aged <40 years.

In summary, intensified surveillance using MRI and mammography is recommended in women at high risk based on the proven much higher sensitivity of MRI in these women compared to mammography or no surveillance.

The benefit of detection at earlier stages (as proven for women at high risk) has to be weighed against the costs for the increased number of histopathological assessments, the high costs of MR-guided biopsies, and costs for MR-guided wire-marking and diagnostic surgery in those cases where MR-guided vacuum-assisted breast biopsy is not available, not reimbursed, or not possible. Furthermore costs for a yet unknown rate of overdiagnoses may need to be considered, especially for MR screening beyond high risk.

Outside of the high-risk population, data are insufficient for recommending MRI screening. Thus, no recommendation for MRI screening exists yet for women at intermediate risk.

For women at average or intermediate risk, no reliable data exist for estimates of cost-effectiveness. When weighing advantages and disadvantages in these women, risks from contrast agent also have to be considered. According to the literature, these risks are at least comparable to (or higher than) risks expected from radiation by mammography.

Overview of Utility and Expenditure for Imaging and Needle Biopsies

See Tables 11.1–11.4.

Table 11.1 Comparative utility of imaging methods according to tasks

Method	Symptomatic disease	Screening average risk	Screening high risk	Assessment of detected lesions
Mammogram	+++	+++	++	+++
Tomogram	+++	++	–	++
Ultrasound	+++	–	–	+++
MRI	+	–	+++	+

MRI, magnetic resonance imaging.

+++, essential; ++, useful; +, not mandatory; –, no role.

Table 11.2 Comparative utility of image-guided needle biopsy methods according to tasks

Method	Symptomatic disease	Assessment of detected lesions (average risk screening)	Assessment of detected lesions (high risk screening)
Ultrasound-guided core biopsy	+++	+++	+++
Fine-needle aspiration	+	+	+
Mammogram-guided VAB	+	+++	+++
MRI-guided VAB	+	–	+++

MRI, magnetic resonance imaging; VAB, vacuum-assisted biopsy.
+++, essential; ++, useful; +, not mandatory; –, no role.

Table 11.3 Comparative expenditure for imaging methods

Method	Equipment, installation and running costs	Time needed of well-trained personnel
Mammogram	++	+
Tomogram	++	+(+)
Ultrasound	+	+++
MRI	+++	+++

MRI, magnetic resonance imaging.
+++, high; ++, moderate; +, low.

Table 11.4 Comparative expenditure for image-guided needle biopsies

Method	Equipment, installation and running costs	Time needed of well-trained personnel
Ultrasound-guided core biopsy	+	+
Fine-needle aspiration	(+)	(+)[a]
Mammogram-guided VAB	++	++
MRI-guided VAB	+++	+++

MRI, magnetic resonance imaging; VAB, vacuum-assisted biopsy.
+++, high; ++, moderate; +, low; (+), negligible.
[a]Exceptional expertise required.

Emerging and Future Imaging Modalities

Introduction

Any transfer of new or evolving breast imaging methods into practical health policies has to answer the following basic questions:

- Will the new method transfer a substantial benefit to the whole population or diseased single individuals compared to older standards regarding better detection or characterization of breast cancer?
- Do negative collateral effects exist that may compromise the intended benefit?
- Can the new method be implemented and controlled at reasonable costs and adequate quality standards?

Physical Principles to Differentiate Benign from Malignant Tumours

Breast cancer lesions present with a variety of different characteristics such as density, stiffness, electrical activity, ultrasound impedance, and necrosis pattern compared to normal tissue. The various tissue resorption and scattering patterns of benign and malignant breast tissue have stimulated research on almost all parts of the electromagnetic and mechanical wave spectrum.

Signal Detection Used by New Breast Imaging Candidates

Absorption, transmission, reflection, emission, and time of flight of energy are the cardinal principles that allow signal detection. The spectrum of energy is further assessed by spectroscopy. For photons and mechanical ultrasound waves, the time to pass through tissue is higher in the presence of scattering than without. The phase shift of waves travelling through scattering tissues can be expressed as phase contrast when compared with normal tissue and be used to enhance the basic signals. Optical imaging separates photons by their time of flight through non-scattering or scattering tissues. Further, phase contrast may enhance edges of tissue with ultrasound and X-ray imaging.

Multiparametric, Multispectral, Hybrid, and Fusion Technology

These terms overlap to some degree and are not used consistently in the literature. Multiparametric imaging combines the various outcomes of one basic technology. One example is modern ultrasound computed tomography that co-registrates and combines the sound information generated by reflection, attenuation, and speed of sound within one ultrasound system to an integrated image.

Multispectral mammographic techniques fuse the results of images that have been generated at different energy levels. The final synthesized image of dual-energy spectral mammography brings together a high resolution and high spectral information to an image that yields more information than any of the source images.

Hybrid technologies are the result of two parental technologies that are combined together, but comprise still the recognizable elements of each parent technology. Examples are combining mammography and ultrasound or digital breast tomosynthesis and microwave nearfield radar imaging.

Fusion technology synthesizes two or more different technologies to something uniquely new. For example, fusion algorithms merge simultaneously recorded absorption (conventional digital mammography), differential phase contrast (phase contrast mammography), and small-angle scattering signals (grating-based X-ray dark-field) that are combined by a single image. Higher edge contrast and indirect information about very small calcifications are the promises of this approach that override the information from the basic mammography.

The current most successful candidate on the run to screening is digital breast tomosynthesis followed by automated breast ultrasound, alternatively named automated breast volume ultrasound, as an adjunct to mammography screening. Both technologies are US Food and Drug Administration-approved for these purposes. Abbreviated MRI as a screening tool can examine six to eight patients per hour and probably will offer higher detection rates than any other approach. In case of suspicious findings an additional T2-weighted sequence could be added immediately.

Evolving technologies have generated studies that are based on highly selected case series and have been prone to selection bias.

Contrast-enhanced digital mammography acquires two images after contrast using the so-called dual-energy technique. Contrast-enhanced digital mammography shows high sensitivity between 96% and 100% at a low specificity between 38% and 77%.

Photoacoustic imaging or optoacoustic imaging applies pulsed laser light, and subsequent thermoelastic conversion of absorbed light to ultrasound. The near-infrared laser impulses are mainly absorbed by haemoglobin in vessels. A short heat-induced expansion and contraction within nanoseconds reaches frequencies of ultrasound. The generated travelling ultrasound waves can be visualized by diagnostic ultrasound.

Dedicated breast computed tomography promises an optimized detection and characterization of calcified ductal carcinoma in situ, and, if combined with contrast media, enhanced detection of masses compared to mammography.

Future technologies will lead to different imaging variants based on electric impedance and spectroscopy, microwaves, Hall effect, dark-field X-ray, and will probably result in the hypersensitive spectral analysis of total photon counting, the future ultimate weapon of breast imaging.

Key Messages

- Triple assessment (clinical examination, imaging, ultrasound ± mammography, and needle biopsy, where indicated) is the method of choice for women with significant breast symptoms.
- Working in multidisciplinary teams is highly recommended for diagnosis and treatment of women with breast diseases.

- Screening should be offered in a fully quality-assured environment in order to optimize the benefit:harm ratio.
- In developing countries, providing adequate care for women with symptomatic disease should have priority over screening, which is not cost-efficient under these conditions.
- The quality criteria for mammography should be systematically monitored in a quality-assured system.
- The role of ultrasound is mainly in the assessment of symptomatic disease and mammography-detected abnormalities and the guidance of needle biopsies.
- The role of MRI in the discrimination between benign and malignant disease is limited. It has an established role in high-risk screening and is useful in rare special situations.
- New methods must be vigorously investigated to determine whether they will be able to improve the already high accuracy of existing diagnostics from a patient and an economic viewpoint.

References

1. American College of Radiology. Practice Parameters Breast Imaging and Intervention. Available at: https://www.acr.org/Clinical-Resources/Practice-Parameters-and-Technical-Standards/Practice-Parameters-by-Organ-or-Body-System
2. Kollmann C et al. Guideline for Technical Quality Assurance (TQA) of ultrasound devices (B-Mode)—version 1.0 (July 2012): EFSUMB Technical Quality Assurance Group—US-TQA/B. *Ultraschall Med* 2012;33:544–549.
3. Willett A et al. *Best Practice Diagnostic Guidelines for Patients Presenting With Breast Symptoms.* Department of Health, UK; 2010. Available from: https://associationofbreastsurgery.org.uk/media/1416/best-practice-diagnostic-guidelines-for-patients-presenting-with-breast-symptoms.pdf
4. D'Orsi CJ et al. *ACR BI-RADS® Atlas, Breast Imaging Reporting and Data System.* Reston, VA: American College of Radiology; 2013. Available from: https://www.acr.org/Clinical-resources/Reporting-and-Data-Systems/Bi-Rads
5. IARC Working Group on the Evaluation of Cancer—Preventive Interventions (2016) *Breast Cancer Screening—IARC Handbook of Cancer Prevention*, Vol. 15. Available from: http://publications.iarc.fr/Book-And-Report-Series/Iarc-Handbooks-Of-Cancer-Prevention/Breast-Cancer-Screening-2016
6. Perry N, Puthaar E editors. *European Guidelines for Quality Assurance in Breast Cancer Screening and Diagnosis*, 4th ed. Office for Official Publications of the European Communities; 2006. Available from: http://www.euref.org/downloads?download=24:european-guidelines-for-quality-assurance-in-breast-cancer-screening-and-diagnosis-pdf

12

The Status of Breast Pathology around the Globe

Shahla Masood, Roberto Salgado, Peter Regitnig, and Rudi Pauwels

Definition of Breast Pathology

Breast pathology, defined as the study of breast disease, is the foundation of breast health care. There is no doubt that the quality of breast health care and the ultimate patient outcomes are directly related to the quality of breast pathology diagnosis. Without accurate diagnostic and predictive information, clinicians are misled and patients suffer from the wrong therapy and consequent adverse clinical outcomes. Therefore, measures should be taken to reduce barriers to providing optimal pathology service around the world.

The Contributions of Pathologists in Multidisciplinary Breast Health/Cancer Care

Advances in science and technology, molecular characterization of tumours, and participation of pathologists in the process of the delivery of integrated breast health care have provided significant change in the role of pathologists. As members of a multidisciplinary team, pathologists have become responsible for providing the most up-to-date morphological and biological information that is required for immediate therapy and long-term follow-up management of their patients. Currently, in a multidisciplinary breast health centre with patient-focused strategies, pathologists are an integral part of the system (Figure 12.1).

Pathologists are expected to establish a diagnosis, classify a neoplasm, differentiate between a primary versus a metastatic tumour, predict response to therapy, provide prognosis, and compose a comprehensive pathology report (Box 12.1).

For many years, the abovementioned roles were based on morphologic examination of the surgically excised samples. However, the introduction of minimally invasive diagnostic sampling procedures such as fine-needle aspiration biopsy and core needle biopsy and the availability of molecular targeted therapy have created a different challenge for practising breast pathologists. It has also been realized that breast cancer is not a single disease, and there are different subtypes of breast cancer with various

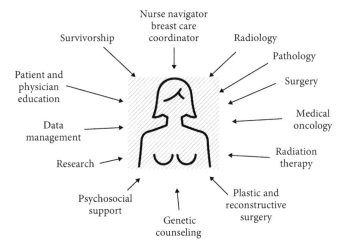

Figure 12.1 Integration of breast health services.

morphological appearances, biology, responses to therapy, and ultimate outcome (Figures 12.2 and 12.3).

Pathologists are expected to identify novel biological markers for diagnosis and/or determination of prognosis of breast cancer patients, and pathologists continue to assist in recognizing changes at the DNA level and consequent changes in gene expression involved in the multi-step process of oncogenes in breast cancer. This is currently exemplified by technologies such as immunohistochemistry, in-situ hybridization, quantitative polymerase chain reaction, oligonucleotide and cDNA microarray, and others which permit localization of hormone receptors, oncogenes, tumour suppressor genes, and many other gene products at the cellular and molecular levels, as well as genetic profiling. The traditional prognostic factors such as tumour size, type, grade, and the status of lymph node metastasis have played an important role in selections of patients for systemic chemotherapy. However, within the good-prognostic groups such as axillary node-negative cases, there are differences in behaviours. Therefore, it is necessary to separate defined prognostic markers into low- and high-risk groups in terms

---

Box 12.1 The changing role of pathologists in multidisciplinary breast care

- Establish a diagnosis
- Classify a neoplasm
- Differentiate between a primary versus a metastatic tumour
- Predict response to therapy
- Provide diagnosis
- Compose a comprehensive breast pathology report

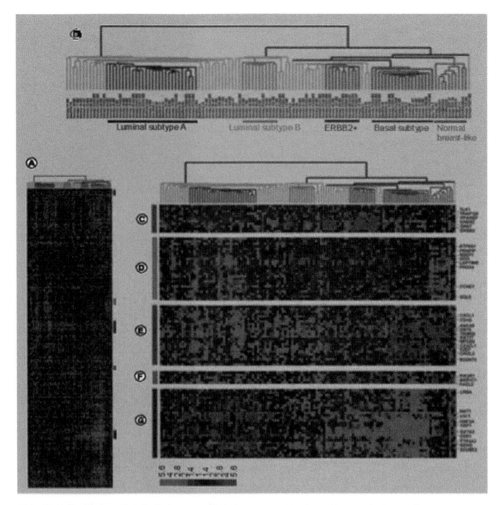

Figure 12.2 Hierarchical clustering of 115 tumour tissues and seven non-malignant tissues by using the intrinsic gene set. (A) A scaled-down representation of the entire cluster of 540 genes and 122 tissue samples based on similarities in gene expression. (B) Experimental dendrogram showing the clustering of the tumours into five subgroups. Branches corresponding to tumours with low correlation to any subtype are shown in grey. (C) Gene cluster showing the ERBB2 oncogene and other co-expressed genes. (D) Gene cluster associated with luminal subtype B. (E) Gene cluster associated with the basal subtype. (F) A gene cluster relevant for the normal breast-like group. (G) Cluster of genes including the ER (ESR1) highly expressed in luminal subtype A tumours. Scale bar represents fold change for any given gene relative to the median level of expression across all samples.

of the probability of recurrence, and to offer adjuvant chemotherapy only to those patients at high risk. Attempts have also been made to identify parameters that can predict response to therapy, because even high-risk patients should be spared treatment, if it can be reliably determined that they would not benefit from that treatment. In order

Slides   *Cytology*   *Histology*

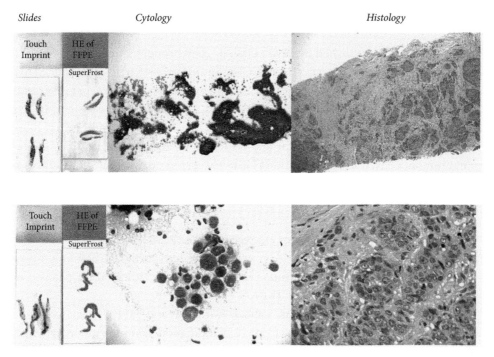

Figure 12.3 Left side: Touch imprint slides aside final histology of formalin-fixed, paraffin-embedded breast carcinomas (HE). Middle: high cellularity and obvious atypia (Diff Quik); both are C5. Right side: HE of core needle biopsies showing breast carcinomas. *Reproduced* courtesy of Dr. Peter Regitnig

to achieve the goal of providing individualized therapy based on specific characteristics of each tumour, further markers have been identified.

These factors relate to important cancer parameters such as cell cycle, proliferation and apoptosis, cell adhesion and invasion, the status of hormone receptors, and expression of oncogenes and tumour suppressor genes. Among various biomarkers, oestrogen and progesterone receptors and HER-2/neu oncogene are recognized predictors of response to endocrine and trastuzumab therapies, respectively. Trastuzumab is a novel immunotherapy, which is considered as the first agent specifically developed for HER-2/neu overexpression in metastatic breast cancer and was the first agent which has successfully demonstrated the application of immunotherapy in breast cancer. Other tests such as Oncotype Dx, a 21-gene assay, and MammaPrint, a 70-gene assay, were recently developed to predict risk for distant recurrence among lymph node-negative and oestrogen receptor-positive breast cancer patients. When to perform prognostic/predictive testing, how to interpret the result, and how to use it to guide therapy requires communication between pathologists and oncologists. This can be achieved by open forum communication, such as tumour conferences and tumour boards, or more individualized case-based discussion.

Molecular Subtypes of Breast Cancer

The seminal article published by Perou et al. in 2000 brought a new understanding of the genetic profiles of breast cancer (1). The authors of that article introduced five subgroups based on 496 genes that differentiate breast cancer into separate groups according to gene expression patterns (Figure 12.2). It could be classified in five intrinsic subtypes (luminal A and B, HER2-enriched, basal-like, and normal-like), corresponding to hormone receptor and HER2 status and further stratifies the luminal tumours based on proliferation (2). It was also reported that these subtypes differed markedly in prognosis and in the repertoire of therapeutic targets they express.

- Luminal A breast cancer, hormone-receptor positive, HER2 negative, and with low levels of proliferation (Ki-67), growing slowly, and having the best prognosis.
- Luminal B breast cancer, hormone-receptor positive, either HER2 positive or negative with high proliferation (Ki-67).
- Triple-negative/basal-like breast cancer, hormone and HER-2 negative, more common in women with BRCA1 gene mutation, more common among younger and African-American people.
- HER2-enriched breast cancer, hormone receptor negative, growing faster, having a worse prognosis, but with successful therapeutic options with targeted therapies, such as Trastuzumab, Pertuzumab, Tyverb and T-DM1.
- Normal-like breast cancer, similar to luminal A disease but with a slightly worse prognosis.

Molecular subtyping of breast cancer is not yet universally incorporated in breast pathology reporting. However, the eighth edition of The American Joint Commission of Cancer, which remains the worldwide basis for breast cancer staging, has adapted the inclusion of prognostic factors such as tumour grade, hormone receptors, and HER-2/neu amplification in addition to TNM classification in breast pathology reporting.

The Essentials/Requirements of Optimal Breast Pathology Reporting

Diagnosis

Rendering an accurate breast pathology diagnosis and providing optimal information about prognostic/predictive factors requires access to a well-established pathology laboratory with skilled and knowledgeable technical staff pathologists. There is no substitution for an accurate diagnosis with respect to securing patient safety and appropriate therapy. It is also essential to take proper measures for establishing effective communication between pathologists and other members of the breast health team. It should be understood that the accuracy of pathology diagnosis is a shared responsibility among pathologists, radiologists, surgeons, and oncologists.

Accurate diagnosis of breast cancer requires knowledge about the type of procedure, pertinent clinical history, and breast imaging findings. These include personal and/or family history of breast cancer and other risk factors, history of any systemic disease, implants, nipple discharge, the site and the size of the lesion, any previous history of radiation and/or chemotherapy, and whether the patient is pregnant or lactating. Associated with a history of other malignancies, the possibility of a metastatic tumour to the breast should be seriously considered. In addition, knowledge about the breast imaging findings make it possible to correlate those with the pathologic features and to recommend resampling of the lesion, if there are any discrepancies between the results. More importantly, proper orientation of the intact tissue sample by the surgeon is critically important for assessing the surgical margins.

Risk Prediction

Identification of borderline breast lesions associated with an increased number of image-detected biopsies is the result of the widespread use of screening mammography. There has been an increase in the diagnosis of high-risk proliferative breast diseases that are considered a morphological risk factor. Recognition of the spectrum of morphological features of these entities is important in identifying high-risk individuals, who may benefit from appropriate risk reduction modalities associated with early breast cancer detection and prevention.

Detection of Tumour Metastasis in Sentinel Lymph Node Biopsy

Assessment of the presence or absence of metastatic tumour cells in sentinel lymph nodes has become an important function of pathologists. This information defines the course of surgical information with respect to the decision about the follow-up total axillary dissection.

Detection of Tumour Cells at Surgical Margins in Lumpectomy Specimens

The status of surgical margins at the time of initial lumpectomy is considered an important predictive factor of tumour recurrence. The accurate assessment of lumpectomy surgical margins by pathologists is directly related to appropriate orientation of the specimen by surgeons followed by proper handling of the sample in the surgical pathology laboratory. Intraoperative assessment of lumpectomy surgical margins by gross examination of the specimen, imprint cytology, and/or frozen section is rapid and cost-effective. This assessment helps to minimize the possibility of local recurrence and reduces the number of unnecessary surgeries for re-excision.

Prognosis: Treatment Planning

Providing individualized therapy for breast cancer patients requires detailed characterization of tumour cells. An optimal breast pathology report includes tumour size, tumour type, histological grading, presence or absence of lymphovascular invasion, the status of surgical margins and the lymph node metastasis, the presence of ductal carcinoma in situ, the status of multicentricity and multifocality, the presence or absence of skin/nipple involvement, and ulceration. The diagnosis of ductal carcinoma in situ requires inclusion of size, nuclear grade, presence or absence of necrosis, and the type of growth pattern.

Prediction of Response to Therapy

Assessment of oestrogen and progesterone receptors by immunocytochemistry is an important predictor of response to endocrine therapy and is currently measured in every newly diagnosed breast cancer. In addition, assessment of HER-2/neu oncogene amplification and overexpression by fluorescent in-situ hybridization and immunochemistry is used to predict the therapeutic response to adjuvant chemotherapy and endocrine therapy and to select patients for trastuzumab immunotherapy.

The Status of Breast Pathology in Different Regions of the World

A majority of the world's population resides in resource-poor countries. These people have limited access to optimal standard of life, quality medical care, long life expectancy, and predictable disease outcome. The gap between the available resources of those who live in countries of limited resources versus those who enjoy a different lifestyle in resource-rich countries is significant. An emerging concern that has received attention at an international level is the status of pathology services in developing countries that also includes the practice of breast pathology. Currently, there is significant variation in the practice of breast pathology at the global level. There are important differences in tissue sampling and processing, interpretation of pathology findings, and analysis of breast samples for biomarkers. Contributing factors for these differences include financial constraints and variation in the level and extent of training of pathology personnel in breast pathology. Implementation of breast pathology guidelines in countries with limited resources is a significant challenge. Availability of pathology laboratories with trained personnel and pathologists is a major obstacle that requires attention. There are still regions of the world that have no/limited access to pathology diagnosis, and often mastectomies are performed based on clinical presentation of a palpable mass or other abnormalities. Development of collaborative relationship among laboratories in different regions of the world may provide an effective alternative.

Building blocks for access to accurate diagnosis of breast lesions by a qualified pathologist require international collaboration. Aside from allocation of financial resources, training of qualified personnel involved in handling, processing, and interpreting pathological findings is the most critical step in this process. This may be achieved by implementation of low-cost interventions that can make a difference. In addition, provisions should be made to educate the heads of governments, health care leaders, administrators, physicians, scientists, health care providers, nurses, social workers, industry, and religious leaders about the value of accurate pathology diagnosis for the delivery of optimal breast care. It should be understood that proper diagnosis of a breast lesion by a qualified pathologist minimizes over- and underdiagnosis as well as the burden of under- and overtreatment. Measures such as the use of fine-needle aspiration biopsy as the initial diagnostic procedure, establishment of regional laboratories that can provide interpretation of cytology/pathology slides, and the use of telepathology for diagnosis and training of personnel and local physicians/pathologists are effective initiatives to consider. Despite resource limitation in low- and middle-income countries, appropriate pathology reporting, tumour staging, quality measures, and the availability of prognostic/predictive information are essential factors for the design of personalized therapy and follow-up management. It should be also recognized that the financial burden of establishing or providing access to breast pathology services is counterbalanced by the cost savings from inappropriate use of resources that result from poor pathology practice. The practice of breast pathology is complex and requires integration of morphology with clinical presentations, risk factors, breast imaging, and the status of biomarkers in order to provide meaningful contribution to patient care.

Ultimately, partnership between resource-rich and resource-limited countries is essential to overcome the current barriers in the delivery of optimal breast pathology services around the globe. To improve access to quality breast pathology practice, there are important caveats to be recognized by those combatting breast cancer. For pathologists, however, this requires a cultural change. To actively participate in this process, pathologists not only need to strive for excellence in breast pathology, but they also need to change from being isolated morphologists to being real-time clinician-scientists who see patients. As patient advocates, pathologists can lead educational efforts directed towards the public, physicians, leaders in the health care community, and the government. As clinicians, more pathologists can become familiar with the performance of minimally invasive procedures. As a pathologist-scientist, a pathologist can better understand the biology of breast cancer and recognize the morphological and biological alterations observed within the spectrum of high-risk proliferative breast disease and premalignant and malignant lesions. In order to achieve these goals, it is critically important to create a worldwide excellence in breast pathology programmes encouraging international collaboration among interested pathologists to form the building blocks for a voluntary breast pathology educational programme. This initiative may be realized by the establishment of 'The International Institute of Breast Pathology', which could serve as a bridge to connect diverse groups of pathologists and healthcare providers who share the same vision of providing a better quality of breast pathology to the women of the world. This institute may be the first step towards introducing innovative approaches for enhancing the knowledge about optimal practice of breast pathology, including the use of telepathology as a global technology that allows for expert information-sharing across the globe.

Essentials/Requirements of the Practice of Breast Cytology

Cytology has been used less often in recent years than in previous decades, when primary diagnoses of breast cancer were performed using fine-needle aspirates (FNA), and at a time when the characterization of tumour receptors was less important. Nowadays, cytology has mostly been replaced by core needle biopsies (CNB), but it still has value in special situations, such as when a less invasive method is preferred to guide further clinical decisions (Table 12.1). Furthermore, in low-resource settings, cytology might be used as an appropriate tool to distinguish benign from malignant processes.

Interpretation of Cytology

Clinical information is necessary: age, location (retro-areolar or peripheral or axillary tail, etc.), clinical appearance (e.g.: palpable, microcalcification).

Table 12.1 Use of cytology

Method	Expected result	Clinical use and key messages
FNA cytology of solid lesion or cyst	Detection of malignant tumour cells or mixture of benign cells (further details possible)	Less used today because of the need for predictive tumour characterization of CNB prior to surgery or primary systemic therapy. Useful in low-resource settings.
FNA cytology of clinically suspect lymph node	Detection of malignant tumour cells	Guiding extent of lymph node dissection, especially if primary systemic therapy is intended without prior sentinel node biopsy
Touch imprint cytology of core needle biopsies	Representativeness of biopsy. Detection of malignant tumour cells without further discrimination between 'in situ' or invasive.	Immediate feedback allows possibility of repeating CNB. Enables clinicians to counsel patients and plan the appropriate treatment (1). Can also be used to immediately order immunohistochemistry for the next morning (this allows being able to provide a full histochemistry and IHC report within 24 h).
Touch imprint cytology of resection margins in breast-conserving therapy or nipple-sparing mastectomy	Detection of malignant tumour cells. No need for differentiation between in-situ or invasive tumour cells.	Larger areas can be examined compared to pure macroscopic or frozen section examination. Immediate further resection avoiding secondary surgery is possible.
Touch imprint cytology of nipple secretion	Occasional detection of intraductal epithelial cell proliferation (papilloma, ductal hyperplasia, in-situ carcinoma).	Any (single-sided) nipple secretion outside of lactation is abnormal and should be examined cytologically. Detection rate of atypical epithelial cells is scarce in such materials and most often dyshormonal regulation is the cause. Nipple secretion cytology has a low sensitivity, but a high specificity.

FNA, fine-needle aspiration; CNB, core needle biopsy; IHC, immunohistochemistry.

People reading cytology, generally pathologists, must be well experienced in order to avoid misinterpretation. Profound knowledge of the histological morphology is important and probably most helpful for the correct interpretation of cytological breast specimens. High-grade breast carcinomas are most often highly cellular and show obvious atypia. However, low-grade carcinomas are more difficult to recognize. Here, the lack of myoepithelial cells within epithelial cell clusters is a hallmark.

The useful of FNA is limited in the diagnosis of in-situ carcinoma, lobular carcinoma, tubular carcinoma, and small non-palpable tumours, and it is also not effective in the evaluation of microcalcifications.

Regarding specimen adequacy, initially the amount of evaluable epithelial cells should be noted. Reasons for inadequacy may be hypocellularity, error in aspiration, spreading or staining, or excessive blood.

Depending on the clinical question, cellularity may already be an important result. For example, if a touch imprint of a CNB harbours no or only a very small number of epithelial cells, the probability of a carcinoma is low, except in cases of lobular carcinomas, which can demonstrate a low cellularity.

The cytological result may be given as either three-tiered (negative, suspicious, or positive) or by the five-tiered C-classification: C1, unsatisfactory; C2, benign; C3, atypia probably benign; C4, suspicious of malignancy; C5, malignant.

Quality Control

Whenever possible, the cytological results should be correlated with further histological results. This enables an easy way to calculate sensitivity and specificity of the method, if the B-classification is used for reporting CNB or with further histology of resections.

The accuracy of FNA depends on three main factors:

1. a sample that is adequate and representative of the lesion;
2. suitable processing and staining without artefacts;
3. accurate interpretation of the cytological material with a clear report conveyed to the rest of the clinical team.

The procedure can fail at any of the stages of preparation (aspiration, spreading, and staining) even before diagnostic interpretation. The confidence and experience of the aspirator are vital for obtaining a satisfactory sample. This part of the procedure, like other parts, should not be delegated to novices.

For FNA, a sensitivity of >70% and a specificity of >90% should be reached. For C5, a positive predictive value of 99% should be reached. Calculations are according to the European Guidelines.

Establishment of Breast Pathology Guidelines in Low- and Middle-Income Countries by Breast Pathology Focus Group of the Global Breast Health Initiative (BHGI)

In response to the need for attention to the significance of access to optimal pathology laboratory facilities in 2005, the leadership of BHGI assembled a panel of interested pathologists, breast cancer clinician specialists, and patient advocates to assess the status of the practice of breast pathology in countries of limited resources and to develop resource-stratified guidelines which emphasized the necessity for accurate pathology diagnosis of breast cancer worldwide. Considering the relative necessity, therapeutic benefit, and cost, four levels were suggested: basic, limited, enhanced, and maximum. The 2005 panel also acknowledged the appropriateness of fine-needle aspiration biopsy (FNAB) as the most economic method for the initial diagnosis and emphasized the necessity of access to optimal cytologic interpretation. In addition, the availability of resources necessary to provide prognostic and predictive factors as well as assessment of the status of axillary lymph nodes were emphasized at different levels within these guidelines. The next step was to determine how to adapt these guidelines into real-time implementation in countries of limited resources and how to identify system changes necessary for this implementation (3).

Special Considerations for Breast Conservation and Sentinel Lymph Node Biopsies

Table 12.2 summarizes the guidelines, process, and quality indicators related to the possibility of offering breast conservation in countries of limited resources. As previously indicated, detailed information about the tumour as well as the status of surgical margins and sentinel lymph nodes are essential to the report.

Accreditation

During the last several years, international breast cancer organizations have focused on the establishment of guidelines that promote an organized approach to providing quality care. Various quality metrics have been developed, and it has become a serious expectation that those engaged in providing breast health care follow the established guidelines. The National Accreditation Program for Breast Centres, the International Serologic Society, and the European Society of Breast Cancer Specialists have adapted guidelines for breast pathology reporting focused on the previously discussed emphasis to assure access to the high quality of breast pathology reporting that our patients deserve. In addition, during the last several years, the practice of breast pathology has changed. Pathologists are no longer required to differentiate between benign and malignant disease, but they are required to recognize the spectrum of borderline breast

Table 12.2 Special considerations for breast conservation and sentinel lymph node biopsy

Guideline	Process	Quality indicator
Pathology report should include the status of margins, the presence and extent of ductal carcinoma in situ, and the presence of lymphovascular invasion	Adopt standardized methods of orienting specimen, and inking and sampling the surgical margins	% of pathology reports include margin status, ductal carcinoma in situ, and lymphovascular invasion
Measures in place to provide intraoperative evaluation of sentinel lymph nodes	Adopt standardized methods for determination of the presence and quantification of ductal carcinoma in situ and lymphovascular invasion Adopt standardized methods for processing and reporting of sentinel lymph nodes	% of diagnostic discordance between intraoperative and final pathologic diagnosis for sentinel lymph nodes

Reproduced with permission from Masood S, Vas L, Ibarra JA, et al. 'Breast Pathology Guideline Implementation in Low- and Middle-Income Countries'. *Cancer*. Volume 113 Volume 8 (Suppl). pp. 2297–304. Copyright © 2008 John Wiley & Sons. DOI: https://doi.org/10.1002/cncr.23833

disease in small tumour samples and provide comprehensive information about the biology of each pathologic entity. These challenges are more conspicuous in countries with limited resources, inadequate number of staff and pathologists, and differences in the stage of breast cancer presentation. Thus, international collaboration is the key to making a difference. The establishment of the International Society of Breast Pathology in 1977 and the integration of breast pathology as one of the main components of BGHI are strong messages of support for the significance of optimal breast pathology practice around the globe.

Current Challenges Associated with the Practice of Breast Pathology

One of the most important obstacles in the practice of breast pathology is the limited understanding of the public about the role that pathologists play in their care and outcome. To some extent, the significance of the role of pathologists has remained under-recognized among the medical community. The issue of pathology becomes real when the patients become aware of a mistake in the diagnosis of their pathology during a review process, or there is a significant discrepancy between the clinical presentation, breast imaging, and the pathology diagnosis. Breast pathology is complex, and there are several look-alikes that are easy to misdiagnose as cancer if the pathologist is inexperienced. These difficult-to-diagnose cases include a variety of atypical proliferative lesions, atypical ductal hyperplasia (ADH) versus low-grade ductal carcinoma in situ (DCIS), lobular neoplasia, papillary lesions, atypical sclerotic lesions, fibroepithelial tumours, mucinous lesions, and the status of microinvasion.

A prominent story appearing in the *New York Times* in July 2010 and entitled 'Prone to Error: Earliest Steps to Find Cancer' alerted the public to breast pathology diagnosis. In this article, patients who were misdiagnosed as suffering from DCIS and who had undergone unnecessary treatment for cancer were profiled, and they shared their stories. One patient recounted having been misdiagnosed with invasive breast cancer, and, when faced with the prospect of a mastectomy, she sought a second opinion. Once her case had been reviewed by three separate expert breast pathologists, they all agreed that there was no evidence of invasive cancer. However, three different diagnoses were given by the three pathologists. One pathologist diagnosed DCIS, with the others diagnosing her case as ADH and apocrine adenosis. Due to the complexity of her case and the differing opinions of the three pathologists, the patient ultimately decided to remain under surveillance, but to postpone any treatment or surgical procedures. After eight years, the patient still had no evidence of cancer.

Errors in breast pathology are not uncommon. Most times, these errors are realized when cases are sent to other medical centres for review, or when a patient requests a second opinion. Once a misdiagnosis is realized, there can be significant changes to treatment planning, and this can cause both relief and anxiety for patients and their families. In some cases, a misdiagnosis can cause years of anxiety. In one case, a patient came for advice on what to do as a high-risk patient, since her mother was a breast cancer survivor, who had been diagnosed at age 35 years while she was eight months pregnant. After the birth of her daughter, her mother had undergone a mastectomy and axillary dissection. Upon reviewing her mother's case, it was determined that there was no clear evidence of cancer, and that her mother had undergone these procedures unnecessarily. Although there was nothing that could be done to reverse what had been done to her mother, the patient was relieved that she was no longer considered high risk for breast cancer.

Quality Assurance and Patient Safety in the Practice of Breast Pathology

Currently, there are no uniform guidelines in place to effectively measure the rate of diagnostic errors in everyday practice of breast pathology. In addition, the fear of disclosure and medicolegal issues are limiting factors in the reporting of diagnostic errors in breast pathology. Therefore, the establishment of quality measures and the monitoring of the status of compliance are critical steps in improving the quality of practice of breast pathology. These quality indicators range from pre-analytic factors, such as fixation and processing of the tissue samples, to analytical factors that begin when the pathologist receives the glass slides, interprets the findings, and renders a diagnosis. The post-analytical factors involve the correlation of the pathology diagnosis with clinical presentation and imaging findings.

Recognition of difficult-to-diagnose cases in breast pathology uses all of the available measures to find the correct answer for every case in breast pathology and is essential in

---

Box 12.2 Suggestions for quality measures in breast pathology

Establishment of quality assurance programmes
- Internal quality measures
  - Consensus slide conference
  - Mandatory second review of cancer cases
  - Mandatory adherence to established guidelines

Second opinion
- The review of outside pathology slides and reports by a local pathologist before the initiation of cancer therapy

Involvement in external quality assurance programmes

---

securing the safety of our patients with different breast diseases. Attempts also should be taken to consider accreditation of breast pathology fellowships in recognition of the significance of additional training in a multidisciplinary integrated environment of care.

There is sufficient evidence suggesting that the time has come to abandon the term of low-grade ductal carcinoma in situ and replace it with the term 'borderline breast disease', completely remove the entire lesion, and offer the patient risk assessment and risk reduction options. This approach is similar to what is now offered as a 'wait and watch' approach for low-grade prostate cancer.

Ultimately, every breast pathology practice should establish their own quality assurance programmes that include internal and external quality measures and second opinions (Box 12.2).

Future Perspective: Can Precision Medicine Be Delivered Sustainably and Affordably?

Clinical studies have shown that mutational lesions and/or gene expression changes within tumours affecting the protein target of a drug may be predictive for the efficacy of that drug. Examples of such predictive biomarkers include classical activating mutations of epidermal growth factor receptor (EGFR) in non-small cell lung cancer, which confer exquisite sensitivity to EGFR tyrosine kinase inhibitors (TKIs), amplification of ERBB2 and/or high-level expression of the encoded receptor tyrosine-protein kinase erbB-2 (HER2) in advanced breast cancer, which are predictive biomarkers for the HER2 antibody, trastuzumab, and BRAF V600E mutations in malignant melanoma in relation to the selection of patients suitable for treatment with the serine/threonine-protein kinase B-raf inhibitors, vemurafenib, and dabrafenib. In addition, tumours with activating mutations in genes encoding downstream components of specific signalling pathways may be insensitive to drugs targeting upstream components, as exemplified by KRAS mutations and the lack of activity of cetuximab and panitumumab in the treatment of metastatic colorectal cancer. The adoption of such biomarkers into routine clinical practice has clearly shown the potential of precision medicine in relation to the identification of subpopulations of patients more likely to benefit from treatment with a targeted agent.

The Bumpy Road to Biomarker Discovery and Drug Development

This wider concept of precision medicine envisages that multi-agent therapies can be customized according to the individual complex genomic signature of a tumour with all the caveats about data quality and processing, but without the normal rigorous clinical testing of efficacy and safety of such combinations to guide physician recommendations. The presumed promise of such individualized customized therapy is that because it is more precise it will be more effective. However, this raises several key questions: if therapy is increasingly individualized, how can it be evidence-based; how can the safety of hundreds of different possible combinations be assessed; how can a predictive biomarker be validated and appropriate cut-offs defined if it is used in hundreds of different contexts to make hundreds of different decisions; how can payees evaluate the value of each individualized treatment plan; and, in an era of precision medicine, how will hospitals or governments budget for a far wider range of treatment plans?

So, while comprehensive molecular profiling of tumours and the collection of corresponding clinical outcome data from patients will lead to substantial research opportunities, and while such profiling may be useful in enrolling patients into adaptive clinical trials, such approaches cannot, at the current time, be used to deliver effective precision medicine according to this wider context. Whether this will be possible in the future remains an open question. Indeed, on a technical level, the issue of tumour heterogeneity is a potentially serious confounding factor in relation to achieving this goal, because if a particular detected mutational event is present in only a minor subclone of tumour cells, targeted therapy against the encoded product is likely to have only marginal effects on the overall viability of the tumour. It may be that multiple agents could be used to target multiple subclones of a patient's tumour, but this would require the derivation of information on appropriate doses of targeted drugs when administered in a huge number of different possible combinations across different settings. In addition, such an approach would most likely carry substantial cost implications for payers, yielding, perhaps, little or no real-world patient benefit in many cases, and creating a situation which might be disastrous for self-funding individual patients faced with difficult treatment decisions at a time when they are at their most vulnerable. The high cost would also essentially restrict precision medicine treatment strategies to high-income individuals in resource-rich counties.

So, although progress will inevitably continue to be made in relation to the development of new drugs, and although new biomarker assays will continue to be developed to predict the efficacy of those drugs, it is difficult to envisage a situation developing in routine practice, in the foreseeable future, where complex genomic profiles will be used to customize multi-agent targeted therapy on an individual patient basis.

Can We Afford Precision Medicine?

Since precision medicine approaches may result in considerably increased treatment costs, are there strategies for current implementation that would mitigate those projected costs? In relation to biomarker test development, regulatory standards should be tightened, so that there is increased confidence that, as new assays are introduced into clinical practice, they deliver what they are intended to deliver with respect to clinical utility. Trial designs for new drugs should also be aimed at the delivery of clinically meaningful outcomes, so that we move away from the situation where drug approvals are based on large phase III trials which deliver marginal statistically significant improvements in outcome, but which are of minimal value to patients. A further way to constrain costs and minimize variations in care is to employ evidence-based clinical pathways that are regularly updated. Although the use of such pathways may be viewed as running counter to a precision medicine approach, they can be adapted to include predictive assays that are highly evidence-based. One further way to constrain the costs of highly priced targeted drugs will be to rigorously explore indication-specific and value-based pricing.

One other aspect that should be considered in relation to the clinical use of genome-level data in a precision medicine context is that physicians will need to have sufficient training in clinical genomics, associated analysis techniques, and risk assessment to enable them to effectively support patients in making informed decisions on possible treatment alternatives (4). This requirement will represent a significant educational challenge (Chapter 8).

Are We Ready to Use Next Generation Sequencing (NGS) in Daily Practice? An Example in Breast Cancer

The currently lower cost and wider availability of NGS technology raise the debate on the use of NGS in clinical routine. However, some proposed treatments based on NGS data are not always evidence-based.

Today, clinicians can choose between large varieties of targeted gene panels offered by gene sequencing companies. Several companies allow the identification of genetic variants based on the sequencing of 200–400 genes, whereas other companies provide restricted gene panels of three to 50 genes for different tumour types. Moreover, oncologists and pathologists do not always have the same point of view regarding the choice of the genes that should be analysed, to say the least.

Targeted gene panels can be separated into two groups: a limited targeted gene panel mainly containing genes with strong scientific evidence for their clinical utility, usually six to 50 genes, or a broad targeted gene panel that also contains genes with weaker scientific evidence for clinical utility, usually more than 50 genes. Several grading approaches exist to define these levels of evidence (OncoKb, CEBM).

For breast tumours, no gene currently has a strong scientific evidence for its clinical utility except perhaps ESR1. However, other molecular tests have enabled improvement in diagnosis and treatment. For example, OncoTypeDX and MammaPrint, which allow separation of breast patients into low and high risk, thus enable change in the clinical management of these patients. Limited targeted NGS gene panels can also be used on the blood to detect germline mutations and predict cancer susceptibility. This test mainly concerns the BRCA1 and BRCA2 genes but also some other genes (Chapter 21).

Until now, some clinical trials have revealed limited benefits. For example, University of Texas MD Anderson Cancer Center, Houston, Texas, conducted a study in advanced breast cancer, wherein 423 patients were enrolled, 283 genomic analyses were feasible, 195 genomic alterations were identified, 55 patients might benefit from personalized therapy, 43 patients were treated, only four had positive responses, and nine had disease stability. This illustrates that the implementation of precision medicine still encounters major obstacles, if these are to be translated to a health care setting (4).

New Technologies as an Enabler for Globally Accessible Molecular Diagnostics

The Rise of Molecular Diagnostics

The world population is expected to grow towards 10 billion by 2050. Rising health care costs and budget constraints today push us towards a more intelligent, proactive approach, where diagnostics provide clinicians with more and better information leading to better treatment outcomes. Health care policymakers, governments, insurers, and other payers are already implementing price control systems that favour early diagnosis, better screening and monitoring, and cost-effective therapies.

The global in-vitro diagnostics market was valued at US$60.22 billion in 2016 and is expected to grow at a compound annual growth rate of 5.5% during the forecast period (2016–2021) to reach US$78.74 billion by 2021 (5).

By application, the largest medical diagnostic segment in 2016 was infectious disease, representing 43% of the medical diagnostic market, followed by oncology (19%), blood screening (13%), genetics (10%), microbiology (9%), and others (7%). Biocartis (www.biocartis.com), an innovative molecular diagnostic company, is attempting to revolutionize molecular testing with a unique proprietary (Idylla) platform. They focus on the two largest segments: oncology (primary focus) and infectious diseases.

The Oncology Molecular Diagnostics Market: Breast Cancer as Largest Share

The global oncology-based molecular diagnostics market is expected to reach US$3,391.0 million by 2022 according to a new report by Grand View Research Inc. (6). Breast cancer accounted for the largest market share in 2014 with revenue estimated at around US$170.0 million. Molecular diagnostic assays for breast cancer prognostics are expected to increase the adoption of molecular diagnostics in the near future.

Bridging the Technology Divide in Molecular Diagnostics

There is an increasing divide between the speed of development of new technologies and the access to these technologies. Looking at hospital settings in 2014, the American College of Surgeons reported that more than 80% of cancer patients are treated locally. This is in distinct contrast with up to 90% of molecular diagnostic tests which are today being sent to an external laboratory, since local testing capabilities are unavailable. Today, due to the technical complexity of molecular diagnostic testing and the fact that most current systems rely on batch-based testing (meaning that a large number of samples requiring the same test are tested in parallel), medical diagnostic testing is currently centralized in specialized molecular laboratories. Consequently, smaller hospitals (lacking the volume of tests for which batch-based systems are designed), or laboratories that are not specialized in medical diagnostic testing, typically send out their samples for analysis by external reference centres. However, this system is being challenged by companies such as Biocartis, which are bringing highly reliable molecular information from virtually any biological sample, in virtually any setting, enabling fast and effective treatment selection in a global world.

References

1. Perou CM et al. Molecular portraits of human breast tumours. *Nature* 2000;406(6797):747–752.
2. Russnes H et al. Breast cancer molecular stratification. *Am J Pathol* 2017;187(10):2152–2162.
3. Gutnik LA et al. Breast cancer screening in low- and middle-income countries: a perspective from Malawi. *J Glob Oncol* 2(1):4–8.
4. Meric-Bernstam F et al. A decision support framework for genomically informed investigational cancer therapy. *J Natl Cancer Inst* 2015;107(7):djv098.
5. In vitro diagnostics market by product (instruments, reagents), technology (immunoassay, clinical chemistry, molecular diagnostics, hematology, urinalysis), application (diabetes, oncology, cardiology, nephrology)—forecast to 2023 | Markets and Markets. Available from: https://www.marketsandmarkets.com/Market-Reports/ivd-in-vitro-diagnostics-market-703.html
6. Oncology molecular diagnostics market worth $3.39bn by 2022. Available from: https://www.grandviewresearch.com/press-release/global-oncology-molecular-diagnostics-market

13

Breast Cancer Surgery

Peter A. van Dam, Cary S. Kaufman, Carlos A. Garcia-Etienne, Marie-Jeanne Vrancken Peeters, and Robert Mansel

Introduction

Ancient Egyptians described breast cancer but considered it as an incurable disease. The first recorded attempt to amputate a breast is attributed to Leonides of Alexandria in the second century AD. By the 1600s, prints in northern Europe show horrible scenes of women undergoing mastectomies by surgeons using forceps, knives, and cauterizing irons. Disinfection and sterilization, dedicated instruments, the use of sterile gloves, and general anaesthesia revolutionized surgery. The first axillary lymph node dissections (ALNDs) as part of the tumour eradication philosophy were performed in 1882 by William Banks, and in the beginning of the 20th century William S. Halstead (Baltimore, MD, USA) reported his radical mastectomy, which became the reference standard for breast cancer surgery during the next decades. Gradually, a less aggressive surgical trend emerged beginning with modified radical mastectomy sparing the pectoral muscles. This was then followed by breast-conserving surgery (BCS) preserving the breast. These evolutions were only possible thanks to breakthroughs in the understanding of the biology of breast cancer in the early 1970s and, the introduction of radiation treatment, and a new era of adjuvant systemic therapy. Then sentinel lymph node mapping was introduced with the hope of reducing the extent of axillary dissection. Finally, oncoplastic surgical techniques appeared to enable breast contour preservation such as skin-sparing mastectomy, in which the skin is conserved to facilitate breast reconstruction (1).

Minimum and Ideal Requirements

Standard breast surgery does not require complex or expensive technology. In principle, it can be performed all over the world in a unit equipped with a surgical theatre, sterilization facilities, a radiology department taking care of marking non-palpable lesions, and a pathology unit. The key to successful breast cancer treatment is a multidisciplinary approach in which the breast surgeon collaborates closely with the other involved breast cancer specialists (2). Compared to other types of surgery such as bowel or vascular surgery, the technical aspects of breast surgery are relatively easy to learn. However, as there are so many aspects in the timing of surgery, neoadjuvant and adjuvant treatment, and reconstructive care of breast cancer patients, there is a need for specialized breast surgeons who can incorporate this in their decision-making and in their input to the team. There is evidence that patients with breast cancers treated in high-volume centres (i.e. more than 150 primary breast cancer surgeries a year) and by specialized surgeons (operating on more than 30–50 new cases a year) have improved survival (2–4). This is not just related to surgical skills but also to a multidisciplinary approach involving specialized radiologists, pathologists, etc. It is likely that the demand for breast surgical oncologists will increase in step with the ageing population. Breast surgical oncologists of the future are more likely to be trained in oncoplastic techniques and thereby provide more comprehensive care.

Best Practice

Current data clearly show that the use of quality indicators (QIs) for breast cancer care, regular internal and external audit of performance of breast units, and benchmarking are effective means to improve the quality of care (2). Adherence to guidelines markedly improves the quality of care, notably regarding adjuvant treatment, and emerging data show that this results in better outcomes. Since quality assurance benefits patients, it will be a challenge for the medical and hospital community to develop affordable quality control systems that do not lead to excessive workloads. The European Society of Breast Cancer Specialists (EUSOMA) started a voluntary certification process in an attempt to improve the clinical performance of dedicated European Breast Centres in 2003 (3,5).

Surgery of the Breast

Surgical removal of the tumour is the cornerstone for treating early stage breast cancer. There are two options for breast surgery: a mastectomy involving removal of the entire breast and BCS removing just the tumour and a small amount of surrounding normal tissue. BCS plus radiation therapy is referred to as breast-conserving therapy, or BCT. In the 1970s, pioneering trials demonstrated equivalent long-term survival rates for patients with early stage invasive breast cancer treated by mastectomy or BCS combined with adjuvant radiotherapy (RT), and the superiority of BCS with radiation compared to BCS alone (6). It is likely that the emergence of adjuvant therapy made a less radical surgical approach of breast cancer possible. After breast conserving surgery, it is important to have a margin of normal breast tissue around the tumour. If cancer cells are found at or near the edges of the tissue removed, additional surgery may be necessary, because positive margins are related to a higher local recurrence rate. In the past, a margin width of 5–10 mm was considered necessary, but recently it was shown that 'no ink on specimen' is sufficient (7). Re-excision rates to achieve tumour-free margins are necessary in up to 20–25% of cases (2). If a large amount of tissue has been removed, and the margins are still involved, mastectomy may be recommended. In general, about two-thirds of patients are treated with BCS and one-third with mastectomy. Certain factors clearly favour mastectomy over BCT, including multiple or extensive tumours in a smaller breast not allowing resection with a nice aesthetic result, and contraindication for RT (e.g. pregnancy or previous RT on the ipsilateral breast). If the breast tumour is large or more advanced, neoadjuvant treatment with chemotherapy, targeted drugs, or sometimes anti-oestrogen therapy may be recommended before surgery. In cases where the tumour area remains large, oncoplastic breast-conserving approaches can be considered. In recent years, mastectomy rates appear to have increased in the USA for a variety of reasons, including larger tumour size, multicentric breast cancer, family history, race, younger age at diagnosis, preoperative magnetic resonance imaging utilization, socioeconomic status, distance from a radiation facility, patient preference, provider preference, and availability of and advances in reconstructive surgery. Some patients will opt to have a mastectomy (often on both sides) to reduce the risk of future breast cancers. This is especially the case in women who carry a breast cancer gene mutation or those with strong family histories (family clusters) or documented high-risk proliferative lesions. Last but not least, patients may have individual preferences for BCS versus mastectomy.

There are several types of mastectomy. A total or simple mastectomy involves removing the entire breast without removing the axillary lymph nodes. In a skin-sparing mastectomy, the nipple and areola are usually removed, but the rest of the skin over the breast is preserved. This is done in conjunction with immediate reconstruction. Standard mastectomies (both simple and skin-sparing) usually involve removing the nipple–areola complex (NAC). However, we have learned that the NAC rarely includes terminal duct lobular units where carcinoma arises in most cases, so it may be safe to preserve either the entire NAC (the nipple-sparing mastectomy) or remove the nipple with the breast tissue but preserve the areola (areola-sparing mastectomy). During a modified radical mastectomy, the breast tissue and the lymph nodes in the axilla are removed. A complete axillary node dissection is necessary only if the cancer has spread to the lymph nodes. Some women undergoing mastectomy may opt to have the opposite (uninvolved) breast removed, and this is known as contralateral prophylactic mastectomy and is performed to reduce the risk of a subsequent new breast cancer, especially in women at a high risk of second breast cancers (such as those with strong family histories or known genetic mutations). However, for most situations there is no proven survival benefit for removing the contralateral breast prophylactically.

Oncoplastic and reconstructive procedures have revolutionized breast cancer surgery considerably over the past decades, and reconstruction of the breast is an important option for women who undergo mastectomy (8,9). There are several options for reconstruction, and all women planning to undergo mastectomy should see a plastic or reconstructive surgeon to discuss these options before having surgery of the breast. Reconstruction of the breast volume itself can be performed with the use of either implants or autogenous tissues. The choice of technique is dictated by a variety of factors that include the size and shape of the native breast, the location and type of cancer, the availability of tissues around the breast and at other sites, the age of the patient, the patient's medical risk factors, and the type of adjuvant therapy. The final decision is often based on the patient's preference. Breast reconstruction may be performed either immediately or after a delay. There is now clear evidence that neither implant-based nor autogenous tissue-based reconstruction has any effect on the incidence or detection of cancer recurrence. Technically, immediate reconstruction allows for the preservation of critical anatomical structures such as the inframammary fold and it maximizes the amount of native skin available for the reconstructive process and, thereby, maximizing the overall aesthetic result. In addition, the preservation of body image, femininity, and sexuality through the immediate reconstruction of a breast can have psychological benefits and significantly reduce postoperative emotional stress. A more detailed review of breast reconstruction and oncoplastic surgery is presented in Chapter 14.

Management of the Axillary Lymph Nodes

Most women with invasive cancer will have an operation to assess the presence of cancer cells in the axillary lymph nodes (10).

ALND involves removing most of the lymph nodes in the axilla. This operation was commonly performed for all women with invasive breast cancer in the past and is associated with complications such as pain and arm swelling (lymphoedema). ALND is now usually performed only for patients when cancerous lymph nodes can be felt in the axilla or when the sentinel lymph node excision reveals multiple nodes containing cancer or a large burden of cancer cells. ALND is also recommended in women undergoing mastectomy who have cancer in their sentinel lymph node, especially if they are not having postmastectomy radiation.

The sentinel lymph node is the first lymph node that receives lymphatic drainage from the breast. The sentinel node for patients with breast cancer is usually located in the axilla, but in some patients may be near the sternum (breast bone) between the ribs (intercostal lymph nodes). In addition, there may be more than one sentinel lymph node. Most patients do not have cancer in their sentinel lymph nodes.

A **sentinel lymph node excision** is performed to stage the axilla and to spare patients an ALND when the biopsy was negative. It is based upon the finding that if the sentinel node does not contain cancer cells, the likelihood that other lymph nodes in the axilla contain cancer cells is very small. To identify the sentinel lymph node, the surgeon injects blue dye, a radioactive material, or a combination of both into the breast. The dye or radioactive material enters the lymphatic channels and flows to the sentinel lymph node. This allows the surgeon to identify and remove the appropriate lymph nodes. The sentinel nodes are subsequently examined under the microscope by a pathologist (10–16).

Data from recently published trials have provided practice-changing recommendations for the indication for ALND. The Z0011 trial, a randomized controlled trial from the American College of Surgeons Oncology Group (ACOSOG), included patients with T1/2 (≤5 cm) lesions who were candidates BCT, who had not received neoadjuvant chemotherapy, and who had one or two positive sentinel nodes (micro- or macroscopic disease). In all, 446 patients were randomized to no further surgical treatment of the axilla (sentinel lymph node biopsy (SLNB) only) and 445 cases to ALND. A recent update with a median follow-up of 9.25 years showed that the cumulative incidence of regional recurrences at 10 years in the ipsilateral axilla was similar between each arm, two patients (0.5%) in the ALND group compared with five patients (1.5%) in the SLNB-only group ($P = 0.28$). Ten-year cumulative locoregional recurrence was 6.2% in the ALND group and 5.3% in the SLNB-only group ($P = 0.36$). The 10-year overall survival was 86.3% in the SLND-only group and 83.6% in the ALND group (hazard ratio (HR): 0.85; one-sided 95% CI: 0–1.16); non-inferiority $P = 0.02$). The 10-year disease-free survival was 80.2% in the SLND-only group and 78.2% in the ALND group (HR: 0.85; 95% CI: 0.62–1.17; $P = 0.32$).

There are additional recent studies also questioning the impact of ALND in early stage breast cancer. A prospective randomized-controlled trial from the International Breast Cancer Study Group (IBCSG), Trial 23-01, included patients with T1/2 lesions with a positive SLNB for micrometastasis or isolated tumour cells and randomized cases to ALND or no further surgical treatment. With a median follow-up of 5 years, there were no significant differences in 5-year disease-free survival (DFS) nor 5-year overall survival ($P = 0.16$, $P = 0.73$, respectively).

The AMAROS (After Mapping of the Axilla: Radiotherapy or Surgery?) trial from the EORTC (European Organisation for Research and Treatment of Cancer) presented a design similar to the Z0011 trial and included patients with T1/2 lesions who had a positive sentinel node (micro or macroscopic disease), but this trial randomized cases to ALND or axillary RT. After a median follow-up of 6.1 years, there were no significant differences in 5-year axillary recurrence, 5-year DFS, and 5-year overall survival between the two groups (95% CI: 0.00–5.27; $P = 0.18$, $P = 0.34$, respectively). The study did show a statistically significant difference in the 5-year incidence of measured arm lymphoedema with 13% after ALND and 5% in the RT group ($P = 0.0009$).

Another recently published trial, the INT09/98 trial, by Agresti and colleagues from the Istituto Nazionale dei Tumori in Milan addressed whether ALND could be safely avoided and whether tumour biology could be adequate to guide adjuvant treatment. This study was not conducted in patients with a positive SLN, but in cases with cT1 cN0 disease and randomized patients to breast conservation with or without ALND. The study was designed before SLNB was routinely introduced in clinical practice. It included cases with tumours smaller than those in the Z0011, 23-01, and AMAROS trials: 98% of the tumours were pT1 with a mean size of 1.5 cm. Patients had clinically negative axilla and were randomized to BCT with or without ALND. All patients received whole breast RT with no attempt to irradiate the axilla. Decisions for adjuvant treatment were based on clinicopathologic factors that took into account information form axillary lymph node status in the ALND group and from an experimental biological panel only in the non-ALND group. After a median follow-up of more than 10 years (127 months), no statistically significant differences were observed in 10-year

DFS with 92.4% in the ALND group versus 91.3% in the non-ALND group (log-rank $P = 0.97$) and 10-year OS with 93.3% in the ALND group versus 91.5% in the non-ALND group (log-rank $P = 0.436$). The study did show a higher rate of axillary recurrence in the non-ALND group (9%) versus the ALND group (0%). Patients with axillary recurrence underwent ALND, and no significant relationship was observed between overall survival and the number of involved lymph nodes in these cases.

What seems clear from older trials and confirmed by the recent studies described above is that lymph node metastases are indicators, but not governors, of survival. Based on initial reports of the Z0011 study in 2010–2011 and subsequently supported by other studies, the National Comprehensive Cancer Network guideline was modified to consider no further axillary surgery in patients who meet all Z0011 selection criteria: T1/2 lesions, one or two positive SLNs, candidates for BCT, and no neoadjuvant chemotherapy. However, the development of clinical guidelines is always a work in progress, so adherence to these recommendations is expected to be gradual.

It is not completely clear how the axilla of patients undergoing neoadjuvant treatment should be managed. There are studies suggesting that, if there were no evidence of lymph node involvement pre treatment (by ultrasound of the axilla, negative fine-needle aspiration cytology, or positron emission tomography), SLNB after finishing the neoadjuvant treatment may be safe, considering that the sentinel node procedure has a higher false-negative rate (about 10–15%) in this setting compared to primary surgery (>5%). If the axilla were invaded clinically as determined by imaging or fine-needle aspiration at initial diagnosis, it is recommended to perform a full ALND after neoadjuvant treatment. Alternatives such as the MARI procedure (marking the axilla with radioactive iodine seeds (MARI procedure)) and targeted axillary clearance are currently under investigation (10–19).

Comments on EUSOMA Quality Indicators
for Breast Surgery

EUSOMA has developed a framework for internal and external audits to monitor breast cancer care in specialized breast units. Clearly defined quality parameters are monitored continuously, and feedback is given on an annual basis to the certified units to optimize adherence to evidence-based guidelines and treatment results. Prospectively collected information on primary breast cancer cases diagnosed and treated in the units must be sent to a central EUSOMA data warehouse for continuous monitoring of QIs to improve quality of care. Before acquiring certification, a unit must submit its data for validation. Units have to comply with the EUSOMA breast centre guidelines (http://www.EUSOMA.org). Certified units are audited annually. The database was started in 2006 and currently includes in excess of 160,000 cases (all breast diseases included) from Breast Units located in Germany, Switzerland, Belgium, Austria, Netherlands, Spain, Portugal, and Italy. We recently assessed time trends in QI's in EUSOMA certified breast units over the period 2006–2015 and present these below.

Proportion of Patients with Invasive Cancer Who Had an Axillary Clearance with at Least 10 Lymph Nodes Examined (2006: 89.7%; 2015: 86.5%; $P = 0.780$)

In the Halstedian philosophy, radical resection of the breast, the pectoral muscles, and en-bloc resection of the regional lymph node areas were regarded as crucial elements in the surgical local control of breast cancer. However, of 1640 women treated in Memorial Hospital from 1940 to 1943, 1458 underwent radical mastectomy with a cancer-free survival at 30 years of only 13% (with 57% of patients dying of breast cancer, 24% of other causes, and 6% lost for follow-up). The failure of radical mastectomy to cure many patients with breast cancer was initially explained as the failure to extirpate all the draining lymphatics of the breast. In the 1950s, it became clear that one-quarter of the lymphatic drainage of the breast is through the ipsilateral internal mammary nodes. To take this into account, the extended radical mastectomy was developed, which is a radical mastectomy combined with removal of the internal mammary and axillary lymph nodes. A prospective randomized trial comparing radical with extended radical mastectomy failed to show any difference in DFS and overall survival. As the extended procedure induced significant perioperative morbidity, mortality, and long-term sequelae, it became obsolete. In the 1970s it was recognized that failure of surgery to control breast cancer was caused by haematogenic dissemination of tumour cells before the operation, which led to the development of adjuvant cytostatic and endocrine treatment. Breast surgery became less radical, BCT emerged, and the role of ALND changed from a therapeutic procedure into a staging procedure with prognostic implications. Limiting lymphadenectomy to a level 1–3 axillary dissection, it was shown that at least ten axillary lymph nodes had to be removed to reliably distinguish lymph node-negative patients from patients with lymph node metastasis. Removing more nodes did not make much difference, but it did increase morbidity. In those days, the lymph node status was crucial for decision-making, because only lymph node-positive patients with early breast cancer received postoperative adjuvant systemic treatment. In the 1980s, the NSABP-B04 and the King's College, Cambridge, randomized trials published their 10-year follow-up results after comparing ALND plus RT with no treatment to the axilla in clinically node-negative patients. In both studies, treating the axilla did decrease the recurrence rate significantly (1.4% for AD, 3.1% for RT, and 14% for no treatment) but did not improve the survival rate in early stage breast cancer patients. As mentioned above, the ACOSOG Z0011 phase 3 randomized clinical trial enrolled patients from May 1999 to December 2004 at 115 sites (both academic and community medical centres). Among women with T1 or T2 invasive primary breast cancer, no palpable axillary adenopathy, and one or two sentinel lymph nodes containing metastases, 10-year OS for patients treated with sentinel lymph node dissection alone was non-inferior to overall survival for those treated with ALND. In both the Z0010 study and the NSABP B-32 trials, decisions regarding adjuvant systemic therapy were taken independently of results of the sentinel node immunohistochemistry analysis. This supports current practice, whereby decisions regarding adjuvant systemic therapy reflect consideration of biological or molecular factors associated with the primary tumour rather than solely based on occult sentinel nodal metastases. It is likely that this QI will become obsolete in the future.

Proportion of Patients with Invasive Cancer ≤3 cm (Total Size Including DCIS) Who Underwent BCS (2006: 73.7%; 2015: 84.7%; $P < 0.001$)

In centres specializing in breast cancer treatment, approximately 60–85% of women with early stage breast cancer are candidates for BCT. In 25 to 50% of women, there are medical, cosmetic, and/or social and emotional reasons for having a mastectomy rather than BCT. Survival outcomes are the same whether BCT or mastectomy is performed. Although there is a trend in the USA of increasing mastectomy rates, this does not seem to be the case in European breast units, where the BCS rate is going up. This may be explained by a multidisciplinary approach and accumulated experience in these units. The use of neoadjuvant chemo- or hormonotherapy may also be a tool to reduce tumour size and to make BCS treatment possible in more cases.

Proportion of Patients with Non-Invasive Breast Cancer ≤2 cm Treated with BCS (2006: 77.9%; 2015: 83.4%; $P < 0.001$)

Ductal carcinoma in situ (DCIS) is a heterogeneous group of diseases that differ in biology and clinical behaviour. Until the 1980s, DCIS represented less than 1% of all breast cancer cases, but, with the increased use of mammography, DCIS now accounts for 15–25% of newly diagnosed breast cancer cases. The natural history of DCIS is poorly understood. The most direct evidence regarding the progression of DCIS to invasive cancer comes from studies where DCIS was initially misdiagnosed as benign and treated by biopsy alone. These studies showed that between 14% and 53% of DCIS treated with excision alone may progress to invasive cancer over a period of 10 or more years. Until a few decades ago, mastectomy was the reference standard of treatment for DCIS, with a reported survival rate of 98–99%. There was a general impression that patients with DCIS were often overtreated. The Van Nuys Prognostic Index (VNPI) was developed in 1996 by Silverstein as a guide for treatment decisions in DCIS patients. The original VNPI was based on tumour size, margin width, and pathologic classification (nuclear grade and comedonecrosis). Scores of 1 (most favourable) to 3 (most unfavourable) were assigned for each of the three predictors. The total VNPI score is the sum of the score of the three predictors and varies from 3 to 9. Depending on the final VNPI score, a specific treatment is recommended. Excision only for patients with VNPI scores of 3 or 4 is defensible due to the low risk of recurrence. Patients with intermediate scores (5, 6, or 7) have a 17% decrease in local recurrence rates with radiation therapy. Mastectomy should be considered in patients with a VNPI score of 8 or

9, because they have extremely high local recurrence rates. The proportion of patients with DCIS who undergo mastectomy has strongly decreased in recent years, however. EUSOMA data show that when one focuses on BCS in patients with DCIS, mastectomy rates can be reduced to 15%. BCS strives for a balance between cosmetic outcomes and negative margins. The earlier statement that free margins of at least 10 mm decrease the risk of ipsilateral recurrence suggested that a more radical excision is recommended, which may lead to poor cosmetic results. In the NSABP B17 and B24 trials, ink-free margins were required, and only 72 (2.8%) out of 2612 patients treated with BCS with and without RT died of breast cancer after 15 years of follow-up. Thus, any net benefit of more widely free margins on the OS of women with DCIS would be extremely small or negligible. With increasing molecular characterization of these preinvasive lesions, optimum risk prediction in the future is likely to be achieved by integration of both conventional and molecular factors, which should be incorporated into a validated predictive model to help with clinical decision-making.

Proportion of Patients with DCIS Who Do Not Undergo Axillary Clearance (2006: 88.8%; 2015: 97.3% %; $P < 0.001$)

DCIS is considered a non-invasive malignancy, but it may also occur in association with invasive carcinoma. The likelihood of lymph node metastases is very low. Although traditionally an axillary clearance was performed in patients with DCIS, the benefit for these patients has never been proven. The need to perform SLNB in patients with DCIS is controversial, and according to recent ASCO guidelines it should not be performed in women with DCIS treated by lumpectomy. However, DCIS is upstaged in 10–35% of cases to microinvasion (DCISM) or invasive breast cancer on final surgical pathology after an initial diagnosis of DCIS on a core or vacuum aspiration biopsy. As a result of the probability of upstaging after initial diagnosis, multiple investigators have stressed the need for SLNB in patients with high-risk DCIS. These include patients aged 55 years or younger, mammographic abnormality greater than 4 cm, high-grade or comedo necrosis on histological evaluation, and the presence of a palpable tumour.

The incidence of a positive sentinel lymph node in DCISM has been reported to be between 3% and 20%. In 2002, de Mascarel et al. published an interesting series of patients with DCISM ($n = 243$) and divided these patients in two distinct pathologic groups: type 1 with isolated cells and type 2 with clusters of cells (20). The clinical behaviour of the type 1 subgroup was similar to DCIS without microinvasion, and the type 2 subgroup resembled invasive ductal carcinoma associated with large areas of DCIS. The positive sentinel lymph node reported for de Mascarel's type 2 subgroup was 10.1% for the type 1 subgroup 0%. However, this study included cases with a >0.1 cm focus of invasion in the type 2 subgroup; given the current classification system, these cases would not be considered microinvasive disease.

Proportion of Patients with Invasive Breast Cancer Who Received a Single Breast Operation for the Primary Tumour Excluding Reconstruction (2006: 80.0%; 2015: 91.2%; $P < 0.001$)

As preoperative histological diagnosis has become a quality indicator for the treatment of patients with early invasive breast cancer, this has markedly improved adequate preoperative planning. In addition, better imaging, the use of magnetic resonance imaging (MRI), ultrasound of the axilla, a multidisciplinary approach, and specialized breast surgeons have all contributed to enable optimal planning of primary BCS, BCS after neoadjuvant systemic treatment, and mastectomy with or without reconstruction. Lumpectomy often fails to achieve clear surgical margins, and on average 20% of patients who undergo BCS will require repeat surgery to achieve an R0 resection. Reoperations potentially have several negative consequences including delayed commencement of adjuvant therapy, worse cosmesis, increased patient anxiety, and higher costs. There are several possible modalities to assess surgical margins intraoperatively in order to reduce breast cancer reoperation rates post BCS. Techniques evaluated include specimen radiography, intraoperative ultrasound, touch imprint cytology, frozen section, and radiofrequency spectroscopy. EUSOMA data show that when a breast unit focuses on this issue, the re-resection rate can be greatly reduced. This can only be achieved by a team approach in which radiologists, surgeons, and histopathologists are heavily involved.

Proportion of Patients with DCIS Who Received a Single Breast Operation for the Primary Tumour Excluding Reconstruction (2006: 63.4%; 2015: 79.9%; $P = 0.006$)

Preoperative assessment of the extent of disease and intraoperative specimen assessment is much more difficult in patients with DCIS compared to invasive breast cancer. Many trials confirm that tumour margins are the most important prognostic factor of local recurrence for DCIS patients treated with BCS alone or with BCS plus RT. DCIS is present in more than 80% of patients diagnosed by mammography screening. Typically, clustered microcalcifications are common in 85–90% of the cases, and other potential findings include circumscribed masses, focal nodular patterns, asymmetry, dilated retro-areolar ducts, ill-defined, rounded tumour, focal architectural distortion, subareolar mass, and developing density. Up to 20% of DCIS remain mammographically occult due to the lack of calcifications and/or small tumour dimensions. Breast MRI has a sensitivity for the diagnosis of DCIS of 77–96% with a high false-positive rate. The risk of ipsilateral recurrence is lower for patients with DCIS treated with BCS upon negative margins.

Proportion of Invasive Breast Cancer Patients with pN0 Who Do Not
Undergo Axillary Clearance (2006: 61.1%; 2015: 96.7%; $P = 0.006$)

SLNB has become the primary means of axillary staging evaluation in patients with clinically node-negative invasive breast cancer, because it is as accurate as ALND but less morbid. The NSABP B-32 trial randomized 5611 patients to receive SLNB alone versus SLNB plus ALND. In this trial, at least one SLN was identified in more than 97% of patients and was positive in 26%. The false-negative rate in the group who underwent ALND was 9.7%. The SLN was the only positive node in 61.5%, and only 0.6% of patients had a positive SLN outside the axilla. The morbidity risk with this procedure is not zero. In both single institutional studies as well as in prospective trials, the sequalae of lymphoedema, paraesthesia, decreased limb use, persistent pain, and seroma have been reported. Validation of the SLNB technique by this trial allowed avoiding ALND for staging purposes in the majority of invasive breast cancer cases.

Look to the Future

It is undeniable that the role of the surgeon managing breast diseases is the subject of continuous evolution moving from the cancer-extirpative surgeon to a deeply informed surgical leader who interacts in a multidisciplinary setting and encompassing tasks for risk assessment, genetic counselling, and new diagnostic approaches. It is also conceivable that further in the future we may identify a subset of tumours that could be managed by some type of non-surgical ablation or medication only. However, it is likely this will apply only to a small subset of cases.

Key Messages

- The role of the breast surgeon has evolved to that of a surgical leader interacting in a multidisciplinary setting and encompassing tasks such as risk assessment and new diagnostic approaches.
- Standard breast surgery does not require complex technology, but it can be performed all over the world in a unit equipped with a surgical theatre and sterilization facilities.
- Patients with breast cancer treated by specialized surgeons and a dedicated multidisciplinary team have a better outcome.
- Breast surgeons in the future are more likely to be trained in oncoplastic techniques and provide more comprehensive care.
- In general, two-thirds of the early breast cancer patients can be treated with BCT.
- Recently practice-changing recommendations were published for the indication for ALND.

References

1. Matsen CB, Neumayer LA. Breast cancer: a review for the general surgeon. *JAMA Surg* 2013;148(10):971–979.
2. van Dam PA et al.; eusomaDB Working Group. Time trends (2006–2015) of quality indicators in EUSOMA-certified breast centres. *Eur J Cancer* 2017;85:15–22.
3. Mikeljevic JS et al. Surgeon workload and survival from breast cancer. *Br J Cancer* 2003;89(3):487–491.
4. Roohan PJ et al. Hospital volume differences and five-year survival from breast cancer. *Am J Public Health* 1998;88(3):454–457.
5. Biganzoli L et al. Quality indicators in breast cancer care: an update from the EUSOMA working group. *Eur J Cancer* 2017;86:59–81.
6. Fisher B et al. Five-year results of a randomized clinical trial comparing total mastectomy and segmental mastectomy with or without radiation in the treatment of breast cancer. *N Engl J Med* 1985;312:665–673.
7. Morrow M et al. Society of Surgical Oncology–American Society for Radiation Oncology–American Society of Clinical Oncology consensus guideline on margins for breast-conserving surgery with whole-breast irradiation in ductal carcinoma in situ. *J Clin Oncol* 2016;34(33):4040–4046.
8. Cordeiro PG. Breast reconstruction after surgery for breast cancer. *N Engl J Med* 2008;359: 1590–1601.
9. Clough KB et al. Mammoplasty combined with irradiation: conservative treatment of cancers located in the lower quadrants. *Ann Chir Plast Esthet* 1990;35(2):117e22.
10. Agresti R et al. Axillary lymph node dissection versus no dissection in patients with T1N0 breast cancer. A Randomized Clinical Trial (INT09/98). *Cancer* 2014;120:885–893.
11. Donker M et al. Radiotherapy or surgery of the axilla after a positive sentinel node in breast cancer (EORTC 10981-22023 AMAROS): a randomized, multicenter, open-label, phase 3 non-inferiority trial. *Lancet Oncol* 2014;15(12):1303–1310.
12. Galimberti V et al. Axillary dissection versus no axillary dissection in patients with sentinel-node micrometastases (IBCSG 23-01): a phase 3 randomised controlled trial. *Lancet Oncol* 2013;14:297–305.
13. Gentilini O and Veronesi U. Abandoning sentinel lymph node biopsy in early breast cancer? A new trial in progress at the European Institute of Oncology of Milan (SOUND: Sentinel node vs Observation after axillary UltraSouND). *Breast* 2012;21(5):678–681.
14. Giuliano AE et al. Locoregional recurrence after sentinel lymph node dissection with or without axillary dissection in patients with sentinel lymph node metastases: long-term follow-up from the American College of Surgeons Oncology Group (Alliance) ACOSOG Z0011 randomized trial. *Ann Surg* 2016;264(3):413–420.
15. Giuliano AE et al. Effect of axillary dissection vs no axillary dissection on 10-year overall survival among women with invasive breast cancer and sentinel node metastasis: the ACOSOG Z0011 (Alliance) randomized clinical trial. *JAMA* 2017;318(10):918–926.
16. Krag DN et al. Sentinel-lymph-node resection compared with conventional axillary-lymph-node dissection in clinically node-negative patients with breast cancer: overall survival findings from the NSABP B-32 randomised phase 3 trial. *Lancet Oncol* 2010;11(10):927–933.
17. Donker M, Straver ME, Wesseling J, et al. Marking axillary lymph nodes with radioactive iodine seeds for axillary staging after neoadjuvant systemic treatment in breast cancer patients: the MARI procedure. *Ann Surg* 2015;261(2):378–382.
18. van der Noordaa MEM et al. Major Reduction in Axillary Lymph Node Dissections After Neoadjuvant Systemic Therapy for Node-Positive Breast Cancer by combining PET/CT and the MARI Procedure. *Ann Surg Oncol* 2018 June;25(6):1512–1520.

19. Caudle AS, et al. Improved axillary evaluation following neoadjuvant therapy for patients with node-positive breast cancer using selective evaluation of clipped nodes: implementation of targeted axillary dissection. *J Clin Oncol* 2016;34:1072–1078.

20. de Mascarel I et al. Breast ductal carcinoma in situ with microinvasion: a definition supported by a long-term study of 1248 serially sectioned ductal carcinomas. *Cancer* 2002;94(8):2134–2142.

14

Reconstructive and Oncoplastic Surgery

Maurício Magalhães Costa, Peter A. van Dam, Mahmoud Danaei,
Paulo Roberto Leal, and Daniel Leal

Introduction

Breast reconstruction has evolved over the last century, especially with the advent of new technologies including anatomical implants, expanders, and, most recently, acellular dermal matrix. The development of techniques ranging from free/pedicle flaps, implant-based reconstruction, fat grafting, and oncoplastic surgery have also played a major part in the success in this field (1,2).

However, recent studies reveal that most women undergoing mastectomy (as many as 80%) are not having breast reconstruction (Figure 14.1). In those areas where a surgeon is not available to perform a reconstruction, it is important that patients are informed about the possibility of some type of reconstructive surgery in a second stage. In many cases, immediate breast reconstruction can at least be started at the time of mastectomy with placement of an implant, expander, or flap. This ultimately helps the patient, emotionally, through the loss of the breast, and in most cases decreases the number of surgical procedures the patient ultimately needs to undergo.

A recent study demonstrated that oncoplastic approaches add to the oncologic safety of breast-conserving treatment, because a larger volume of breast tissue can be excised, and wider negative surgical margins can be obtained. Oncoplastic techniques are especially indicated for large tumours, for which standard breast-conserving approaches have a high probability of leaving positive margins associated with heightened local recurrence risk and/or creating unacceptable deformity of the breast.

The surgery should be performed by someone with the required training, either a plastic or oncoplastic surgeon, and this is an important quality assurance issue for the patient. Immediate breast reconstruction is gaining wide acceptance; however, secondary reconstruction is also a valid instrument, and in many cases it is a reference standard procedure. There is increasing demand for patient-reported outcome instruments in cosmetic and reconstructive breast surgery research and clinical practice. The conceptual framework includes six domains: satisfaction with her breasts, overall outcome, process of care, psychosocial, physical wellbeing, and sexual wellbeing.

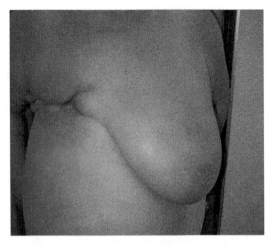

Figure 14.1 Bad aesthetic result after right mastectomy. Large contralateral breast causes cervical discomfort.

Breast Reconstruction: Minimal and Ideal Requirements

Even though breast reconstruction has a clear benefit on patient's quality of life after mastectomy, more than 60% of women still do not have it performed (3,4). The decision to have breast reconstruction includes various factors which may be linked to sociodemographics, ethnic backgrounds, or medical conditions. The decision is personal and is made according to the patient's perspective of her body image, sexuality, and self-esteem. Education of the patient is of utmost importance, and all reconstructive options should be discussed. Breast cancer patients considering breast reconstruction should know that they have both a voice and a choice.

Patient–doctor interaction is an important factor in the decision concerning the choice of mastectomy and reconstruction. The reconstruction audit in the UK showed that the rate of mastectomy and reconstruction varied from 23% and 75%, while immediate reconstruction varied from 8% to 43% (5).

Prior to the mastectomy, the patient should have a consultation with the plastic surgery team to evaluate if she is an eligible candidate for immediate or delayed breast reconstruction. Mastectomy with immediate breast reconstruction may protect breast cancer patients from a period of psychosocial distress, poor body image, and diminished sexual wellbeing compared with those waiting for delayed breast reconstruction (6).

As a disadvantage, immediate breast reconstruction may be a larger surgery requiring a longer recovery time. Also, if the patient experiences any kind of complication (wound dehiscence, haematoma, flap loss) it may postpone her adjuvant therapy. A patient may want to delay reconstruction until after all treatments have been completed. Many women feel that delaying reconstruction gives them time to focus on treatments and research the type of reconstruction that best suits their needs.

Immediate breast reconstruction is often performed with an expander or an implant, particularly with the recent popularity of skin- and nipple-sparing mastectomy for early invasive or in-situ disease or even prophylactic mastectomies. The rate of immediate breast reconstruction with implant is increasing by an average of 5% per year, since it promotes great oncological safety combined with an acceptable complication rate (7,8).

Autologous reconstruction after breast cancer surgery is not a common procedure, unless a large skin resection is mandatory for oncological reasons, or the patient does not want implants. Reconstruction with autologous tissue is often reserved for delayed or salvage procedures in the case of local recurrence, previously irradiated patients, or patients having a prophylactic (bilateral) mastectomy (Figure 14.2). Even though implant-based reconstruction is gaining popularity, when compared to autologous reconstruction it has lower rates of patient satisfaction and long-term aesthetic results (9).

Adjuvant therapy is another concern regarding breast reconstruction, especially postmastectomy radiotherapy. Randomized studies have demonstrated that postmastectomy radiotherapy may decrease local recurrence and increase survival for patients with positive axillary lymph nodes (10). The surgical planning for immediate breast reconstruction with implants should always include an expander in case of a different scenario. The indication for adjuvant radiotherapy is dynamic and may change perioperatively. Radiotherapy is known to increase the surgical complication rate, including capsular contracture, and to decrease the aesthetic result of implant-based reconstruction (11). Fat grafting can help improve skin quality on the irradiated tissue and may be an excellent tool for these patients (12) (Figure 14.3).

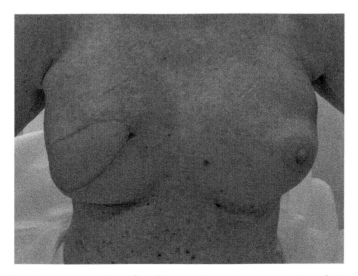

Figure 14.2 Breast reconstruction after skin-sparing mastectomy using a latissimus dorsi myocutaneous flap.

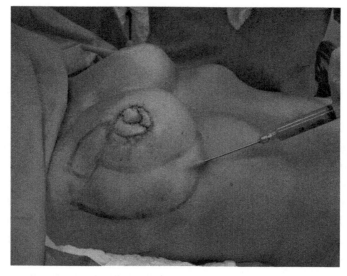

Figure 14.3 Breast reconstruction using lipofilling to correct a volume defect after breast cancer surgery.

Quality of Implant (Saline/Silicone)

Whereas some surgeons recommend silicone implants for their natural feeling and appearance, studies using the BREAST-Q provide evidence that can be used to help guide patients in their decision-making process (8). In augmentation patients, Gryskiewicz et al. demonstrated that patients who received silicone implants were more satisfied with their overall outcome than patients who received saline (13). In breast reconstruction patients, multiple studies have demonstrated similar findings with higher overall satisfaction, psychological wellbeing, sexual wellbeing, physical function, and satisfaction with their surgeon in patients receiving silicone implants in comparison to saline. In the past, there have been some scandals with non-approved implants having an increased risk (up to 500%) of leaking and which were implicated in several deaths due to systemic toxicity. Local governmental regulations on the use of prosthetic material are essential to guarantee high-quality breast protheses for patients.

Emerging Modality: Oncoplastic Surgery

The term oncoplastic surgery was introduced in 1998 with the aim of developing surgical techniques with oncological objective and linked to concepts of the plastic surgery. Therefore, patients might have effective treatment with smaller aesthetic and psychological damages. Oncoplasty describes an evolving area of breast surgery that applies principles of surgical oncology and plastic and reconstructive surgery to the management of women with breast cancer. The main aims are to reduce the rate of

(a)   (b)

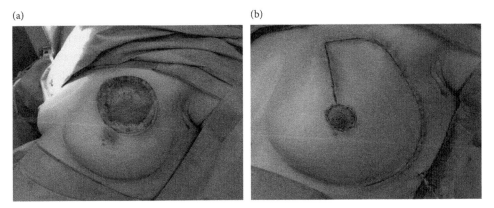

Figure 14.4 The use of a mammary flap rotation technique to correct a large defect after wide local excision of a breast cancer.

mastectomies, reduce the rate of re-excisions, and improve the quality of cosmetic outcomes with breast-conserving surgery (BCS) (Figure 14.4).

Pietro Berrino presented a very interesting classification of the deformities after BCS (14):

- Type I: distortion and malposition of the nipple–areola complex (NAC) related to scar contraction and fibrosis (significant in 53%);
- Type II: tissue deficiency: skin, subcutaneous, glandular (significant in 33%);
- Type III: breast retraction, severe asymmetry (significant in 16%);
- Type IV: severely irradiated breast, important retraction and fibrosis, NAC malpositioned (significant in 9%).

The individual therapeutic procedure is worked out and planned together with the patient. Taking into account the exact localization and topography of the tumour, a decision is made on a promising application of neoadjuvant chemotherapy, the choice of neoadjuvant chemotherapy, the choice of surgical intervention, and the corresponding postoperative treatment. The patient's needs and desires are of paramount importance, but the surgical approach should be balanced with oncological safety. Not all patients are good candidates for having oncoplastic surgery. The ideal candidate would be a woman with a small tumour in a good location (in the area of resection of a breast reduction marking, for example) with wide margins.

Clough et al. classified the breast defects and oncoplastic procedures according to the response to reconstruction (15). Thus, patients with a type I breast deformity have a normal-appearing breast with no deformity. However, there is asymmetry in the volume or shape between breasts, and this was managed by a contralateral breast surgery. However, type II patients have deformed breasts, and this was treated by an ipsilateral breast surgery or flap reconstruction. Type III patients have either major deformity with fibrosis, and these were treated with total mastectomy and reconstruction.

Some controversy remains as to whether the oncological or the plastic surgeon should perform oncoplastic surgery. In most countries and in most large breast centres, a multidisciplinary approach with both oncological and plastic surgeons working together is the reference standard for the reconstructive cases. But the scenario is variable and depends on many different factors. However, most breast cancer patients worldwide do not receive any kind of breast reconstruction. So, there is a trend in many countries to change this reality with the creation of a super-specialist breast surgeon, who has a double qualification both as a plastic and oncological surgeon and who can perform oncological and reconstructive cases. Also, a breast surgeon with oncoplastic skills could handle the simplest reconstructive cases.

Best Practice: Breast Reconstruction and Quality Control

Health care quality is the degree to which health care services for individuals and populations increase the likelihood of desired health outcomes (16). Understanding the relationship between quality, cost, and accessibility of health care is mandatory to measure the quality of care level. Breast reconstruction as a quality measure for breast cancer care is a complex analysis. There are many variables determining whether the patient can be reconstructed. These include the patient's preference, the surgeon's preference and skills, and the available technology. Cultural and sociodemographic factors may also be included in that analysis. However, it is well described that offering breast reconstruction for a mastectomy patient may improve quality of life and thus quality of care (6).

Assessment of outcome is very important for the measurement of quality of care. In oncology, the most common outcomes measured are usually disease-free survival and overall survival. Understanding the patient as a biopsychosocial model, improving the patient's overall survival will not be beneficial if she has a poor quality of life. So, quality of life, body image, and patient satisfaction are taken into account in the measurement of quality control for breast reconstruction.

There is a concern regarding the measurement of quality of care in plastic surgery, where the results are usually measured by the presence of complications, number of revision surgeries, and patient satisfaction with the aesthetic results. Although complications are not frequent, the concept of beauty is subjective, and the surgeon's view of a good result may not agree with that of the patient. Double-blinded studies in surgery are difficult to design, because surgeons can rarely be blinded. The majority of published articles in plastic surgery compare cohorts of patients having different reconstructive procedures, and this does not fit the criteria for a randomized controlled trial. Standardized and validated outcome assessment instruments such as scales and questionnaires should be used in the search for more objective and reliable results.

In order to quantify pre- and postoperative patient satisfaction and health-related quality of life for reconstructive and cosmetic breast surgery, a validated questionnaire was created: the BREAST-Q (17). The conceptual framework included six domains: satisfaction with breasts, overall outcome, process of care, psychosocial wellbeing, physical wellbeing, and sexual wellbeing. The BREAST-Q contains three modules (augmentation, reconstruction, and reduction), each with a preoperative and postoperative version. By applying the questionnaire, a measure can facilitate comparisons of different surgical techniques from a patient perspective and provide a reference point for comparisons between studies and surgical populations.

The key for having optimal breast cancer care lies in the multidisciplinary team. Surgical planning can only be perfect if the patient has already had a good breast-imaging study and preoperative diagnosis. The best option for reconstruction, including the placement of incisions, should be discussed exhaustively with the patient and between plastic and oncological surgeons. The surgical procedure should be performed by an experienced surgeon who has full training to manage all case scenarios.

Surgical Training

Oncoplastic surgery is an essential factor in maintaining quality for care, but there is still no standardized training programme. Although oncoplasty is not a specialty nor even a technique, there are some independent teaching programmes around the world.

Oncoplastic surgery has four levels of competence:

- Level 1: unilateral and displacement techniques, aesthetic skin incisions, de-epithelialization of areola margins, glandular mobilization and reshaping techniques, and purse string suture of central quadrant reconstruction;
- Level 2: bilateral and replacement techniques, breast reduction, mastopexy, Grisotti flap, and nipple and areolar reconstruction;
- Level 3: expander and implant techniques, immediate breast reconstruction with temporary expanders or implants, and contralateral symmetry procedures;
- Level 4: autologous flap techniques, either pedicle or free tissue transfer or a combination of both techniques.

Breast surgeons should be prepared to work with levels 1 and 2, but the ideal is to have a full training to manage all case scenarios.

As the demand for breast reconstruction steadily increases and the key to optimizing care is the multidisciplinary approach, an inter-specialty training programme with plastic and breast surgeons developed to equip surgeons with the combined skills of oncological and reconstructive techniques would be an excellent development.

Future Perspectives

The future of breast reconstruction may be associated with new technologies and advances in regenerative medicine. With the studies on fat grafting and its regenerative potential mediated by stem cells, we will soon be able to reconstruct an entire breast with only fat. The development of three-dimensional (3D) printing and tissue engineering is also promising for plastic surgeons. New implant materials, textures, and shapes may diminish the rate of capsular contracture and complications in implant-based reconstructions.

Virtual reality and 3D imaging for preoperative planning are already a reality in some breast centres. These technologies may be useful for patient education at the preoperative consultation. In the future, oncoplastic surgical techniques will become essential to the basic practice of versatile breast cancer surgeons, and all the women with breast cancer will have the opportunity to have reconstruction. In low- and middle-income countries, the breast surgeons are being trained in reconstructive surgeries and are offering this alternative for their patients.

The binomial of oncological safety and cosmesis is currently the regent for successful surgical treatment. Quality control in breast reconstruction is difficult to quantify, but great quality care lies in a multidisciplinary team, a well-trained surgeon, and an educated patient.

Key Messages

- All breast cancer patients must be informed about the possibility of having some type of reconstructive surgery.
- The reconstruction must be performed by a specialist with the required training, either plastic or oncoplastic.
- The decision for a breast reconstruction is personal and will be made based on the patient's perspective of her body image, sexuality, and self-esteem.
- Breast cancer patients considering breast reconstruction should know they have both a voice and a choice.
- The future of breast reconstruction will be associated with new technologies and advances in regenerative medicine.

References

1. Al-Ghazal SK et al. Comparison of psychological aspects and patient satisfaction following breast conserving surgery, simple mastectomy and breast reconstruction. *Eur J Cancer* 2000;36(15):1938–1943.
2. Veronesi U et al. Twenty-year follow-up of a randomized study comparing breast-conserving surgery with radical mastectomy for early breast cancer. *N Engl J Med* 2002;347(16):1227–1232.
3. Reuben BC et al. Recent trends and predictors in immediate breast reconstruction after mastectomy in the United States. *Am J Surg* 2009;198:237–243.
4. Alderman AK et al. Use of breast reconstruction after mastectomy following the Women's Health and Cancer Rights Act. *JAMA* 2006;295:387–388.
5. Caldon LJM et al. Clinicians' concerns about decision support interventions for patients facing breast cancer surgery options: understanding the challenge of implementing shared decision-making. *Health Expect* 2010;14:133–146.

6. Zhong T et al. A comparison of psychological response, body image, sexuality, and quality of life between immediate and delayed autologous tissue breast reconstruction: a prospective long-term outcome study. *Plast Reconstr Surg* 2016;138:772.

7. Albornoz CR et al. A paradigm shift in U.S. Breast reconstruction: increasing implant rates. *Plast Reconstr Surg* 2013;131:15.

8. Munhoz AM et al. Clinical outcomes following nipple-areola-sparing mastectomy with immediate implant-based breast reconstruction: a 12-year experience with an analysis of patient and breast-related factors for complications. *Breast Cancer Res Treat* 2013;140:545–555.

9. Olson J et al. Nipple sparing mastectomy in patients with prior breast scars: is it safe? *Ann Plast Surg* 2017;77:22–27.

10. Yueh JH et al. Patient satisfaction in postmastectomy breast reconstruction: a comparative evaluation of DIEP, TRAM, latissimus flap, and implant techniques. *Plast Reconstr Surg* 2010;125:1585–1595.

11. Recht A et al. Postmastectomy radiotherapy. Clinical practice guidelines of the American Society of Clinical Oncology. *J Clin Oncol* 2001;19(5):1539–1569.

12. Vandeweyer E and Deraemaecker R. Radiation therapy after immediate breast reconstruction with implants. *Plast Reconstr Surg* 2000:106(1):56–58.

13. Gryskiewicz J and LeDuc R. Transaxillary nonendoscopic subpectoral augmentation mammaplasty: a 10-year experience with gel vs saline in 2000 patients—with long-term patient satisfaction measured by the BREAST-Q. *Aesthetic Surg J* 2014;34(5):696–713.

14. Berrino P et al. Postquadrantectomy breast deformities: classification and techniques of surgical correction. Plastic Reconstr Surg 1987;79(4):567–572.

15. Clough K et al. Improving breast cancer surgery: a classification and quadrant per quadrant atlas for oncoplastic surgery. *Ann Surg Oncol* 2010;17(5):1375–1391.

16. Rigotti G et al. Clinical treatment of radiotherapy tissue damage by lipoaspirate transplant: a healing process mediated by adipose-derived adult stem cells. *Plast Reconstr Surg* 2007;119:1409–1422; discussion 1423–1404.

17. Agency for Healthcare Research and Quality. Available from: https://www.ahrq.gov/

15

Radiation Therapy

Philip Poortmans, Marion Essers, Sandra Hol, Lawrence B. Marks,
and Orit Kaidar-Person

Introduction

Radiation therapy (RT) is a cornerstone of treatment in the post-lumpectomy breast and post-mastectomy settings. Over the last few decades, there have been several advances in clinical areas (e.g. more accurate patient selection based on tumour- and patient-related characteristics and more accurate treatment volume delineation) as well as in the field of technology (e.g. treatment planning and delivery). More recently, biological factors are entering clinical practice. Using evidence-based estimates from the literature, the number of patients receiving RT for breast cancer is expected to increase in Europe by approximately 16% from 2012 to 2025 (1).

Postoperative RT is applied to reduce the probability of local–regional recurrences of breast cancer following surgery. The Early Breast Cancer Trialists' Collaborative Group (EBCTCG) meta-analyses of prospective randomized trials demonstrated that postoperative RT improves local control, disease-free survival, and overall survival for patients with early stage breast cancer in the case of lymph node involvement and/or in the framework of breast-conserving therapy (2,3). In view of the impressive improvement of the outcome after diagnosis and treatment that has been obtained over the last decades, current research also focuses on de-escalation of treatments for low-risk patients (4).

RT reduces the risk of all types of recurrence, and the greatest effect is observed for local and regional control. While the risk for distant metastases is also reduced, the competing risks for recurrences outside of the irradiated volumes limit the impact that local RT can have on overall survival. With the increasing use and effectiveness of adjuvant systemic therapy, the potential for improvements in local–regional control to improve overall survival might increase (5).

Side-effects of treatments, related to comorbidity and age-related disease conditions, have a well-demonstrated influence on patient outcomes. Their reported rates are confounded by insufficient standardized reporting and the interaction with surgery and systemic treatments. In early stage, low-risk, node-negative breast cancer patients, this may, for example, lead to a possible choice between radiation or endocrine therapy based on the risk for side-effects rather than based on the expected efficacy. Therefore, in all circumstances, the full range of factors that contribute to the risks related to tumour progression as well as to the occurrence of side-effects should be individually discussed with every patient. The personal scope of the patient, including her

Box 15.1 The proper sequence for treatment preparation highlights that the technique itself is a tool to fulfil pre-set requirements

Defining the indication for radiation therapy
Defining the target volumes
Prescribing the dose
Setting the dose objectives for the target volumes and the dose constraints for the
    organs at risk
Target and organ at risk volume delineation
Treatment planning

expectations for her future life, should be considered as possible decisive factors in this shared decision-making process.

To de-escalate the use of RT, a critical appraisal is required not just of patient selection, but even more importantly for target volume selection, target volume size, and dose (5) (Box 15.1). While a boost to the primary tumour bed can be indicated for patients with a high risk of local recurrence, accelerated partial breast irradiation might be offered to low-risk patients as an attractive low-burden treatment approach. With the decreasing surgical approach towards the axillary lymph nodes, combined with the encouraging results from the recent regional nodal RT trials, de-escalation of the total treatment includes a selective substitution of surgery by RT to the lymph node regions.

Minimal and Optimal Requirements

In general, patients with cancer, and notably patients with breast cancer, often have several treatment options and need to be evaluated by a multidisciplinary team before final treatment recommendations are made. Treatment recommendations should take into consideration patient-related factors (e.g. age and comorbidities), disease-related factors (e.g. pathology features and stage), and the patient's own preferences (6). RT, being an integral part of the treatment of most non-metastatic breast cancer patients and contributing to the management in the metastatic setting (e.g. palliation, pain relief), requires a broad understanding by the entire breast team on the indications for RT for breast cancer patients.

Technological advances, such as patient imaging set-up and correction before and during treatment, immobilization, target volume definition, improved treatment plans, and respiratory control during treatment have led to more accurate treatment planning and techniques to deliver therapeutic radiation doses more precisely to the target tissues while reducing the doses (and subsequent risks) to the surrounding normal tissues, and thereby improving the therapeutic ratio of RT. Similarly, progress in our understanding of the optimization of radiation fractionation regimens and target volumes definition have reduced the treatment burden for breast cancer patients, for example, by shortening radiation courses and introducing partial breast irradiation (PBI). However, many of these advances tend to *increase* the complexity of treatment and thus might increase the risk of an error (7). Consequently, a comprehensive understanding of the utility and hazards of these advances and an open, collaborative relationship between the members of the multidisciplinary radiation oncology team (i.e. radiation oncologist, medical physicist, radiation therapist, technician, nurses, etc.) are required to ensure high treatment quality. All members of the radiation oncology team need to have appropriate training and support peer review, standardization, incident reporting, and ongoing quality assurance as a means to enhance the culture of safety and quality of care. These concepts are especially important as we embrace new technologies (8).

Equipment, Personnel, and Patient Load

Cancer is a growing global problem and is not restricted to high-income countries. Therefore, there are several ongoing global initiatives to assure treatment availability

Table 15.1 Requirements for infrastructure, staffing, and workload, as defined by the Radiation Oncology Group of the European Organisation for Research and Treatment of Cancer

	Before 2009	Since 2009
Human resources: workload		
FTE radiation oncologists per department	Minimum 2.5	Minimum 3
Patients treated per year/FTE radiation oncologist	Maximum 300	Maximum 250
FTE qualified radiation physicists per department	Minimum 1.3	Minimum 2
Patients treated per year/FTE radiation physicist	Maximum 500	Maximum 500
Radiation technologists per treatment unit	Minimum 2	Minimum 2
Equipment: numbers		
Simulator (classical and/or CT scanner)	Minimum 1	Minimum 1[a]
Megavoltage treatment units[b]	Minimum 2	Minimum 2
Equipment: workload[c]		
Patients per year/megavoltage unit	Maximum 700	Maximum 600
Patients per year/conventional simulator	Maximum 1500	Maximum 1200
Patients per year/CT simulator	–	Maximum 2400

CT, computed tomography; FTE, full-time equivalent.
[a]Including access to a CT scanner.
[b]Preferably aged <10 years.
[c]Based on normal working hours.

Reproduced with permission from Budiharto T et al. 'Profile of European radiotherapy departments contributing to the EORTC Radiation Oncology Group (ROG) in the 21st century'. *Radiotherapy and Oncology.* Volume 88, Issue 3, pp. 403–10. Copyright © 2008 Elsevier Ireland Ltd. DOI: 10.1016/j.radonc.2008.05.013 (10).

and quality, and these include task forces specialized for breast cancer. The Global Task Force on Radiation Therapy for Cancer Control (GTFRCC) defined the role of, and the global needs for, RT (9). Several countries and study groups defined minimum criteria for the infrastructure and staffing of a radiation oncology department as well as their participation in clinical studies (10,11) (Table 15.1).

The needs for RT in Europe are estimated to rise over a decade by 16% with a variation of less than 5% to more than 30% among European countries. The expected relative increase by 2025 for breast cancer is 10% (12).

The optimal timing of RT after surgery has not been well defined, but there is a fair amount of data to guide us. Clinical trials that reported the benefit of postoperative radiation after breast-conserving surgery typically restricted the maximum interval between surgery and the start of RT to 6–8 weeks. Although there is not much data about the minimum acceptable time from surgery to the beginning of external beam radiation, 3–4 weeks following surgery to initiate RT should allow for adequate healing of the breast and axillary area and for the patient to have adequate arm mobility to facilitate treatment planning. A further reduction seems feasible in view of the decreasing use of axillary surgery and as demonstrated to be feasible by the intraoperative (partial breast) irradiation studies.

Best Practice

General

The mortality:incidence ratio of breast cancer decreased from 1:2.5 in the 1970s to 1:6 more than three decades later (13). This can be attributed to a combination of earlier (and perhaps increased) diagnoses and improved treatment. Therefore, we have to re-think some of the conventional treatment paradigms and to consider the interaction between local–regional and systemic treatments. In low-risk patients with a very good outcome after one of the treatment options, parameters such as side-effects and quality of life should be used to assist the patient in making an individualized treatment choice. By contrast, high-risk patients will benefit most from a positive interaction between both treatment modalities by individualizing their combination. Thanks to advances in both our knowledge of the biology of breast cancer and RT techniques, the occurrence and the severity of late side-effects have been sharply reduced. Many factors, several of which might be modulated, may influence RT-induced morbidity.

Radiation Therapy Fractionation Schedules

Various fractionation schedules have been used for whole breast irradiation in randomized clinical trials, ranging from a total of 40 Gy in 16 daily fractions to 54 Gy in 30 daily fractions (with or without a boost to the tumour bed). A very common conventional fractionation schedule used for whole breast is 50 Gy in 25 fractions.

Several randomized trials evaluated shorter courses of radiation (hypofractionation) of 15 or 16 fractions of 2.66 or 2.67 Gy in 3 weeks, mainly in patients undergoing breast-conserving surgery (without nodal RT) (14). These studies report similar disease control rates compared to conventional fractionation at a follow-up of around 10 years. No significant differences regarding toxicities such as cardiac disease were noted, while cosmesis was even better for the hypofractionation protocols compared to conventional fractionation in the START A/B trials. A tumour bed boost was not consistently used in these clinical trials. Further reduction of the treatment duration was tested in the FAST randomized trial, which compared two hypofractionation schemes (28.5 Gy in five fractions and 30 Gy in five fractions, both over 5 weeks) versus a conventional regimen (50 Gy in 25 fractions over 5 weeks) for node-negative patients aged >50 years with tumours <3 cm. At a median follow-up of 3 years, the 28.5 Gy schedule was equivalent to the conventional fractionation regarding breast appearance, while acute skin toxicity (during radiation) grade >2 (using RTOG toxicity scale) occurred more often in the conventional fractionation group compared to the hypofractionation group (15). Subsequently, the FAST-FORWARD trial, which compared two schemes of hypofractionated RT (27 Gy in five fractions and 26 Gy in five fractions over 1 week) versus 40 Gy in 15 fractions over 3 weeks, was launched. Acute skin reactions are mild with all three schedules used (16). After including more than 4000 patients, a sub-study of this trial recently started to evaluate the same fractionation schedules for axillary/periclavicular irradiation.

There is not much published data regarding hypofractionation to the chest wall, although some patients were included in the abovementioned trials (for example, 15% of the patients participating in the START A/B trials). No specific adverse effects were noted with radiation in the post-mastectomy group. None of the patients underwent breast reconstruction prior to irradiation.

Prospective data about hypofractionation for elective nodal irradiation is relatively scarce, though no studies have reported increased recurrence or complication rates compared to the standard fractionation.

Older RT techniques have resulted in relatively heterogeneous doses with 'hot spots', where the delivered dose exceeded the prescription dose (often by ≈15%). With the higher prescribed doses per fraction used with hypofractionation, the delivered doses to these areas of 'hot spots' could be even higher. Modern RT techniques are better able to deliver homogeneous doses, reduce the size/magnitude of 'hot spots' of higher doses, and are thus likely increase the safety of hypofractionation. Therefore, hypofractionated schedules are being increasingly adapted for broader indications and target volumes (4).

Total Dose

Since most local recurrences occur in the same quadrant of the primary tumour, the concept of a 'boost' dose to that region after whole breast irradiation was introduced. Several trials evaluated the role of the boost delivery and demonstrated that it reduces the risk of local recurrences by about 40% at long-term follow-up (17). However, no improvement in overall survival was seen, and cosmetic outcomes are worse after boost delivery. As the absolute rates of local–regional recurrences decline (likely following better diagnostic tools, patient selection, systemic therapies, surgery, and RT), the role of the boost dose also declines, but it remains clinically relevant especially for high-risk patients (4).

Partial Breast Irradiation

Partial breast irradiation has been introduced as an alternative treatment to conventional whole breast radiation in selected patients with early stage low-risk breast cancer. A major advantage of PBI is the shorter treatment time (as it usually implies an accelerated schedule) compared with the standard fractionation and less exposure of dose to normal tissues. The concept of PBI is supported by the observation that the majority of in-breast tumour recurrences following lumpectomy without whole breast irradiation occur at or near the initial tumour bed. The RT techniques used to deliver PBI include interstitial brachytherapy (e.g. via multiple interstitial catheters), intracavitary brachytherapy (e.g. via a single or multi-catheter balloon placed inside the lumpectomy cavity), intraoperative radiation (e.g. via megavoltage electrons or low-energy photons), and external beam radiotherapy (e.g. via electrons or photons). Typical regimens include the delivery of 34.5–38.5 Gy in 10 fractions or 30 Gy in five daily fractions, both in 1 week for fractionated schedules and 20–21 Gy in one fraction for intraoperative treatments.

Most studies evaluating the role of PBI in low-risk breast cancer patients reported good local control rates of 1–1.5% at 5 years for well-selected patients, and these are similar to local control rates following whole breast irradiation (18). However, many of these studies had relatively short follow-up for favourable breast cancer patients, considering that most patients also receive adjuvant endocrine therapy.

Cosmetic results after PBI vary from one study to another, and this points to the importance of details regarding techniques and doses for partial breast irradiation. Possible explanations for this variation are that the volume of the breast receiving a significant proportion of the prescribed dose should be more restricted and that the twice-daily schedule does not allow for complete inter-fraction recovery (thereby increasing the relative biological effect). In the Florence study, which used a once-a-day fractionation schedule for PBI and limited the dose to the non-target parts of the breast, cosmetic results were very favourable (18). Outside of clinical trials, patients who fulfil ESTRO and ASTRO recommendations for PBI (19) could be offered this time-sparing approach.

Simultaneous Integrated Boost

New radiation treatment planning and delivery techniques allow for dose painting as a means to deliver higher radiation doses to the tumour bed concurrently with whole breast irradiation (i.e. not subsequent to whole breast irradiation as is conventionally done and as was done in the major boost trials). Such a 'concurrent boost', introduced in the framework of a clinical trial around 2005, offers dosimetric as well as overall treatment duration advantages (4). While preliminary results are encouraging, and there is broad introduction in some regions, additional prospective data (e.g. RTOG 1005) might also be awaited.

Proton Radiation Therapy

Photon beams (i.e. X-rays) deposit dose throughout their entire path through the patient (i.e. upstream and downstream from the target). Conversely, proton beams deliver dose in a more defined range of depths (i.e. only upstream of the target, and there is essentially no 'exit' dose). Tissues at specific depths are targeted by careful selection of the proton beam energy, and of specific target thicknesses treated by varying that energy (i.e. 'spreading out the Bragg peak'). Theoretically, there are potential advantages for proton beam over conventional photons for many tumour sites, including breast. However, there has been only limited study of proton beam therapy in patients with breast cancer. Further, proton therapy is not widely available, and it is associated with expensive infrastructure and operating costs. In addition, since the uncertainties with protons are generally larger than with photons, it is possible that they may even result in worse outcomes. Therefore, proton beam treatment should currently be reserved for limited and well-defined indications (e.g. very challenging geometry and resultant clear cardiac risks as well as, possibly, re-treatments. There are several technical and clinical issues that need to be better addressed before this approach should become routinely applied for patients with breast cancer (20).

A Glimpse at the Future for Radiation Therapy in Breast Cancer

RT has evolved into a very effective, and increasingly less toxic, modality. Additional expected advances include the following:

- Multidisciplinary patient- and tumour-based selection of an individualized combination of local and systemic treatments including the sequence and the extent.
- Individualized risk-adapted target volume selection: whole breast or partial breast; which part of the regional lymph nodes; boost to the primary tumour bed or to other high-risk zones.
- Individualized anatomy-based target volume delineation.
- Delineation of organs at risk based on international standards and on actual risks for side-effects.
- Improvements in individualized treatment-planning procedures based on dose objectives for target volumes and dose constraints for organs at risk.

- Further alterations in fractionation schemes including fraction size as well as risk-based dose adaptation.
- Generalization of improved patient positioning including respiratory control such as gating and breath hold.
- Improvements in set-up verification during treatment delivery and leading, also, to adaptive treatment strategies.
- Registration of treatment outcome for all treated patients and analysis of this 'big data'.
- Personalizing the delivered total dose based on assessments of tumour and normal tissue responses defined on tissue samples obtained before or during the early phase of RT.

Key Messages

- The radiation oncologist should actively contribute as a member of the multidisciplinary team evaluating/treating breast cancer patients from the initial phase of the diagnostic–therapeutic pathway.
- Postoperative RT decreases local–regional recurrence in the post-lumpectomy or post-mastectomy settings by 75–85%; patients at a higher risk for local recurrences experience a greater absolute benefit.
- Postoperative RT in the post-lumpectomy or post-mastectomy settings can decrease any/all-site recurrences, and breast cancer-related and overall mortality.
- Generally, postoperative RT is recommended in the post-lumpectomy setting for axillary node-negative and node-positive patients to decrease local recurrence, breast cancer-related mortality, and overall mortality.
- Generally, postoperative RT is recommended in the post-mastectomy setting for axillary node-positive patients to decrease local–regional recurrence, breast cancer-related mortality, and overall mortality.
- Modern RT starts with careful consideration of treatment positioning/immobilization, target volume delineation and treatment volume-based prescription. The available treatment techniques serve the goal of optimizing dose distributions, but its use is not an objective by itself (Figure 15.1).
- Patients treated in trials starting in the 1990s and later generally have no increased treatment-related mortality at 10 years. With contemporary radiation techniques, short- and long-term side-effects are expected to be further reduced.
- The interaction between local–regional and systemic treatments is complex. Most of the benefit of RT on survival is expected for low-risk patients, who do not receive systemic therapy, and high-risk patients, who receive effective systemic therapy. As the efficacy of systemic therapies increases, the ability of local–regional therapy to improve survival may *increase*.

- Lowering the burden of RT can be done via reducing the total dose, the number of fractions, and/or the size of the target volumes.
- While RT might be omitted for low-risk patients receiving endocrine therapy, the administration of 3 weeks of radiation instead of several years of endocrine therapy should be evaluated in a prospective clinical trial.
- Decreasing the extent of surgical treatment to the axilla in node-positive patients suggests that 'less therapy' could be adequate for the axilla. However, recent studies suggest that regional nodal irradiation may improve outcomes, so reductions in planned nodal therapy should be done carefully.

References

1. Borras JM et al. How many new cancer patients in Europe will require radiotherapy by 2025? An ESTRO-HERO analysis. *Radiother Oncol* 2016;119(1):5–11.
2. Darby S et al. Effect of radiotherapy after breast-conserving surgery on 10-year recurrence and 15-year breast cancer death: meta-analysis of individual patient data for 10,801 women in 17 randomised trials. *Lancet* 2011;378(9804):1707–1716.
3. McGale P et al. Effect of radiotherapy after mastectomy and axillary surgery on 10-year recurrence and 20-year breast cancer mortality: meta-analysis of individual patient data for 8135 women in 22 randomised trials. *Lancet* 2014;383(9935):2127–2135.
4. Poortmans P et al. Over-irradiation. *Breast* 2017;31:295–302.
5. Poortmans P. Postmastectomy radiation in breast cancer with one to three involved lymph nodes: ending the debate. *Lancet* 2014;383(9935):2104–2106.
6. Del Turco MR et al. Quality indicators in breast cancer care. *Eur J Cancer* 2010;46(13):2344–2356.
7. Malicki J et al. Patient safety in external beam radiotherapy—guidelines on risk assessment and analysis of adverse error-events and near misses: introducing the ACCIRAD project. *Radiother Oncol* 2014;112(2):194–198.
8. Marks LB et al. The challenge of maximizing safety in radiation oncology. *Pract Radiat Oncol* 2011;1(1):2–14.
9. Atun R et al. Expanding global access to radiotherapy. *Lancet Oncol* 2015;16(10):1153–1186.
10. Budiharto T et al. Profile of European radiotherapy departments contributing to the EORTC Radiation Oncology Group (ROG) in the 21st century. *Radiother Oncol* 2008;88(3):403–410.
11. Dunscombe P et al. Guidelines for equipment and staffing of radiotherapy facilities in the European countries: final results of the ESTRO-HERO survey. *Radiother Oncol* 2014;112(2):165–177.
12. Defourny N et al. Cost evaluations of radiotherapy: what do we know? An ESTRO-HERO analysis. *Radiother Oncol* 2016;121(3):468–474.
13. GLOBOCAN 2008: Cancer incidence and mortality worldwide. Available from: https://www.iarc.fr/en/media-centre/iarcnews/2010/globocan2008.php
14. Yarnold J. Changes in radiotherapy fractionation-breast cancer. *Br J Radiol* 2018:20170849 [Epub ahead of print].
15. Agrawal RK et al. First results of the randomised UK FAST Trial of radiotherapy hypofractionation for treatment of early breast cancer (CRUKE/04/015). *Radiother Oncol* 2011;100(1):93–100.
16. Brunt AM et al. Acute skin toxicity associated with a 1-week schedule of whole breast radiotherapy compared with a standard 3-week regimen delivered in the UK FAST-Forward Trial. *Radiother Oncol* 2016;120(1):114–118.
17. Bartelink H et al. Whole-breast irradiation with or without a boost for patients treated with breast-conserving surgery for early breast cancer: 20-year follow-up of a randomised phase 3 trial. *Lancet Oncol* 2015;16(1):47–56.

18. Livi L et al. Accelerated partial breast irradiation using intensity-modulated radiotherapy versus whole breast irradiation: 5-year survival analysis of a phase 3 randomised controlled trial. *Eur J Cancer* 2015;51(4):451–463.
19. Kirby AM. Updated ASTRO guidelines on accelerated partial breast irradiation (APBI): to whom can we offer APBI outside a clinical trial? *Br J Radiol* 2018;91(1085):20170565.
20. Mast ME et al. Whole breast proton irradiation for maximal reduction of heart dose in breast cancer patients. *Breast Cancer Res Treat* 2014;148(1):33–39.

16

Systemic Therapy

Didier Verhoeven, Etienne Brain, François P. Duhoux,
Gilberto Schwartsmann, and Fatima Cardoso

Introduction

Systemic breast cancer treatment is defined as the use of drugs that spread throughout the body such as is the case with cytotoxic chemotherapy, endocrine therapy, targeted therapy, and, more recently, immunotherapy. Evidence for the efficacy and safety of these treatments is obtained through clinical trials, which usually start at advanced stages of the disease. Limited literature is available concerning quality indicators in systemic treatment of breast cancer. Although population-level studies focusing on quality of care of systemic therapy are increasing, gaps remain, and further studies are warranted (1).

Before 2005, underuse of chemotherapy, non-evidence-based schedules, and variability in dose intensity were the most common findings. More recently, the American Society for Clinical Oncology publication, 'Choosing Wisely: top five cancer-related tests, procedures and treatments many patients do not need', stressed the overuse of chemotherapy and overburdening of society with unnecessary costs (http://www.choosingwisely.org).

Increasing attention is being paid to the reporting of patient outcomes in a standardized way. By involving physician leaders, outcome researchers, and patient advocates, standard sets of health outcomes for breast cancer have recently been defined (see Chapter 6).

The average age of breast cancer diagnosis is 63 years, and this highlights the marked increase of breast cancer incidence with age. Most people dying of breast cancer are aged >65 years. This stands in sharp contrast with just 9% of patients included in clinical trials aged ≥65 years. The lack of evidence of the advantage of systemic treatment in many older patients makes a geriatric assessment increasingly necessary to fine-tune and adjust the strategy to the health status.

For each breast cancer patient, a multidisciplinary specialized team with a lead oncology specialist responsible for coordinating treatment modalities must be present. Depending on the stage of the disease and local organization, this will usually be either the breast surgeon or the medical oncologist.

A Canadian study analysed the quality improvement priorities for women receiving systemic therapy for early breast cancer. It identified computerized electronic order entry for chemotherapy, emergency room visits or hospitalizations during chemotherapy, and timely receipt of the treatment as the quality measures with the largest potential for improvement (2).

Five indicators of systemic treatment have been identified by the European Society of Breast Cancer Specialists (EUSOMA) (see Chapter 4). These indicators were all identified by expert opinions. Quality indicators must be reliable, relevant, interpretable, actionable, and measurable (see Chapter 3).

In the US, the Quality Oncology Practice Initiative published its quality measures in 2013 (3). In China, a set of quality indicators on systemic treatment was developed by Han Bao using the existing US indicators (4). These indicators must enhance patient-centred decisions, supply information to providers and institutions driving transparency and improvement, and make comparative research possible.

Defining Quality Indicators of Systemic Treatment

Structure Indicators

Education: A Global Curriculum
The best way to improve the use of systemic treatment for breast cancer is by promoting medical and clinical oncology in as many countries as possible. Adherence to the European Society of Medical Oncology (ESMO)/ASCO Global Curriculum in Medical Oncology ensures that patients have an equal chance of receiving treatment by well-trained physicians, respecting a multidisciplinary approach, wherever they live. The fundamental pillar is 5 years of training with a minimum 2 years of internal medicine and 2 years of medical oncology (see Chapter 8). In developing countries, in the absence of a medical oncologist, systemic treatment could be given by other specialists with at least one year of training in systemic treatment. Even so, every effort must be made to train medical oncologists. A separate chapter was included in the global curriculum to understand the challenges of cancer delivery in low-resource environments. The ability to discuss the World Health Organization (WHO) Essential Medicine List for Cancer and familiarity with the concept of resource-stratified treatment guidelines must be obtained. Medical oncologists must be able to coordinate all aspects of the use of multi-modal drug treatment. They must have an in-depth understanding of the prognostic and predictive clinical and molecular factors contributing to the best treatment. They must be able to perform specialist assessment, treatment, and counselling including genetics, prevention, early detection, and screening without forgetting the need for referrals to highly specific supportive carers beyond the first level of such treatments.

Day Clinic Facilities
Delivery of chemotherapy continues to shift from the inpatient setting to ambulatory day services. Rapid access to treatment in a separate oncology unit or department of service dedicated to the administration of systemic treatment for cancer patients is required. Availability of trained oncology nurses and patient navigators is needed.

Staffing of chemotherapy nurses is a top priority for cancer centres, although no optimal standard nurse:patient ratio can be stated (see Chapter 19).

Dedicated Pharmacy Facilities

A close collaboration with dedicated pharmacy facilities must be present. The oncology pharmacy plays a critical role in discussing pharmaceutical treatment and supervising the preparation of oncology drugs. Experience in the interactions with other drugs and dose adjustments according to age, liver, and kidney functions is required. In Europe, they must comply with the European QuapoS guidelines (European Society of Oncology Pharmacy, http://ww.esop.eu). Cytostatic and other oncology drugs must be handled and prepared in a designated area which meets the criteria with which pharmacies must comply. It must take place under the supervision of an oncology pharmacist in accordance to the Ljubljana Declaration of 2006: 'The close cooperation between oncology physicians and oncology pharmacists is vital for optimal patient care. The multi-professional approach will deliver best practice to patients within a clinical governance framework. Professional, close, and timely collaboration will ensure economic use of resources and improve patient safety.' Recommendations for safe handling represent a reasonable and practical set of procedures that the intended users should implement to minimize opportunities for accidental exposure. They are not limited to just one point of care. They cover the entire chain of cytotoxic handling from the time such agents enter the institution until they leave and are delivered to the patient or disposed of as waste. They encompass personnel protective equipment, transport, storage, drug preparation, transport after preparation, drug administration, home care, management of waste, accidental exposure, spills management, and environmental cleaning (5). They also include checking that treatment use agrees with approved indications, especially for inpatient use, and this contributes to cost control.

Process Indicators (Box 16.1)

Access to Appropriate Advice by Experts in Systemic Treatment (with Timeline)

The time between the diagnosis of breast cancer and the start of treatment (surgery or systemic treatment) is very important for patients to ensure efficacy and avoid anxiety. The maximum amount of time between the patient's first appointment in the system and treatment start must be between 4 and 8 weeks.

A report of the treatment delivery to patients following local or national or international guidelines is key for quality control. Insight into treatment as well as schedule and the dose intensity administered is required. Ideally, a database is present in each breast centre. The percentage of the whole breast cancer population of the centre receiving chemotherapy, endocrine therapy, and antibodies (e.g. trastuzumab, pertuzumab, T-DM1) must be registered to give insights into the prescription pattern of the centre. In addition, this percentage must be obtained for the different subgroups: triple-negative patients, HER2-positive patients, and oestrogen receptor

Box 16.1 Ideas for identification of process quality indicators for systemic treatment (suggested by the authors, to be adapted according to local guidelines and registration possibilities)

Documented plan for systemic treatment/chemotherapy

1.1 Dose–route–time interval

1.2 Height–weight–body surface area

1.3 Availability of histological diagnosis, TNM classification with determination of grade, hormonal receptors status, HER2 status and a proliferation marker (Ki67) (before decision of systemic treatment)

1.4 Serotonin antagonist and corticosteroids with moderately and highly emetogenic chemotherapy

1.5 Staging: % PET-CT if stage I or II (negative indicator)

1.6 % patients (early and metastatic) discussed at the multidisciplinary tumour board

Signed informed consent

2.1 Discussing also fertility preservation with patients in reproductive age before starting therapy

2.2 Genetic counselling if increased risk of hereditary cancer

Wellbeing, quality of life

3.1 Assessed by second visit (adjuvant treatment)

3.2 % complications of chemotherapy resulting in hospitalization

3.3 % of patients dying in known location—hospice, hospital

3.4 % of patients administered chemotherapy in the last 2 weeks of life

3.5 % of device infections

3.6 % of patients returning to normal activity of daily living, one year after treatment

3.7 % of patients maintaining professional activity during treatment and after treatment

Receiving optimal therapy by patients aged <70 years, stage 1 (T1c) to 3, within 4 months of diagnosis and 1 year after diagnosis

4.1 % of chemotherapy: all the patients/and triple negative for breast cancer

4.2 % trastuzumab if HER2 positive/in general/and if T1a (last one is negative indicator)

4.3 % hormone therapy if ER or PgR positive within 1 year of diagnosis/and in general

4.4 % receiving at least 5 years of adjuvant endocrine therapy

4.5 % of patients receiving adjuvant chemo if T1a, ER+ and HER2– (negative indicator)

Geriatric patients (aged >70 years)

   5.1 % geriatric patients with geriatric screening

   5.2 % of geriatric patients (>75 years) with documented geriatric assessment (if screening is positive)

   5.3 % receiving adjuvant chemotherapy if ER+

   5.4 % receiving adjuvant chemotherapy if triple negative

   5.5 % of patients receiving trastuzumab in adjuvant setting without chemotherapy (negative indicator)

   5.6 In adjuvant setting, % of patients receiving the whole duration of treatment as planned

Optimal systemic treatment for metastatic patients

   6.1 % of ER+ patients whose first-line therapy is endocrine treatment (versus chemotherapy)

   6.2 % of single agent chemotherapy (versus combination)

   6.3 % of geriatric patients who need dose adjustment in the 3 months after start of chemotherapy and/or targeted treatments

   6.4 % intravenous bisphosphonate or denosumab for multiple bone metastases

Locally advanced and inflammatory breast cancer

   7.1 %patients who received multidisciplinary treatment with primary neo-adjuvant chemotherapy

(ER)-positive patients. Figure 16.1 shows, as an example, the administration of chemotherapy and endocrine treatment in Belgian hospitals. Although the administration of endocrine treatment seems equally distributed at around 80%, much more variation is seen for chemotherapy (6). Reimbursement modalities can change the use of treatments, but not always in a rational way (e.g. limitations of reimbursement to intravenous administration and not by oral use) and this may lead to overuse of certain modalities and underuse of others. This underscores the importance of obtaining a detailed picture of the use of ambulatory versus inpatient treatments according to their administration schedule, oral, subcutaneous, or intravenous.

Equity in Systemic Treatment

With respect to confounding factors such as race, income, and location, equity in systemic treatment must be recognized as an important aspect of quality. An analysis of breast cancer mortality in the USA based on SEER data has repeatedly shown important differences between Caucasian, African-American, Asian, and Hispanic patients, partly due to ethnic considerations, but also due to socioeconomic resources, barriers to care, and many other factors (7). Recently, a racial/ethnic disparity was identified in adjuvant endocrine therapy adherence explained by socioeconomic status and out-of-pocket medication costs (8).

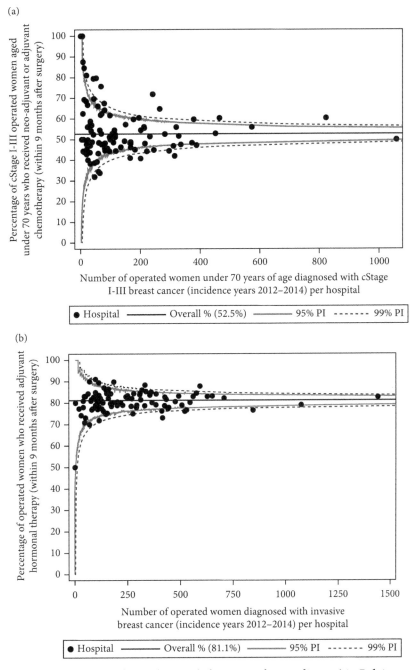

Figure 16.1 (a) Percentage chemotherapy (adjuvant and neo-adjuvant) in Belgian hospitals before or after surgery. (b) Percentage endocrine therapy.

Thanks to the support of VIP[2] (Vlaams Indicatoren Project voor Patiënten en Professionals—Flemish Region), AviQ (Agence pour une Vie de Qualité—Walloon Region) and COCOM (Common Community Commission—Brussels-Capital Region)

Outcome Indicators 'Fulfilling the Purpose'

Different ways of looking at the final results of our treatments are possible depending on the patients' and doctors' visions. Although overall survival remains the keystone, more attention is now placed on quality of life (QoL).

Overall Survival

Overall survival (OS) remains the reference standard as an endpoint in breast cancer trials. The level of evidence supporting a relationship between OS and potential surrogate endpoints is low. For early breast cancer, long-term follow-up up of at least 10 years is necessary, especially for the luminal-like subtype. Health-related quality of life (HRQoL) constitutes an alternative endpoint which ensures earlier assessment of direct clinical benefit for the patient (9). Crosslinking data from cancer registries with individuals in the broader population may help obtain survival data in a country, but this is subject to legal approval by national authorities, as is done in Belgium (Figure 16.2). Nevertheless, these data may be misleading, because of the problem with recognizing all influencing factors and the need for large numbers with a long follow-up.

Health-Related Quality of Life

Patient satisfaction surveys after treatment must include the percentage of reply to survey in order to be reliable. Patient-reported outcome measurements (PROMs)

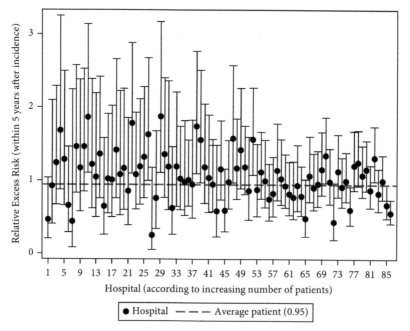

Figure 16.2 Relative excess risk of death in breast cancer patients as a function of the treating Belgian hospital (represented by a black dot; numbered according to increasing number of patients).

With permission of the Belgian Cancer Registry.

capture a patient's perception of their health (symptoms, anxiety, unmet need); patient-reported experience measurements (PREMs), capture a patient's perception of their experience with health care or services (integrated care, waiting times, communication, etc.) (see Chapter 6). Recent advances in technology provide possibilities for collecting PROMs and PREMs electronically using simple, but to the point, questionnaires. This could play a major role in shared decision-making. Nevertheless, technological problems, reimbursement barriers, and standardization have prevented, thus far, the wide use of these methods. Although maintaining a good QoL may be more important in the metastatic setting due to the poor median survival which remains at 2–3 years, with some exceptions in cases of HER2+ or some HR+ cancers, HRQoL assessment has been better studied in early stages. Specific measurements were developed by various research groups, such as the European Organisation for Research and Treatment of Cancer QLQ C-30 scale (http://www.eortc.org/tools). This questionnaire consists of multi-item and single scales. It includes functional scales (physical, emotional, social, and cognitive), symptom scales (fatigue, nausea, and pain), global health status and other items (dyspnoea, insomnia, appetite, constipation, diarrhoea, and financial items). This tool is currently being updated to become a questionnaire of 45 items (BR45). Other QoL scales are available, such as the WHO Quality of Life (WHOQOL-100), developed by the WHOQOL Group with 15 international field centres, aiming to be applicable cross-culturally. No specific tools for QoL measurements in the metastatic setting exist, and this leads to very limited evaluation of the impact on QoL for many interventions. Care should be oriented not only to physical, but also to functional, social, psychological, and spiritual domains. Also, few quality measurements for end-of-life care are available. All patients with advanced breast cancer should receive dedicated palliative care services early enough in the disease course, i.e. concurrent with active treatment, in order not to be implemented too late and, thereby leading to feelings of abandonment and loss. An optimal collaboration with interdisciplinary palliative care services must be established. Palliative care means patient- and family-centred care that optimizes QoL by anticipating, preventing, and treating suffering. Of note, such a policy will also cause a reduction in direct breast cancer costs (10) (see Chapter 18).

Safety

Chemotherapy administration is a highly error-prone process. The number of systemic treatments is rising. Most cytotoxic drugs have a narrow therapeutic range, and dose adjustments are often needed. Medication delivery is a multi-step process, and each step is a potential source of error. Recent studies have shown about 3–10% of potentially harmful errors, even with the use of a computerized physician order entry system. To build a system that prevents errors, the following measures can be taken (11):

- recognize that mistakes occur and review them for education;
- create a culture of preventing errors with co-workers;
- maintain accurate orders of chemotherapy and systemic treatment;
- continual staff training;

- identification of patients;
- focus on pharmacy concerns.

In 2015, the American Society of Health-System Pharmacists (ASHP; http://www.ashp.org) defined guidelines on preventing medication errors with chemotherapy and biotherapy (12).

Many errors are due to high patient load and inattention of the prescribers to omissions in prescription:

- incorrect dose;
- abbreviations;
- incorrect instructions;
- incorrect drug;
- no signatures.

Toxicity

Patients receiving treatment for cancer may experience many side-effects, and clinicians should be aware of these. Many problems are due to inappropriate use of medication. Future challenges are identifying the appropriate dosing of cytotoxic agents to maximize therapeutic efficacy while limiting both acute and long-term side-effects. Some important toxicities to monitor are listed below.

- Infection of an intravascular device.
- Hospitalization due to acute toxicity of treatment.
- Long-term toxicities in survivors (e.g. leukaemia after anthracycline use, cardiac failure after trastuzumab, neuropathy after taxanes).

Minimal and Ideal Requirements

WHO Essential Medicines List (EML)

Global drug spending grew by about 9% in 2015, outpacing overall health expenditures and economic growth. Total spending was US$887 billion in 2010 and will be US$1430 in 2022 (http://www.statista.com). In the Netherlands, three recent recommendations called for transparency of pharmaceutical research cost, adequate public return, and public investment and testing of new business models (13). The model EML maintained by WHO plays a central role in global health policy. The 'drugs to be available' included in the EML are defined as follows: 'they satisfy the health care needs of the population' and 'they must be available at all times and at a price the community and the individual can afford'.

The WHO list of essential antineoplastic agents for breast cancer (March 2017) was (14):

- Supportive: ondansetron, metoclopramide, dexamethasone, filgrastim, zoledronic acid.

- Cytostatics: capecitabine, carboplatin, cyclophosphamide, docetaxel, doxorubicin, 5-fluorouracil, methotrexate, paclitaxel, vinorelbine.
- Endocrine treatment: aromatase inhibitors, leuprorelin, tamoxifen.
- Antibodies: trastuzumab.

Multidisciplinary Discussion

All decisions related to systemic therapy should be taken in a multidisciplinary meeting (MDM) or tumour board. Characteristics of the MDM are discussed in Chapter 10.

Guidelines

Guidelines are evidence-based statements to deliver high-quality care in early, locally advanced, and metastatic breast cancer. Many international and national organizations have defined 'their' guidelines for breast cancer: ESMO, ASCO, National Comprehensive Cancer Network (NCCN), National Institute for Health and Care Excellence (NICE), European School of Oncology (ESO)-ESMO ABC Consensus Guidelines, Sankt-Gallen Consensus Guidelines, etc. All these organizations claim that their guidelines are widely recognized, are free to consult, and that they should be used as the standard for clinical oncology by clinicians, and payers. Ideally, they are regularly updated with availability of 'proven' new treatments. They must be based on reliable statistics with clear endpoints. In case of conflicting results or multiple similar studies, meta-analyses are helpful, such as those published by the Early Breast Cancer Trialist Group (EBCTG). Pitfalls and usual biases are the unpublished data and a frequent lack of analysis of QoL. A regular discussion of the guidelines among the separate breast units for local implementation remains essential to reach the right appropriation. Constant efforts should be made to harmonize the different guidelines covering the same topics. A consensus meeting, such as the Sankt-Gallen Conference and the ESO-ESMO ABC Conference can help decision-making in cases where no clear guidelines are available (see Chapter 9).

Follow-up

A minimal follow-up, including regular medical consultations and (yearly) mammography, is recommended by most international guidelines. Who should be consulted, and how frequently, must be decided depending on the availability of nurse practitioners, primary care physicians, medical oncologists, or breast surgeons. No specific exams are required besides mammography and ultrasound of the breast, except if treatment is ongoing, or if monitoring and management of side-effects is necessary. Supportive and survivorship issues must be discussed. The dosing of tumour markers for the detection of relapse has no proven benefit. Special and first attention must be put on complaints, symptoms, and compliance to treatments, especially concerning endo-crine therapy (15). A regular bone densitometry is useful in case of aromatase inhib-ition. Follow-up is recommended up to 10 years in case of endocrine therapy and must address long-term QoL problems and after effects issues.

High-Value, Patient-Centred Care

The International Consortium for Health Outcomes Measurement (ICHOM) takes a unique approach to defining health care outcomes. First, they involve patients directly in the process, as the ones who experience health outcomes first-hand. Then, they bring together leading physicians from across the globe who specialize in treating breast cancer. These physicians hold diverse perspectives and are pioneers in their respective countries. Finally, the ICHOM team acts as a facilitator as physicians and patients dis-cuss, and agree upon, defining the outcomes that matter most to them (see Chapter 6).

A good example of patient-centred outcomes is 'number of days spent at home in the last 6 months of life' (16):

- 180 days minus all days spent in inpatient facilities (including hospice unit).

WHO Priority Medical Devices for Cancer Management of Systemic Treatment

Along with the EML, WHO has also defined an essential list of medical devices. For breast cancer patients, implantable medical devices and modalities to give intravenous perfusion are important (http://www.who.int/medical_devices).

Needs in Workforce

A systematic assessment of future human resources is needed, as is the determination of the actions required to meet those needs. There is an ongoing joint effort between WHO and ESMO to define workforce needs in Europe and worldwide. The 2017 WHO cancer resolution is a landmark document, because it calls for the implementation of national cancer plans, population-based cancer registries, a world cancer report, and a well-trained oncology workforce. ASCO has called for an increased use of non-physician practitioners, research in care delivery efficiency, and efforts to recruit new oncologists. Physicians dedicating up to 25% of their time to non-direct patient care activities decreases specialists' availability and adds to dissatisfaction and burnout (17).

Best Practice

Tailored Therapy

Tailored therapy has become a term popularly used (and misused) with respect to cancer therapy. Tailor-made therapy should not be confused with implementing simple prognostic or predictive factors. In general, the latter do not define direct biological targets, but rather biological parameters revealing a variable statistical correlation to outcome. The definition of tailored therapy should include targeted therapies based on identification of individual therapeutic targets. Starting out as a non-selective therapy a century ago and following the identification of oestrogen receptor (ER) as a predictive marker, endocrine therapy in breast cancer has been the ultimate targeted, or tailored, cancer therapy since the 1970s. More recently, therapies targeting HER2 have revolutionized treatment for tumours overexpressing HER2 and accounting for nearly one-fifth of all breast cancer tumours. With the introduction of the poly ADP ribose polymerase (PARP) inhibitors, we are now in the process of tailoring treatment for patients carrying BRCA1- and BRCA2-defective tumours. Although much more research in this area is warranted, the results achieved up to now suggest a tailored therapy for most breast cancer patients in need of systemic treatment based on three major molecular groups (luminal, HER2+, and triple negative).

Patient Selection

In theory, a similar discussion should also be applied to anticancer and 'less targeted' strategies, in general, including options such as cytotoxic therapy. On the one hand, parameters such as tumour size, lymph nodes involved, the histological grade, Ki67 expression, as well as gene expression profiles provide moderate statistical correlates to outcome, but they do not define accurate biological targets. They approach, mostly, proliferation (proxy for chemosensitivity) and ER (proxy for endocrine sensitivity). Although recent studies showed the advantage of genomic testing, such as the 70-gene signature test (18), MamaPrint, OncotypeDx (19), or Prosigna, the economic situation of many countries currently makes online breast calculators a reasonable alternative. An estimation of women's survival odds at 10 years with or without taking endocrine or chemotherapy can be found at Oncotype DX http://www.oncotypeiq.com or by using the calculator called Predict (http://www.predict.nhs.uk).

Geriatric Oncology

Cancer incidence increases with age, but it is not a direct effect of age. Rather, the increase in life expectancy gives time for oncogenesis to develop. Ageing also favours both specific sensitivity to carcinogenic factors and decrease of cellular mechanisms controlling homeostasis, especially immune and endocrine functions. Breast cancer is not an exception to the rule. Its incidence peaks currently at age 65 years, and more than 60% of patients will soon be diagnosed after age 70 years according to the projections for the next two decades. Several studies have shown that management of breast cancer in elderly patients does not always reach high-quality standard. Over- and undertreatments are indeed very common and reflect enthusiasm for futile or 'at risk' treatments (often found in oncology) and ageism, respectively. The key points are the competing causes for mortality exerted by multimorbidities, which increase by incidence and severity with age and make non-breast cancer causes of mortality prominent as well as the risk of side-effects. Therefore, the main challenge is to prioritize health problems and adjust strategies, which cannot be simply a copy of what has been developed and approved in younger adults. Older patients are at higher risk of side-effects, especially for treatments with narrow benefit:risk ratio such as chemotherapy. If this can derive sometimes from pharmacokinetic alterations, it also may reflect the decline of many organ functions with no direct translation on pharmacokinetics, which then, incorrectly, appear safe.

The first non-opposable step is a screening for frailty through a short scale or questionnaire. Many tools exist, and debates regarding the selection of the best one are useless. One of the most popular and disseminated tools in Europe is the G8, developed after the Oncodage programme in France. It is built with eight items derived mostly from the MNA, added to some polypharmacy and self-rated health status assessments, and to an age stratum. It has a high sensitivity and specificity (77% and 64%, respectively) and requires 3 min to be completed by a physician or nurse. When impaired (G8 ≤ 14/17), a detailed geriatric assessment is recommended. Whenever possible, the screening tool should be followed by an estimation of life expectancy using a short-term (e.g. Carey, Walter) or a long-term (e.g. Lee, Schonberg) scale depending on the clinical setting (metastatic or adjuvant respectively) as found on the website: http://www.eprognosis.org.

When triggered by an impaired screening tool, geriatric assessment allows review of many different domains of interest (nutrition, cognition, depression, functional status, etc.). It allows stratification of the elderly population from a 'fit' group or Balducci 1 (close to the younger adult population) to an 'unfit' one or Balducci 3 (close to a group candidate for best supportive care). However, between these stands the most important group in numbers, often referred to as 'intermediate' or Balducci 2, encompassing very different situations of patients, vulnerable or frail, depending whether fragility is reversible or non-reversible.

Geriatric assessment may help predict and anticipate toxicity. Two major scores have been described for the use of chemotherapy (CRASH score and CARG score). Both of these accurately discriminate the risk of serious adverse events with standard chemotherapy regimen, when the usual performance status (Eastern Cooperative Oncology Group, WHO, or Karnofsky index) are unable to do so (20).

Most importantly, geriatric assessment allows identification of specific 'geriatric' defects that are 'targetable' by geriatric interventions in order to maximize the benefits of the selected anti-cancer treatment. Oriented geriatric interventions decided according to the geriatric assessment can then be extremely helpful to ensure access to the right care in safe and cost-conscious conditions. Indeed, as the molecular portrait of the tumour allows treatment personalization based on actionable targets, geriatric assessment allows treatment personalization based on a more holistic view of the patient.

This strategy is strongly advocated by the International Society of Geriatric Oncology as mentioned in its 10 priorities (21).

Value of Treatment

'Value and cost are among the biggest issues in healthcare today.' ESMO developed a clinical benefit scale (ESMO Magnitude of Clinical Benefit Scale) depending on the clinical setting due to the difference in calculating the clinical benefit in the curative versus non-curative setting (22). The highest weight is assigned to trials having adequate power for the relevant benefit, and an adjustment is made for the magnitude of benefit. The scale is based on the premise that cure takes precedent over deferral of death or progression, and that OS and QoL take precedence over surrogate endpoints such as disease-free survival, progression-free survival, or response rate.

For treatments with a curative intent, a survival improvement of more than 5% with at least 3 years of follow-up is taken into account. For treatments without curative intent, comparison is made between outcomes in OS or, if not available, in progression-free survival; the median outcome is also taken into consideration. In case of OS more than 12 months, a hazard ratio must be documented, for example, less than 0.7 with a relative gain of more than 5 months.

Very importantly, the scale is then adjusted according to QoL and toxicity and can be downgraded or upgraded by a value of 1.

ASCO has also published a framework for assessing the value of new cancer treatments based on clinical benefit, side-effects, and cost. The framework was constructed to enable comparisons of a new treatment with the prevailing standard of care. In the curative setting, a clinical benefit score is generated with points being awarded depending on the hazard ratio for death (OS) or disease-free survival if no OS score is reported. Balanced with a toxicity score, a 'net health benefit' score is calculated (23). The fourth step is to calculate the cost of the regimen and to wrap it up in a summary: clinical benefit–toxicity–net health benefit and cost.

These two tools allow regulators and administrations to prioritize reimbursements in settings with limited resources. Although both tools were recently updated, they display different results, and more harmonization is desirable.

Safety of Medication

Careful treatment of cancer is critical for patient safety. Anticancer drugs present a narrow therapeutic index with potentially lethal adverse events. A dedicated pharmacist must be present. Many studies have highlighted the benefit of computerized prescription in oncology. The electronic health record (EHR) can help the integration of the quality measurements in daily practice, reduce the time of implementation, and make the indicators more patient-centred. EHR systems could also be very helpful in low- and middle-income countries.

However, computerized prescription may lead to the emergence of new errors defined as e-iatrogenesis that can result in unintended consequences. Unfortunately, prescription software errors are more common than they should be, especially in a high-risk field such as oncology. Such errors, and their putative patient consequences, may occur following software upgrading. Thus, even if software publishers routinely realize regression tests for the new versions, recurring security alerts from health authorities remain necessary. Software upgrades should be performed as regularly as possible, and all software users should perform these control tests (24).

Clinical Trial Participation

The percentage of patients enrolled in clinical trials is sometimes considered as a quality indicator (EUSOMA) depending on the hospital environment. The accepted opinion in the oncological community is that patients are better off when treated within the context of a clinical trial.

Arguments in favour are improved access to innovative medication and adherence to state-of-the-art guidelines. One report showed that recurrence-free survival was significantly better in patients included in clinical trials. Clinical trials guarantee appropriate care with optimal endpoints, but there is little unbiased evidence of outcome improvement.

Possible reasons for better outcome are experimental treatment effects, participation effect, a prognostically favourable subset, the method of data gathering, publication bias, and the fact that these studies are mostly performed by motivated experts.

All breast centres must have the opportunity to collaborate in research. Not only early phase studies are needed. It is also interesting to evaluate long-term effects and the value of treatments in daily practice. In addition, the participation of all centres to cancer registries and the evaluation of 'big data' is extremely valuable. The ASCO Cancer LinQ initiative wants to learn from the 97% of NO research patients in order to enhance cancer diagnosis and treatment (http://www.cancerlinq.org). The aim is to empower the oncology community and improve quality of care and patients' outcomes through transformational data analytics (see Chapter 24).

Emerging Modalities

The paradigm for treating breast cancer has changed enormously over the last decade. Several targeted therapies, e.g. anti-HER2 agents and endocrine therapies, have greatly improved patient outcomes. A much more detailed understanding of the underlying biology that drives malignant progression and metastases has yielded other novel targets including PI3K/mTOR, CDK4/6, and PARP, which are currently being tested clinically. Omitting and de-escalation of chemotherapy has been proposed, and studies suggest that this may be possible in selected cases.

Developing a new funding model that drives consistent, equitable, and high-quality care for patients receiving systemic treatment with reimbursement not as a function of amounts of administered intravenous chemotherapy, but as a function of adequately treated patients (according to guidelines), and with similar reimbursement criteria for oral and intravenous drugs, endocrine, biologicals, and cytotoxic agents must be promoted.

The role of psycho-oncology and communication skills are evolving and considered crucial to help patients face their diagnosis and difficulties during therapy (see Chapter 20). More attention must go to teaching professionals how to speak with, and to listen to, their patients and their families, and to helping professionals cope with their own feelings.

Looking into the Future

In January 2015, US President Barack Obama launched the Precision Medicine Initiative, an effort to accelerate a new era of medicine focused on delivering more tailored health care. The initiative tries to develop better approaches to preventive and curative treatments. It will help patients gain access to their health information and consider each individual specifically. The aims are bringing new, effective technologies faster to the market, designing drugs tailored to a specific treatment, and building a large database of more than 1 million US volunteers.

Researchers have shown that genetic changes normally found through a biopsy can also be detected in a blood sample. Several types of these so-called 'liquid biopsies' are being evaluated, namely circulating tumour cells, circulating DNA or RNA, and exosomes. As a simple blood draw is much less invasive than a tissue biopsy, liquid biopsies may revolutionize treatment and outcome monitoring in the near future. Next generation sequencing will also likely become standard for breast cancer, making molecular tumour boards critical for interpretation.

A similar evolution is seen with the introduction of molecular and functional imaging. The accent is on the characterization of tumours and their underlying biology. Information about tumour response will be provided beyond anatomic measurements such as RECIST (Response Evaluation Criteria in Solid Tumours). Examples are dynamic contrast-enhanced magnetic resonance imaging, positron emission mammography, positron emission tomography–computed tomography with specific markers, for example, for ER and HER2.

The primary care workforce needs to be rethought with an expanded role for nurses and primary care physicians. The shortage of cancer experts is already causing major problems, mostly in developing countries, and is expected to worsen.

Creation of networks is needed to better organize treatments and the usage of the resources. Since the 1990s, the cancer networks model has been adopted widely as a best practice for organizing and delivering high-quality care for patients. Cancer networks have been developed across European countries, at the local or regional level, as well as at the international level for rare cancers. In Europe, the processes leading to the creation of service delivery networks typically implies a reconfiguration of healthcare services to a network-based perspective, but preserves the autonomy of the network participant organizations. Although some cancer networks have resulted from top-down mandated policy strategies (macro-strategy), most have derived from bottom-up agreements and inter-organizational board governance (meso-strategy). Much work is needed to make these constructions acceptable, especially financially, for all partners (25).

Finally, systemic treatment decisions must be taken even more during multidisciplinary meetings of the Breast Units.

Key Messages

- Overuse of systemic treatment can overburden patients with unnecessary toxicity and society with unnecessary costs.
- Structure indicators are education, day clinic, pharmacy facilities, and existence of specialized Breast Units.
- Uniform guidelines are necessary to identify reliable process indicators.
- PROMs and participation of patient advocates are necessary to increase patients' satisfaction and match better their expectations and concerns.
- Systemic treatment is a high-risk process with many potential side-effects.
- Long-term OS remains the reference standard outcome endpoint in breast cancer with QoL gaining substantial importance.
- WHO provides a list of minimal required cancer medicines for all patients worldwide.
- Geriatric assessment can provide personalized, high-quality care for older patients.
- Value-based, clinical benefit of systemic treatment and cost are among the biggest issues in breast cancer care today. ESMO Magnitude of Clinical Benefit Scale and ASCO Framework of Value are important and valuable tools.
- Precision medicine may provide the best care for every breast cancer patient in the future.

References

1. Shen S and Krzyzanowska MA. Decade of research on the quality of systemic cancer therapy in routine care: what aspects of Quality are we measuring? *J Oncol Pract* 2015;11(1):55–61.
2. Enright K et al. Setting quality improvement priorities for women receiving systemic therapy for early-stage breast cancer by using population-level administrative data. *J Clin Oncol* 2017;35:3207–3214.

3. McNiff MPH. The quality oncology practice initiative, American Society of Clinical Oncology. *J Oncol Pract* 2013;2(1):26–30.

4. Han Bao et al. Developing a set of quality indicators for breast cancer in China. *Int J Qual Health Care* 2015;27(4):291–296.

5. Easty AC et al. Safe handling of cytotoxics: guideline recommendations. *Curr Oncol* 2015;22(1):e27–e37.

6. Verhoeven D et al. Identification and calculation of quality indicators in systemic treatment in breast cancer. *Eur J Cancer* 2018;92 Suppl 3:S93.

7. Wheeler S et al. Disparities in breast cancer treatment and outcomes: biological, social and health system determinants and opportunities for research. *Oncologist* 2013;1:986–993.

8. Farias A and Xianglin L. Association between out-of-pocket costs, race/ethnicity and adjuvant endocrine therapy adherence among Medicare patients with breast cancer. *J Clin Oncol* 2017;35:86–95.

9. Basch E. Patient-reported outcomes—harnessing patients' voices to improve clinical care. *N Engl J Med* 2017;376:105–108.

10. Ferrel B et al. Integration of palliative care into standard oncology care: American Society of Clinical Oncology Practice Guideline Update. *J Clin Oncol* 2017;35:96–112.

11. International Society on Oncology Pharmacy Practitioners Standards Committee. ISOPP standards of practice. Safe handling of cytotoxics. *J Oncol Pharm Pract* 2007;13:1–81.

12. American Society of Health-System Pharmacists. ASHP Guidelines on preventing medication errors with chemotherapy and biotherapy. 2015. p. 231–256.

13. Moon S. Powerful ideas for global access to medicines. *N Engl J Med* 2017;376;6:505–507.

14. World Health Organization. WHO Model Lists of Essential Medicines. 2018. Available from: http://www.who.int/medicines/publications/essentialmedicines/en/

15. de Azambuja E et al. BSMO task force on breast cancer survivorship. *Belg J Med Oncol* 2013;7(5):142–155.

16. Groff A et al. Days spent at home: a patient-centered goal and outcome. *N Engl J Med* 2016;375:17.

17. Leon-Ferre RA and Stover DG. Supporting the future of the oncology workforce: ASCO medical student and trainee initiatives. *J Oncol Pract* 2018;14(5):277–280.

18. Cardoso F et al. 70-Gene signature as an aid to treatment decision in early-stage breast cancer. *N Engl J Med* 2016;375:717–729.

19. Sparano JA et al. Adjuvant chemotherapy guided by a 21-gene expression assay in breast cancer. *N Engl J Med* 2018;379:111–121.

20. Kim J and Hurria A. Determining chemotherapy tolerance in older patients with cancer. *J Natl Compr Can Netw* 2013;11(12):1493–1502.

21. Extermann M et al. Main priorities for the development of geriatric oncology. A worldwide expert perspective. J Geriatr Oncol 2011;2(4):270–273.

22. Cherny N et al. ESMO-Magnitude of Clinical Benefit scale version 1.1. *Ann Oncol* 2017;28:2340–2366.

23. Schnipper L et al. American Society of Clinical Oncology statement: a conceptual framework to assess the value of cancer treatment options. *J Clin Oncol* 2015;33:2563–2577.

24. Ministry of Health and Long-Term Care Ontario. *Quality-Based Procedures Clinical Handbook for Systemic Treatment*. March 2014.

25. Prades J et al. Managing cancer care through service delivery networks: the role of professional collaboration in two European cancer networks. *Health Serv Manag Res* 2018;31(3):120–129.

17

Primary Care Physicians

Inge Kriel, Geertruida H. de Bock, Sabine Siesling, and Annette J. Berendsen

Introduction

Worldwide, primary-care-driven systems are important for the promotion of good organized health care. In light of this importance, their increasing shortage, especially in low- and middle-income countries, is becoming a critical problem. Primary care physicians (PCPs) play an essential role in the care and management of patients with breast cancer in any setting, but their contribution is especially valuable in a developing country setting. The PCP is often the first medical practitioner involved in the process of breast cancer diagnosis. The cancer may be detected on a routine screening mammography, or the patient may seek the advice of her PCP for a self-detected irregularity in her breast. The PCP will then refer the patient to a radiologist, a breast surgeon, or a breast centre for further diagnosis and a definitive proposal for management. During the active management of the breast cancer, the patient will continue to see her PCP for acute illness, side-effects of treatment, psychological issues, and management of chronic underlying medical conditions such as hypertension, diabetes, COPD, and, in some countries, hypothyroidism.

Patients usually have a good rapport with their PCP. In many cases, this health care professional has a long history of managing the medical conditions of their patients' entire families. Consequently, patients can feel safe and comfortable with their PCP, and they trust that this individual has their best interests at heart and will give them sound medical advice. The PCP supports the patient and family through the diagnosis of breast cancer and continues to see the patient during remission. In fact, the PCP is often the only health care professional who sees the patient prediagnosis all the way through remission or palliation.

Communication between the family physician and the specialist is vitally important to ensure holistic patient management. The specialist focuses on the management of the breast cancer, whereas the generalist assesses and manages the complex interplay between pre-existing chronic medical conditions and the breast cancer. The biopsychosocial model is the cornerstone of general practice. This ensures that the psychological and social stressors which may significantly impact the patient's overall health are addressed in addition to the physical aspects of the disease. Even if the actual disease process is contained, the patient's health may suffer if the above stressors are not adequately handled.

The PCP can identify emotional and psychological stressors and provide valuable emotional support to patients and their families. Referrals to a psychologist or psychiatrist may be necessary in cases where the patient (or family) is unable to cope with the psychological impact of the diagnosis. Unresolved psychological issues may negatively impact definitive management of the breast cancer, since patients may refuse further interventions or choose harmful alternative therapies instead of conventional medicine. Specialists often do not have the time to address social issues that may impact cancer treatment. The PCP is often aware of potential social pitfalls that may negatively affect treatment, because these issues may have been identified in prior consultations. Patients may also feel more comfortable discussing these concerns with their PCP than with a specialist, whom they have only just met. Financial constraints, lack of family support, and transportation issues have all been implicated as potential causes for non-adherence to treatment. If these issues are not identified and managed appropriately, adherence is unlikely to improve.

In South Africa, 'oncology care physicians' are PCPs who have undergone further training in the management of oncology patients, and as such they are uniquely skilled in addressing oncological issues in addition to general medical conditions. In this way, the PCP can be more involved in all aspects of oncology care from diagnosis all the way through survivorship care. Preliminary studies have shown no difference in the quality of survivorship care provided by an oncologist compared to a PCP who has done further training in oncology care. A well-written specialist letter including a follow-up protocol must be guaranteed (1). With the advent of newer treatment modalities, survival rates have improved, and, as a result, breast cancer survivors are increasing exponentially. This is good news, but this success means that there is now an ever-growing shortage of oncologists to deal with the increasing number of survivors. Generalists, therefore, will need to play an increasingly important role in managing these patients during the survivorship phase (2).

The PCP plays an important role in managing breast cancer patients in all phases of the disease: prediagnosis, diagnosis, during treatment, after-treatment survivorship care, care for elderly, and care for terminally ill patients (3). Availability and shortage of PCPs are also an important issue, especially in developing countries. Time spent during a consultation with the PCP (15–20 min), as well as the waiting time for a consultation, can be considered as a quality indicator of the local health system (4).

The General Practitioner's Role in Breast Cancer Management

Prediagnosis

High-risk individuals can be identified, so that high-risk screening can be implemented. These individuals can also be counselled regarding the various options

available to them in the field of genetic testing. The pros and cons of risk-reducing surgeries can be discussed with these patients, so that they are able to make well-informed
decisions concerning their breast health. Many patients are bombarded with false and
inaccurate information via social media and the Internet. The PCP can provide patients
with scientifically sound information, so that patients can adopt a healthy lifestyle to
help prevent breast cancer.

Diagnosis

Diagnosis of breast cancer aims to detect small tumours without lymph node metastasis, which can be treated well with a good prognosis without large negative cosmetic
results after surgery. To detect breast cancer at an early stage, women should be aware of
their risk for breast cancer and should be educated in awareness and self-examinations.
In some countries, a nationwide screening programme exists (see Chapter 11) for
which women are invited to participate. Often, the patients receive their first referral
from their PCP.

A genetic predisposition for breast or ovarian cancer is possible (i.e. BRCA I–II gene)
in young women (aged <40 years). Here, the PCP can inform the patient and relatives
about the possibility of genetic counselling.

During Treatment

During treatment, a pro-active attitude of the PCP is recommended. Patients will continue to see their family physician for management of chronic medical conditions.
These conditions may be exacerbated by their oncological treatments, and it is important that the PCP actively excludes and manages any potential interactions between
oncological treatments and their pre-existing medical conditions. Acute illness may
also plague the breast cancer patient whose immunity is suppressed. It is important that
patients are counselled not to take common over-the-counter influenza preparations
and vitamin supplements which may counteract their oncological treatments. The PCP
can treat many side-effects of treatment and help patients with psychological issues.
The PCP may act as a coordinator of care between patient and specialist (patient advocacy) and act as a lifestyle coach.

After-Treatment Survivorship Care

Oncology care physicians must understand the physiological impact, patients personal risk for recurrent disease, and the most important long-term side-effects of oncological treatments: surgery, chemotherapeutic agents, radiation, and endocrine agents.
The management of these effects is particularly important for improving quality of

life and adherence during the post-treatment phase known as survivorship care (see Chapter 20).

A good knowledge of the effects of the different oncological treatment modalities such as surgery, chemotherapy, and radiotherapy is mandatory. Most especially, the role of endocrine agents must be understood. The efficacy of selective oestrogen-receptor modulators (e.g. tamoxifen) to decrease breast cancer recurrence and breast cancer mortality rate in oestrogen receptor-positive early breast cancers is well documented. However, adherence is poor among breast cancer patients; only 50% take it for the entire 5 years (5). This is largely due to poor education regarding the benefits of endocrine therapy, the prolonged duration of treatment (5–10 years), as well as the side-effects which may adversely impact quality of life. Hot flushes, mood swings, joint aches, muscle cramps, and sexual dysfunction might all be effectively managed in order to improve compliance.

Oncology care physicians in South Africa (not known in Europe) have an excellent understanding of generalist practice and as such are able to differentiate between potential side-effects of medication and the possible manifestation of new non-oncological medical conditions. A good example of this is a patient who defaulted her tamoxifen treatment due to perceived side-effects. These side-effects, however, were actually symptoms of hypothyroidism. Adequate management of the hypothyroidism improved her symptoms and, consequently, improved her adherence to the endocrine therapy.

Several models of survivorship care are suggested:

- Primary care led
  - Has been shown to be just as effective as secondary care led, and more cost-effective, for early breast cancer.
- Secondary care led
  - Nurse-led remote follow-up: telephone/post/Internet.
- Shared care
  - Varying degrees of primary care involvement.
  - Some evidence for increased patient and provider satisfaction, provider confidence, and patient perception of care.
  - Primary care-based oncology nurse.
- Patient navigator
  - Not all patients want to navigate.
  - Persons who want to make their own choices are more highly educated, adult, and emotionally more stable.

Palliative and End-of-Life Care

Patients who cannot be cured for their breast cancer receive palliative treatment. During this phase, the breast cancer is often spread to other organs, there is no cure possible, but in case of breast cancer many patients can live a normal life for many years.

In this situation, support is important. In case there are no reasonable treatments, the PCP must be closely involved in the end of life care and be near the patient in order that they may together make the difficult decisions to prepare patients and their family for the coming death (see Chapter 18).

PCP-led oncology care furthermore has the following benefits:

- Cost-effective: reduced financial burden as consultations are less expensive than specialist consultations.
- Easily accessible: patients can discuss worrisome new symptoms (that may or may not be related to their cancer) with their PCP instead of the oncologist, who is overburdened with newly diagnosed patients.
- Patients may feel more at ease discussing their concerns with their PCP than burdening their oncologist with trivial complaints.
- Increased duration of consultations with more time to spend on health promotion.
- Holistic approach: the focus is on managing the patient as a whole, instead of just managing the cancer, and this includes physical, psychological (some), and social aspects of cancer care.
- Provision of continuous care.
- Care for co-morbidities.
- Safety net: the PCP can, in addition to the oncologist, screen for symptoms of recurrence or development of any new cancers and late effects.
- Improved adherence through patient education.
- Coordination of care between patient and other agencies.
- Provide lifestyle support.
- Care for family members.

Challenges in Management of Breast Cancer Patients

Care for the Elderly

The geriatric population may be especially challenging when it comes to breast cancer management. These patients often suffer from a myriad of chronic medical conditions and take several chronic medications daily. They may be medically unfit for surgery, certain chemotherapeutic agents, or even radiation. Cardiovascular status in the elderly may be too compromised to withstand potential cardiotoxicity with anthracycline therapy. Radiation-induced pulmonary fibrosis could potentially tip the scales in an individual with pre-existing impaired respiratory function. Aromatase inhibitors may further exacerbate osteopenia, which is a common ailment in the elderly population (see Chapter 16).

Furthermore, potential interactions exist between their chronic medication and chemotherapeutic agents or endocrine therapy. Chronic anti-inflammatories prescribed for osteoarthritis may impair efficacy of certain chemotherapeutic agents used in breast cancer (6), and certain antidepressants (namely fluoxetine, paroxetine and bupropion) cannot be safely taken together with tamoxifen (5). A further concern is that it may be difficult to distinguish side-effects of oncological agents from general complaints of senescence, namely, joint aches, fatigue, and visual disturbances. It is therefore crucial that the family physician and specialist work closely together to ensure that the breast cancer management does not impact the patient's overall health to the extent that the patient succumbs to medical conditions other than the breast cancer, and that a patient's complaints are taken seriously and not merely brushed off due to old age.

Psycho-Oncological Care

Long-term psychological distress was observed in breast cancer survivors (6). A Dutch study showed severe symptoms of depression and anxiety visible up to 10 years after their diagnosis. The PCPs are most important in recognizing this problem (Chapter 20).

Alternative Therapies

The advancement of technology has presented health care professionals with a new challenge: patients are more informed and well-read than before the advent of the Internet and search engines. Patients, unfortunately, do not all have the necessary scientific background to verify the information presented to them. They may be vulnerable to unscrupulous individuals attempting to swindle them with promises of natural cures for cancer. Sweeping claims of the avarice of multibillion-dollar pharmaceutical companies have turned many patients away from conventional medical treatments to poorly researched alternative therapies. Many patients assume that natural therapies are safe and have no deleterious effects. Not only are some of these therapies ineffective, some may be detrimental to the patient's health. PCPs play an important role in educating patients about the potential risks of alternative therapies. Patients need to be advised on complementary therapies that are evidence-based and that will enhance conventional treatments and general wellbeing.

Conclusion

It is clear that PCPs, particularly those with a special interest in oncology care, can make an important contribution to the overall health and wellbeing of breast cancer patients and can improve the quality of care given to these patients. This is not only significant in developing countries, where the burden of disease is enormous and a shortage of health care professionals prevails, but also in developed countries. An improved integration between primary and secondary care with clearly defined roles and responsibilities is key. This requires clearly defined roles, good communication, adequate education, rapid access back to secondary care, and a well-functioning IT system.

Key Messages

- PCPs play a vitally important role in the whole treatment pathway and to support patients during difficult treatment decisions.
- More needs to be done to encourage PCPs to undergo additional training in oncology care, especially in a developing country setting, so that this under-utilized resource can be harnessed to provide the highest level of care to our patients.
- The PCP can identify emotional and psychological stressors and provide valuable emotional support to patients and their families.
- Communication between the family physician and the specialist is vitally important to ensure holistic patient management.
- PCPs must play an expanded role in the care of survivors.

References

1. National Cancer Survivorship Resources Center. Cancer survivorship e-learning series for primary care physicians. Available from: http://gwcehp.learnercommunity.com/elearning-series
2. Grunfeld E et al. Routine follow up of breast cancer in primary care: randomised trial. *BMJ* 1996;313(7058):665–669.
3. Rubin G et al. The expanding role of primary care in cancer control. *Lancet Oncol* 2015;16:1231–1272.
4. Irving G. International variations in primary care physician consultation time: a systematic review of 67 countries. *BMJ Open* 2017;7:10.
5. Bonfill X et al. Long-term effects of continuing adjuvant tamoxifen to 10 years versus stopping at 5 years after diagnosis of oestrogen receptor-positive breast cancer: ATLAS, a randomised trial. *Lancet* 2013;351:305–315.
6. Maass S et al. The prevalence of long-term symptoms of depression and anxiety after breast cancer treatment: a systematic review. *Maturitas* 2015;82(1):100–108.

18

Palliative Care and End-of-Life Care

Carole Bouleuc and Christine Langenaeken

Introduction

For a proper discussion of the role of palliative care (PC), it is important to clarify terminology. According to the World Health organization (WHO) palliative care (PC) is an approach that improves the quality of life of patients and their families facing the problem associated with life-threatening illness, through the prevention and relief of suffering by means of early identification and impeccable assessment and treatment of pain and other problems, physical, psychosocial and spiritual. The 'palliative' phase of the disease (as opposed to 'curative') refers especially to goals of care as cure or prolongation of survival is no longer possible. For advanced disease we use the definition of proposed by the American Society of Clinical Oncology (ASCO), 'Patients with advanced disease are those with distant metastases, late stage disease, cancer that is life-limiting and/or with a prognosis of six to twenty-four months' (1). The term 'end of life/terminal phase' will be used for patients with poor performance status (Eastern Cooperative Oncology Group performance status 3–4), refractory to oncological treatment, and with a life expectancy of 6 months or less. The term 'palliative' will be used to refer to either the phase of the disease, specific aspects of patient care or the sort of care team involved.

Minimum Requirements for High-Quality Palliative Care

Minimum requirements for high-quality PC are integration of PC into standard oncological care (SOC), an educated workforce, and access to essential drugs.

Integrating PC into Standard Oncological Care

Historically, PC focused on terminal illness. It has recently been appreciated that patients with advanced disease too may benefit from PC. In the landmark study by Temel et al. (2), 151 patients with metastatic non-small cell lung cancer were randomized to SOC with or without early consultation with the PC team (2). At 12 weeks, an improvement in quality of life (QoL) and reduction in anxiety and depression were observed in the early PC group. In the subgroup of patients who had died at the time of analysis, a greater percentage in the group assigned to standard care received aggressive end-of-life care. Fewer patients in the standard care group had resuscitation preferences documented in the electronic medical record. Rates of hospitalization and emergency department visits were lower in the early PC group. In the standard care group, fewer patients were admitted to hospice, admissions to hospice occurred more frequently within 3 days of death, and duration of stay was shorter. Despite receiving less aggressive end-of-life care, patients in the early PC group had an increased overall survival. The benefit of integrating PC has been studied extensively and was reviewed in a recent meta-analysis (3). Based on a review of the relevant literature and expert consultation, ASCO issued a recommendation in favour of integrating PC into SOC in 2012 and published an update in 2017 (1,4).

A summary of the 2017 ASCO guideline update is provided in Box 18.1.

Box 18.1 American Society of Clinical Oncology guideline on integration of palliative care—2017 update

---

Recommendation
- Patients with advanced disease should be referred to palliative care specialists taking care of the patients early on, alongside the trajectory of oncological therapy (chemotherapy, radiotherapy, etc.)
- Palliative care should be delivered by multidisciplinary teams with consultation and services available for both inpatient and outpatient settings
- The goals of palliative care teams should include the following:
  - Rapport, relationship, and trust building with the patient and family caregivers
  - Symptom, distress, and functional status management
  - Exploration of understanding and education of illness and prognosis
  - Clarification of treatment goals
  - Assessment and support of coping needs
  - Assistance with medical decision-making
  - Coordination with other care providers
  - Provision of referrals to other care providers as indicated
- Family members and caregivers should also be able to benefit from palliative care team support

Adapted with permission from Ferrell BR et al. 'Integration of palliative care into standard oncology care: American Society of Clinical Oncology Clinical Practice Guideline Update'. *Journal of Clinical Oncology.* Volume 35, Issue 1, pp. 96–112. Copyright © 2017 American Society of Clinical Oncology. DOI: 10.1200/ JCO.2016.70.1474

A number of essential elements need to occur in order to fully integrate PC into standard practice:

- awareness and education of providers and the public;
- coordination through networking;
- evaluation of the impact of palliative care on patient and provider satisfaction;
- evaluation of the economic impact;
- ensure sustainability of the model with adequate reimbursement and linkage of performance to quality indicators.

For patients with metastatic breast cancer, there may be different ways of integrating PC into SOC according to the patients' supportive care needs and the palliative care resources available: first, the solo model in which the oncologist provides the whole of oncological care and PC; second, the referral model in which the oncologist refers the patient to other care providers as needed, including the PC support team, and takes care of the coordination; and third, the integrated model, where the oncologist focuses on the antitumour treatment and the PC physician takes care of symptom control, psychosocial support, and coordination (5). Whatever model is chosen, all oncologists should have basic knowledge of PC.

Best Practices

Specialist Palliative Care Referral

Referral criteria for specialist PC should be established, because it is neither possible nor advisable that PC specialists take over the entire care of the patient with advanced disease.

A list of potential criteria for outpatient PC specialist referral was generated by an international panel of experts (6). Twenty unique categories were identified: six were commonly cited for referral, two were time-based criteria (cancer trajectory, prognosis), and four were needs-based criteria (physical symptoms, performance status, end-of-life care planning, and psychosocial distress). Major referral criteria are summarized in Table 18.1.

There was also consensus on a large number of minor referral criteria. Although these were developed for secondary or tertiary care hospitals, consensus was reached on many of criteria suggesting that some universal patient phenotypes may be appropriate for PC irrespective of health care systems or boundaries.

Prognostication of Survival

Prognosis is a key element for caregivers in guiding the management of advanced/terminal disease. Prognostication is a process rather than an event, as prognostic factors

Table 18.1 Major palliative care referral criteria

• Time-based	• Cancer trajectory	✓ Progressive disease despite second-line therapy ✓ Within 3 months of advanced cancer diagnosis for patients with median survival of 1 year or less
• Needs-based	• Distress	✓ Severe physical symptoms
	• Psychosocial distress	✓ Severe emotional symptoms ✓ Request for hastened death ✓ Spiritual or existential crisis
	• Neurological	✓ Delirium ✓ Spinal cord compression ✓ Brain or leptomeningeal metastases
	• Care/End-of-life care planning	✓ Assistance with decision-making or care planning
	• Other	✓ Patient request

Reproduced with permission from Hui, D. et al. 'Referral criteria for outpatient speciality palliative cancer care: an international consensus'. *The Lancet Oncology*. Volume 17, Issue 12, pp. 552–559. Copyright © 2016 Elsevier Inc. DOI:https://doi.org/10.1016/S1470-2045(16)30577-0.

may evolve over the course of the disease. Prognostic accuracy for a given factor/tool varies by the definition of accuracy, the patient population, and the predicted timeframe. The exact timing of death cannot be predicted with certainty.

Clinician prediction of survival is the most commonly used approach to estimate prognosis. The accuracy of clinicians' estimates is heterogeneous, but evidence suggests that these predictions are frequently inaccurate, and no subgroup of clinicians is more accurate than any other. In clinical practice, survival is often estimated using the 'Surprise Question', 'Would I be surprised if this patient would die within the coming year?' Not surprisingly, estimates based on the Surprise Question have an accuracy ranging from poor to reasonable and were reported in a recent meta-analysis (7,8).

Both clinical and biological factors have prognostic value in advanced disease and at the end of life. The main clinical factors are summarized by the four 'D's: decreased performance status, dysphagia and anorexia–cachexia syndrome, delirium, and dyspnoea. Performance status is one of the most important, albeit with great inter-observer variability. Biological factors include a number of inflammatory markers, e.g. C-reactive protein, leucocytosis and lymphopenia, hypo-albuminaemia (indicating malnutrition), hypercalcaemia, hyponatraemia, and elevated lactate dehydrogenase (9).

A number of prognostic scores have been constructed using these factors, the most reliable ones being the Palliative Prognostic Score, Palliative Prognostic Index, Glasgow Prognostic Score, and Barbot's score (10).

Patient–Clinician Communication in Palliative Care

Effective patient–clinician communication about prognosis and end-of-life care preferences has important benefits for patients, their families, and the health care system. When patients are aware of their short life expectancy, they more often make informed decisions about end-of-life care. Understanding a bad prognosis will allow some patients to address unresolved concerns and leave a legacy for loved ones, e.g. through letters or videos. It has been demonstrated that early PC improves patients' understanding of their prognosis and elicits end-of-life care wishes.

For caregivers, prognostic information strongly influences decisions with regard to pursuing further oncological treatment, taking part in clinical trials, advanced care planning, and end-of-life decisions.

Most metastatic cancer patients want detailed prognostic information, but they prefer to negotiate the extent, format, and timing of the information they receive from their oncologists.

Strategies for effective end-of-life communication include: being open and honest, having ongoing, early conversations, communicating about treatment goals, and balancing hope and reality. Unless complete frankness is explicitly requested, a communication strategy that allows patients to dictate most of the flow or avoid prognostic information is acceptable. For patients at the end of life or in terminal phase, such a 'strategy of necessary collusion' preserves hope by acknowledging uncertainty and allowing information to emerge over time. 'Prepare for the worst and hope for the best' is probably the less harmful way of discussing a short-term prognosis.

Guidelines for patient–clinician communication have been developed (4,11). Training courses appear to be effective in improving health care professional communication skills, e.g. related to information gathering and support (12).

It is important to introduce communication training early on in the curriculum; early exposure to end-of-life conversations will help students 'learn to drive'.

Barriers to implementing these strategies are due to patient, physician, and institutional factors. Physician factors include difficulty with treatment and palliation, personal discomfort with death and dying, diffusion of responsibility among colleagues, using the 'death-defying' mode, lack of experience, and lack of mentorship. Patient factors include patients/families being reluctant to talk about end of life, language barriers, and younger age. Institutional factors include stigma around PC, lack of protocol on end-of-life issues, and lack of training for oncologists on how to talk to patients about end-of-life issues.

Advanced Care Planning

Proper end-of-life management implies advanced care planning (ACP). This includes designation of a trusted person, advance will directives, and discussion of the patient's preferences for end-of-life care. The timing and quality of these conversations are of paramount importance. They are key determinants of the patient's trajectory at the end of life and have an impact transcending the 'do not resuscitate' order.

Choosing the right moment is more important than the mere fact of the conversation taking place. The decision whether or not to continue anticancer treatment and the conversation with the patient and family are some of the most difficult tasks for the oncologist. The following recommendations made in France after broad multidisciplinary expert consultation are broadly applicable:

- the oncologist must take the known prognostic criteria into account;
- discussion at multidisciplinary staff meetings is helpful in evaluating the patient's therapeutic needs and setting reasonable objectives;
- the conversation about interrupting or stopping chemotherapy should focus on resistance of the disease to treatment and potential clinical improvement due to the disappearance of side-effects;
- a discussion about the continuation of therapy should focus on symptom control;
- uncertainty on the patient's life expectancy could be helpful in maintaining some hope.

The content of ACP conversations needs to be well documented in the patient's medical record. Patients participating in ACP have a lower likelihood of receiving aggressive care at the end of life, dying in the hospital, and an increased likelihood of being admitted to hospice.

Patients found the following to be important in ACP conversations:

- the doctor knows their personal history;
- a relative be present;
- the conversation be conducted in a delicate way and after prior patient consent.

Recommendations by the European Association for Palliative Care include the adaptation of ACP based on the readiness of the individual, targeting ACP content as the health condition worsens, and using trained non-physician facilitators to support the ACP process (13). A clinical practice guideline on ACP was developed by the European Society of Medical Oncology (ESMO) (14).

End-of-Life Care

Aggressive care at the end of life refers to over-usage of chemotherapy (within 14–30 days prior to death), insufficient use of palliative services (no admission to palliative care unit, or untimely, i.e. less than 7 days before death), and over-usage of acute care (i.e. increased rate of emergency consultations, short-term hospitalizations, admission to intensive care unit) (15).

In a French trial evaluating 279,846 patients who died in hospital, 19.5% had chemotherapy in the last two months of life, and 11.3% in the last two weeks (16). Female sex, older age, and an increased number of comorbidities were independently associated with a decreased risk of receiving chemotherapy. In a secondary analysis of the Temel trial (2), those receiving early PC had half the odds of receiving chemotherapy within 60 days of death, a longer interval between the last dose of chemotherapy and death, and higher enrolment in hospice care for more than one week.

Aggressive end-of-life care has a negative impact on the QoL of both patient and family. Involving the PC team in end-of-life management may be helpful in facilitating no-treatment decisions, reduce the risk of aggressive measures, and facilitate transfers to PC units.

Quality Indicators

In the development of quality indicators in PC, the focus has been on developing outcome indicators with regard to physical, psychosocial, and spiritual needs of patients as well as on the needs of the (bereaved) family, thus being in line with the WHO definition. In the literature, most outcome and process indicators refer to physical, psychological, and ethical aspects of care and care for the terminally ill. There is a scarcity of indicators of social and spiritual aspects.

Quality indicators often cover one specific setting or target group, e.g. home care. In the Netherlands and Flanders, a set of 33 indicators for palliative patient care and 10 indicators for support for relatives before and/or after the patient's death was developed and tested, and these are applicable for all settings in which PC is being provided for adult patients (17). In the 2013 update by the same research group on behalf of EURO IMPACT, new developments were mainly quantitative in nature with a substantial number of new indicators being found.

Managing Diversity

The impact of culturally different beliefs and attitudes regarding matters of health, illness, and death on individual health care professionals and health care systems is well recognized. In PC, cultural competence refers to the set of knowledge and practical skills needed to properly deal with patients and families belonging to different cultures with regard to supportive and end-of-life care.

Goals of care may vary according to the cultural context. Location of PC may also vary in different cultures and should take into account the availability and engagement of (family) caregivers.

Barriers to High-Quality Palliative Care

A resource-stratified practice guideline for palliative care has been developed by ASCO and provides recommendations for model of care, staffing requirements, roles, and training needs of team members; it also outlines standards for provision of psycho-social support, spiritual care, and opioid analgesics (18).

A number of barriers to PC development in low-and middle-income countries have been identified. These include the absence of PC in national policies, lack of partnership working, insufficient PC education for health care professionals and volunteers, poor public awareness, gaps in access to adequate PC, ACP and essential pain relief medicines, and cultural barriers.

Budget is important for PC in different ways: it is required for education and infrastructure, training of health care professionals, reimbursement, and access to essential medicines. One issue is whether to allocate budgets mainly to end-of-life care or also to include people with advanced disease. The supportive and palliative care indicators tool (SPICT™), a guide to identifying people with one or more advanced illnesses, deteriorating health and a risk of dying with these conditions, as well as for assessment and care planning, might be helpful in setting priorities.

Emerging Modalities

Medical decisions at the end of life have become increasingly frequent. Shifting attitudes in western societies towards secularism and an emphasis on individual autonomy and personal control have supported the movement to legalize assisted dying.

Assisted dying refers to assisted suicide or euthanasia. It has been legalized in some form in five European countries (the Netherlands, Belgium, Switzerland, Germany, and Luxembourg), six US states (Oregon, Washington, Vermont, Montana, California, and Colorado), and Canada. Provision of assisted dying in a health care facility imposes specific institutional obligations to ensure effective and appropriate delivery, to support and protect families and health care providers, and to educate staff about the practice (19).

Assisted dying has met with much controversy, yet its increasing prominence in the public space is not only a threat but also an opportunity. Both the delivery and education process in the home care and institutional setting have enhanced transparency and accountability regarding medical practices at the end of life, and these have encouraged more open conversations about wishes, fears, and preferences.

Palliative sedation is another controversial issue; it is sometimes referred to as 'slow euthanasia'. However, palliative sedation is defined as the use of sedatives to lower a person's consciousness to the degree that is required to alleviate refractory symptoms at the end of life. There are two important aspects that distinguish palliative sedation from assisted dying: first, the principle of proportionality (dosing as required to achieve symptom control) and, second, the goal (symptom control, not death). At an individual, institutional, and policy level, it is essential to be clear about goals and intentions. ESMO Guidelines are available (20), and on the websites of the Flemish Federation of Palliative Care and the Dutch Comprehensive Cancer Center, the latter having an English version (21).

Key Messages

- Integrate palliative care into standard oncological care.
- Ensure timely referral for palliative care, discussion of prognosis, and ACP.
- Avoid chemotherapy near the end of life.
- Work on palliative care awareness in both the public eye and at the policymaking level.
- ACP should be the rule rather than the exception with sufficient infrastructure available to all.
- There is a need for adequate and appropriate legislation and reimbursement.

References

1. Ferrell BR et al. Integration of palliative care into standard oncology care: America Society of Clinical Oncology Clinical Practice Guideline Update. *J Clin Oncol* 2017;35:96–112.
2. Temel JS et al. Early palliative care for patients with metastatic non-small cell lung cancer. *N Engl J Med* 2010;363:733–742.
3. Haun MW et al. Early palliative care for adults with advanced cancer. *Cochrane Database Syst Rev* 2017;12:6.
4. American Society for Clinical Oncology. Supportive care and treatment related issues. Available from: https://www.asco.org/practice-guidelines/quality-guidelines/guidelines/supportive-care-and-treatment-related-issues
5. Partridge AH et al. Developing a service model that integrates palliative care throughout cancer care: the time is now. *J Clin Oncol* 2014;32(29):3330–3336.
6. Hui D et al. Referral criteria for outpatient specialty palliative cancer care: an international consensus. *Lancet Oncol* 2016;16:e552–559.
7. White N et al. How accurate is the 'Surprise Question' at identifying patients at the end of life? A systematic review and meta-analysis. *BMC Med* 2017;15(1):139.
8. White N et al. A systematic review of predictions of survival in palliative care: how accurate are clinicians and who are the experts? *PLoS One* 2016;11(8):e0161407.
9. Maltoni M et al. Prognostic factors in advanced cancer patients: evidence-based clinical recommendations—a study by the Steering Committee of the European Association for Palliative Care. *J Clin Oncol* 2005;23(25):6240–6248.
10. Hui D. Prognostication of survival in patients with advanced cancer: predicting the unpredictable? *Cancer Control* 2015;22(4):489–497.
11. T. Gilligan et al. Patient-clinician communication: American Society of Clinical Oncology Consensus Guideline: *J Clin Oncol* 2017;35:3618–3632.
12. Moore PM et al. Communication skills training for healthcare professionals working with people who have cancer. *Cochrane Database Syst Rev* 2013;28:3.
13. Rietjens JA et al. Definition and recommendations for advance care planning: an international consensus supported by the European Association for Palliative Care. *Lancet Oncol* 2017;18:e543–551.
14. European Society of Medical Oncology. Clinical Practice Guidelines on Supportive Care. Available from: https://www.esmo.org/Guidelines/Supportive-and-Palliative-Care

15. Earle CC et al. Aggressiveness of cancer care near the end of life: is it a quality-of-care issue? *J Clin Oncol* 2008;26(23):3860–3866.

16. Rochigneux P et al. Use of chemotherapy near the end of life: what factors matter? *Ann Oncol* 2017;28(4):809–817.

17. Claessen SJJ et al. A new set of quality indicators for palliative care: process and results of the development trajectory. *J Pain Sympt Manage* 2011;42(2):169–182.

18. Osman H et al. Palliative care in the global setting: ASCO Resource-Stratified Practice Guideline. *J Global Oncol* 2018;4:1–24.

19. Li M et al. Medical assistance in dying—implementing a hospital-based program in Canada. *N Engl J Med* 2017;376:2082–2088.

20. Cherny NI. ESMO clinical practice guidelines for the management of refractory symptoms at the end of life and the use of palliative sedation. *Ann Oncol* 2014;25(3):iii43–iii52.

21. Oncoline. Available from: https://www.oncoline.nl/index.php?

19

Nursing Issues

Victoria Harmer and Cathy Hughes

Specialist Nursing in Breast Care

Specialist nursing in breast care is an example of extending nursing practice to meet patient need. These senior nurses would have undertaken additional studies in breast care and have, or be working towards, masters or doctoral-level qualifications. They should be experts in evidence-based nursing with an ability to problem-solve, reflect, analyse, think critically, and have the skills to communicate the complex information given to patients and their families in breast clinics to facilitate informed decision-making. The specialist nurse should assess patients holistically and present their fears and concerns to the multidisciplinary team.

Specialist nurses should also provide strong leadership and positively impact the training and development of other staff in order to provide patient-centred, safe, and effective solutions to the ever-changing demand for high-quality healthcare (1).

Patient advocacy groups have ranked specialist nurses higher than other health and social care professionals with regard to understanding their needs, being transparent and honest, designing and implementing care pathways, and obtaining patient feedback (2).

However, in the UK there are no official regulations for nurses in advanced roles, and there is no legally specified training other than specialist training associated with a specific task, e.g. colposcopy. Liability is provided by employers, once they have examined competencies, work instructions, and standards of care (3). Specialist nurses need support from their multidisciplinary team to develop safe patient pathways embedded with quality nursing care and to ensure that any service development or role extension is adopted successfully (4). Currently, there are three main types of breast care specialist nurses: clinical nurse specialist, nurse practitioner, and consultant nurse.

Clinical Nurse Specialist

There are four central threads to the clinical nurse specialist (CNS) role (5):

- expert practice;
- patient advocacy;
- holistic assessment and referral;
- service development.

In the UK, the breast care CNS is generally introduced to the patient at diagnosis and is responsible for providing information and support to patients and their families throughout their breast cancer trajectory. European standards recommend that patients have nurse counselling at the time of primary treatment and direct access to a breast care nurse specialist for information and support with treatment-related symptoms and toxicity during the treatment, follow-up, and rehabilitation (6).

The CNS will case-manage the patient and their families while they are undergoing ever-changing treatment pathways and will support complex decision-making and discussion of options, often representing the one constant throughout care pathways using differing treatment modalities. The CNS has a key role in limiting unwanted consequences of treatment and in the identification of disease progression as well as providing expertise over a range of environments for a number of different domains of care (Box 19.1).

The impact of the CNS can be measured in quality and experience of care, safety, productivity and efficiency, and leadership. Patients treated at hospitals with more CNSs have a better experience, receive better emotional support, and benefit from healthcare professionals working well as a team. Timely interventions can deflect expensive care episodes and promote efficacy (7,8). The benefits of a CNS include reduced waiting times, avoidance of unnecessary and unplanned hospital admissions, reduced postoperative length of stay, reduced treatment drop-out rates, freeing up of consultant time, innovative service delivery and improvement, delivering services at the point of need, and educating health and social care professionals (9).

Box 19.1 Clinical domains of practice associated with the clinical nurse specialist

---

Breast screening programme

Benign breast conditions

Family history, genetics, and risk prediction

Newly diagnosed and metastatic breast cancer patients: clinical and emotional support

Breast surgery, reconstruction, prophylactic surgery, and prosthesis fitting

Patients undergoing systemic treatment, chemotherapy, radiation therapy, and endocrine treatment

Management of treatment side-effects: menopausal symptoms, lymphoedema, wounds, psychological distress, treatment-induced fertility issues, hair loss, and sexual complaints

Social issues, financial aspects, and patient advocacy

Survivorship: recovery, rehabilitation, and follow-up (including lifestyle changes)

Nurse Practitioners

Nurse practitioners (NPs) focus on direct clinical assessment, diagnosis, and treatment, as well as health education and disease prevention. Although aspects of CNS and NP roles overlap in relation to leadership, patient and staff education, and service improvements, the breast NP role tends to be grounded in the diagnostic pathway.

The extended remit of the NP often incorporates functions traditionally allocated to physicians, such as performing breast examinations, taking a history, and ordering diagnostic tests. Evaluation of effectiveness, safety, and patient satisfaction with the NP role, although limited, has been encouraging (10).

Consultant Nurses

The consultant nurse (CN) was introduced in the UK in the 1980s and is at the pinnacle of the clinical nursing career ladder (11). There are four components to the CN role:

- expert practice;
- professional leadership and consultancy;
- education, training and development, and service improvement;
- research and evaluation.

Consultant nurses possess the skills and competencies of the CNS but with greater breadth, depth, and complexity. They have a clinical role that ensures clinical credibility and effective role-modelling, but they also focus on the whole service, developing research, service improvement, education, and acting as an expert resource. The CN should have completed, or be studying for, a relevant Doctorate.

The CN should be a transformational leader who fosters widening participation and collaboration, and who contributes to national and international strategies and policies as an expert in their field. The knowledge, skills, expertise, personal qualities and attitudes, and processes of a CN are illustrated in Box 19.2.

Hospital and Community Care

Healthcare and therapies traditionally delivered in hospital are increasingly being delivered in the community, and more drugs are now being administered orally. Consequently, thorough assessment of a patient's ability to self-manage with enough information and support requires new ways of working across boundaries and remotely. For patients to effectively receive care closer to home, there needs to be good communication with healthcare professionals who work in the community. Appropriate support structures need to be in place (12).

Box 19.2 The consultant nurse's knowledge, skills, expertise, qualities, attributes, and processes

Knowledge, skills, and expertise in integrated sub-roles
- Nursing practice as a generalist/specialist
- Research and evaluation in practice
- Practice development and the facilitation of structural, cultural, and practice change
- Education and learning in practice
- Consultancy: clinical to organizational
- Management, leadership, and strategic vision

Personal qualities and attributes
- Being patient-centred
- Being available, accessible, generous, and flexible
- Being enthusiastic
- Being self-aware and attuned to others
- Being a collaborator and a catalyst
- Having a vision for nursing and health care
- Being a strategist and demonstrating political leadership
- Academic criteria

Processes
- Transformational leadership processes
  - Developing a shared vision
  - Inspiring and communicating
  - Valuing others
  - Challenging and stimulating
  - Developing trust
  - Enabling
- Processes of emancipation
  - Clarifying and working with values, beliefs, and assumptions; challenging contradictions
  - Developing critical intent of individuals and groups
  - Developing moral intent
  - Focusing on the impact of the context/system on practice as well as practice itself
  - Using self-reflection and fostering reflection in others
  - Enabling others to 'see the possibilities'
  - Fostering widening participation and collaboration by all involved
- Practising expertly as a practitioner, researcher, educator, consultant, and practice developer
  - Role modeller
  - Facilitating individual, collective, and organizational learning
  - Facilitating change, practice, and service development

Reproduced with permission from Manley K, Tichen A. 'Becoming and being a nurse consultant: towards greater effectiveness through a programme of support'. London: Royal College of Nursing; 2012

Cancer Survivorship

Many more people are living longer following cancer treatment, and many of these cancer survivors experience long-term side-effects from previous treatment or from the cancer itself. Indeed, cancer survivors have significant unmet needs, and specialist nurses are increasingly their key accessible professional and point of contact. Specialist nurses act as an expert resource to support the process of returning to normal, or a new normal (normalization). They support cancer survivors in developing the skills to self-manage while ensuring that they also understand any red flag symptoms, which should be promptly reported to their healthcare provider (4,13).

Metastatic Breast Cancer

There are increasing numbers of nurses dedicated to the management of metastatic breast cancer. These specialist nurses provide support and information to people with life-limiting disease. These patients often need to revisit the cancer landscape and adjust their expectations (14). Seamless care across boundaries is important in this setting to achieve personal goals and a realistic view of the future.

Workforce

The extension of nursing roles will impact workload. In addition, treatments are becoming more numerous and sophisticated, and it is often the specialist nurse's remit to explain, communicate, and manage patient care. The Independent Cancer Taskforce in England documented the need for all cancer patients to have access to a CNS or key worker to coordinate and plan care. They note, however, that there should be a strategic review of workforce deficits and the skills mix required to deliver a modern high-quality service (15). The number of CNSs in breast care has remained the same in England since 2007, despite an 18% increase in the number of new breast cancer cases (16). Therefore, there is a definite need for the number of specialist nurses to be addressed, in order that quality of care is not compromised (4).

There is a global shortage of nurses, although this is most acute in developing countries. The average nurse:population ratio in high-income countries is almost eight times greater than in low-income countries, and there is a link between the number of nurses and health outcomes (17). Developed countries are able to attract nurses from less developed countries with offers of better pay and working conditions. The ongoing trend in nurse shortages is worrying for the provision of healthcare and patient safety.

Key Messages

- A specialist nurse is knowledgeable in breast cancer disease, its treatment modalities, and available support.
- There are three main types of specialist nurse in breast care: clinical nurse specialist, nurse practitioner, and consultant nurse.
- A specialist nurse will coordinate care, act as patient advocate in the multidisciplinary team, and is vital in communicating aims of treatment, potential adverse effects, and assessing the patient throughout the trajectory.
- A specialist nurse has been shown to improve patient experience and outcomes of care and indicates a higher-quality service in Europe and the UK.
- Effective patient assessment optimizes treatment and care.
- There is significant variation in the global provision of specialist nurses with fewest in developing countries.
- Not addressing a global shortfall in the nursing workforce will likely result in a worsening health care system.

References

1. Francis R. *Report of the Mid Staffordshire NHS Foundation Trust Public Inquiry—Volume 3: Present and Future, Annexes.* London: The Stationery Office; 2013.
2. Royal College Nursing/National Voices. *Local Healthcare Commissioning: Grassroots Involvement? A National Survey of Health Advocacy Groups.* London: RCN/National Voices; 2009.
3. Dean E. Proving the value of advanced roles. *Nurs Stand* 2013;27(25):18–20.
4. Harmer V. Nursing issues and the role of the specialist nurse in breast care. In Wyld L et al., editors. Breast Cancer Management for Surgeons. Cham: Springer; 2018. p. 681–688.
5. National Cancer Action Team. *Excellence in Cancer Care: The Contribution of the Clinical Nurse Specialist.* London: NCAT; 2010.
6. Biganzoli L et al. Quality indicators in breast cancer care: an update from the EUSOMA working group. *Eur J Cancer* 2017;86:59–81.
7. Vidall C et al. Clinical nurse specialists: essential resource for an effective NHS. *Br J Nurs* 2011;20(17):S23–27.
8. Griffiths P et al. Is a larger specialist nurse workforce in cancer care associated with better patient experience? Cross-sectional study. *J Health Serv Res Policy* 2013;18(S1):39–46.
9. Royal College of Nursing. *Specialist Nurses: Changing Lives, Saving Money.* London: Royal College of Nursing; 2010.
10. Peate I. The physician's associate. *Br J Nurs* 2016;25(10):533.
11. Manley K and Tichen A. *Becoming and Being a Nurse Consultant: Towards Greater Effectiveness Through a Programme of Support.* London: Royal College of Nursing; 2012.
12. Harmer V. Many issues must be tackled to move care into the community. *Nurs Times* 2013;109(22):11.
13. Armes J et al. Patients' supportive care needs beyond the end of cancer treatment; a prospective, longitudinal study. *J Clin Oncol* 2009;27:6172–6179.
14. Ghandourh WA. Palliative care in cancer: managing patients' expectations. *J Med Radiat Sci* 2016;63:242–257.

15. The Independent Cancer Taskforce. *Achieving World-Class Cancer Outcomes. A strategy for England 2015–2022. Executive Summary.* London: NHS England; 2015.

16. Breast Cancer Care. Breast cancer cases rise but number of specialist nurses stays the same. 2015. Available at: https://www.breastcancercare.org.uk/about-us/news-blogs/news/breast-cancer-cases-rise-number-specialist-nurses-stays-same

17. Buchan J and Calman L. *The Global Shortage of Registered Nurses: An Overview of Issues and Actions.* Geneva: International Council of Nurses; 2005.

20

Psycho-Oncological Care and Survivorship

Luzia Travado, Jane Turner, Julia H. Rowland, Barry D. Bultz, and Paul B. Jacobsen

Introduction

Cancer and its treatment have a significant impact on the quality of life of patients, their families and caregivers. As many as 45% of cancer patients and survivors experience high levels of cancer-related distress (1), and they may develop more serious psychological problems such as adjustment disorders, anxiety disorders, and depression (2). These conditions negatively impact clinical outcomes such as treatment compliance, survival, and quality of life, requiring specialized psychosocial care (3). Psychosocial problems can also affect the patient's family, cause increased emotional distress among the patient's caregivers, and may continue into palliative care and the bereavement period with greater risk of complicated or traumatic grief among relatives. Patients' and their families' psychosocial needs must be a central component of high-quality comprehensive cancer care.

The specialty of psycho-oncology addresses the range of psychosocial, behavioural, spiritual, and existential dimensions that the patient and family may face throughout the cancer care continuum. A primary goal of psychosocial oncology is to ensure that all cancer patients and their families receive optimal psychosocial care at all stages of the disease including post-treatment or during survivorship. To achieve the best clinical outcomes for breast cancer patients, it is recommended that patients' psychosocial needs be regularly assessed, and that psychosocial oncology services delivered by specialized professionals are available in cancer care facilities to address those needs as an integral part of quality comprehensive cancer care (4). In this chapter, we discuss the importance of screening for distress, evidence of the benefit of tailored psychosocial interventions, and the emerging focus on survivorship, which moves beyond distress to address promotion of wellness. The chapter concludes with discussion about guidelines to assist clinicians and with an overview of progress in Europe and across the world.

The Developing Focus on Psychosocial Needs and Assessment

In 1993 the first National Forum on Breast Cancer in Canada was convened and attended by approximately 1,000 multidisciplinary health care providers, government officials, politicians, and advocacy groups. A member of the audience posed a question to an expert panel. The question was simple: 'In your opinion, what do you think has been the single biggest advancement in breast cancer?' The universal response was: 'The inclusion of whole patient cancer care.' One panel member (a psychologist and cancer survivor) then stated that in the care of the breast cancer patient: 'You can't treat the breast without treating the heart.'

To date, comprehensive cancer care has a varied history depending on location. In English-speaking countries (Australia, Canada, the USA, and Great Britain) over the last 30 years, accreditation bodies, cancer societies, and professional organizations have responded to demands from patients and advocacy groups and have begun to embrace the standard of incorporating psychosocial care into cancer care. A particularly compelling rationale for the inclusion of psychosocial care programmes has been the number of large-scale research studies of cancer patients demonstrating the prevalence rates of morbid distress as affecting between 30% and 45% of patients evaluated and an estimated 32% for early breast cancer patients (1,2). Moreover, the distress rates increase with progression of the disease, and the distress rate for those with advanced breast disease is an estimated 60% (5).

In North America, the Institute of Medicine recommended that, irrespective of the type of cancer, whole patient symptom management should be a requirement, there should be zero acceptance of pain, and the identification of psychosocial needs, screening, and the integration of psychosocial services should be seen as standard requirements for best practice in cancer care.

In 2009, the International Psycho-Oncology Society (IPOS; http://www.ipos-society.org) proposed a new standard for quality cancer care endorsed by the Union for International Cancer Control and 76 other international organizations and scientific societies related to cancer treatment and care (6), updated in 2014, which states:

- Psychosocial care should be recognized as a universal human right.
- Quality cancer care today must integrate the psychosocial domain into routine cancer care.
- Distress should be measured as the 6th Vital Sign after temperature, blood pressure, pulse, respiratory rate, and pain (7).

In 2013, the Union for International Cancer Control revised the World Cancer Declaration to include the codification of distress along with pain, stating in Target 8:

- Effective pain control measures and distress management will be available to cancer patients in all countries.

However, detection of distress and psychological morbidity in the past has tended to rely on 'clinical acumen' or 'expert intuition'. Given the findings from the prevalence studies and the acknowledged error (generally underestimation) when relying on clinical acumen alone, oncology practices have begun to systematically address the impact cancer has on the lives of individual patients through screening patients for distress (8).

Still relatively new in cancer care delivery, systematic screening using structured and validated measures for distress, now being referred to as the 6th Vital Sign, is becoming standard practice in comprehensive cancer care (9).

Brief, standardized, screening questionnaires used in cancer care can help identify factors impacting physical, emotional, spiritual, and practical patient concerns related to the diagnosis and treatment of cancer. While distress screening is evolving into a standard practice, no single measure has gained complete support by the cancer community. There is, however, consensus for measures to be brief. Two examples are the single-item Distress Thermometer, and the Canada-endorsed minimum data-set, the 10-item Edmonton Symptom Assessment Survey (10). Both questionnaires are easy to administer, and both have an accompanying problem checklist which includes common problems that cancer patients may be facing in a number of areas, namely practical, familial, emotional, religious/spiritual, or physical.

Studies are beginning to surface concerning the benefits, and limitations, of broad hospital-based screening for distress. Our research has demonstrated that screening of individual patients is an effective tool that is easy to administer and when followed-up can improve clinical care (11). The real challenge is not whether to screen, but rather how health care providers can respond to the patient's distress, and what referrals and interventions may be appropriate for the individual. Medicine has learned to rely on the metrics of a patient's condition by measuring vital signs. Oncology care looks at biomarkers, tumour size, blood counts, genetics, etc. Due to the advances in psychosocial oncology, and specifically the rapid uptake of distress screening, it is time to advance quality management by promoting screening for distress as the 6th vital sign for all patients diagnosed and living with cancer (9). This policy has already been adopted in several countries as reflected by Accreditation Canada and the American College of Surgeons' Commission on Cancer in the USA. Evidence about specific psychosocial interventions that are of benefit for the distressed patient is described in the next section.

Efficacy of Psychosocial Interventions for Women with Breast Cancer

A range of psychosocial interventions have been shown to be effective and efficient in preventing and reducing distress, psychosocial morbidity, and the emotional and psychological burden of having and/or living with cancer. Interventions are also effective in improving patients' quality of life, the ability to deal with the demands of treatment, and to cope with uncertainty (12). Improvement in survival has also been noted.

Systematic reviews and meta-analyses are generally recognized as the premier ways of summarizing the existing empirical evidence about a research question. In this section, we consider the findings of systematic reviews and meta-analyses for the following question: what is the evidence of the benefits of psychosocial interventions for women with breast cancer?

Several systematic reviews and meta-analyses have sought to answer this question, or variants of it. They differ largely in terms of their scope with regard to the populations included (mixed cancers or breast cancer specific) (12), the interventions (exercise or more general psychosocial and behavioural interventions) (13), and outcomes assessed (ranging from broad psychosocial concerns and quality of life to specific concerns such as pain or sexual concerns). We have selected two systematic reviews and meta-analyses to discuss here based on their focus on women with breast cancer, on a well-defined set of psychosocial interventions, and on a range of psychosocial and quality-of-life outcomes.

Duijts and colleagues conducted a systematic review and meta-analysis to determine the effects of behavioural interventions and physical exercise on psychosocial functioning and quality of life in women with breast cancer (13). Inclusion was restricted to randomized controlled trials published until March 2009 which had sufficient quantitative data to calculate effect sizes. The final set included 39 studies of behavioural interventions (ranging from yoga programmes and educational programmes as well as more traditional mental health interventions such as problem-solving therapy and relaxation training), 14 studies of exercise, and three studies of both behavioural interventions and exercise. Our discussion focuses on studies of behavioural interventions. Most studies comprised women with non-metastatic disease and were conducted during the active phase of treatment.

Effect sizes were reported using Hedges' g. According to convention, effect size statistics of 0.2 are considered small, 0.5 medium, and 0.8 large. Significant ($P < 0.05$) effects were found for a benefit of behavioural interventions on fatigue, depression, anxiety, and stress. However, the magnitude of these effects all fell below the medium size threshold.

Matthews and colleagues conducted a systematic review and meta-analysis to determine the effects of psychosocial interventions on psychosocial functioning and quality of life in women with breast cancer (14). Inclusion was restricted to studies published through 2015 of women who had received primary breast cancer surgery for non-metastatic disease. A total of 32 articles were included in the review, of which 22 articles described randomized controlled trials. The types of intervention evaluated included cognitive–behaviour therapy, psychoeducation, mindfulness-based stress reduction, and supportive–expressive therapy.

Once again, effect sizes were reported using Hedges' g. Significant effects were found for the benefit of psychosocial interventions on quality of life, depression, anxiety, body image, distress, mood disturbance, and sleep disturbance. Similar to the other systematic review and meta-analysis, the magnitude of these effects (with the exception of a larger effect for sleep disturbance) all fell below the medium size threshold. It should also be noted that the results for sleep disturbance, along with those for body image, mood disturbance, and distress are based on a limited number of studies, which raises concerns about the robustness of these findings.

Taken together, the results of the two systematic reviews and meta-analyses consistently demonstrate that psychosocial interventions have a statistically significant but relatively modest-sized effect on mental health outcomes such as anxiety and depression. Moreover, results suggest that psychosocial interventions can have a positive impact on other symptoms commonly experienced by women with breast cancer (e.g. fatigue and sleep disturbance).

There is reason to believe, however, that the impact of psychosocial interventions may be greater for a subset of women with breast cancer. One factor to consider is that, to date, most studies of psychosocial interventions for cancer patients have recruited participants regardless of their baseline level of psychological wellbeing. By including many patients who may be experiencing little or no psychological distress, the observed effects of psychosocial intervention may be 'watered down'. Moreover, this approach to providing psychosocial interventions is inconsistent with guidelines for psychosocial care of people with cancer, which generally recommend using mental health interventions with patients who screen positive for problems in psychological wellbeing.

The impact that the baseline level of psychological wellbeing can have on observed benefit of psychosocial interventions was demonstrated in a systematic review and meta-analysis that included patients with all forms of cancer (12). In this work, the authors reported effect sizes separately for all studies and for just the subset of studies that preselected participants according to increased distress. Among the larger group of studies, the effect sizes (Cohen's d) for depression and anxiety were 0.33 and 0.38, respectively, values which are consistent with those reported in the two systematic reviews and meta-analyses discussed previously (13). However, when restricted to just those studies that preselected participants based on increased distress, the effect sizes for depression and anxiety were 0.53 and 0.56, respectively. In summary, there is good reason to believe that psychosocial interventions can have a medium-sized effect on mental health outcomes when administered according to guidelines that suggest reserving these interventions for cancer patients experiencing heightened psychological distress (14).

Moving Beyond Distress to Encompass Wellness— Attention on Survivorship

No discussion about the psychosocial needs of those diagnosed with cancer is complete without consideration of what happens after treatment ends. Up until the latter part of the last century, little attention was accorded the long-term or late consequences of cancer, because most patients were not expected to survive their disease. Efforts in this earlier period were focused on helping people who were dying of cancer, not on those living through or beyond it. However, this picture has changed substantially over the past two decades.

Whereas some low-resource nations still struggle with 5-year survival rates that fall below 50%, the majority can expect to see growing numbers of their population become long-term cancer survivors. Since this population has continued to grow globally, its members have taught us two important lessons. First, transitioning to recovery and life after cancer treatment—also referred to as the survivorship period—is a unique part of the cancer control continuum and brings its own set of challenges and opportunities. Second, the cancer experience does not end when treatment ends. Many cancer survivors experience long-term psychosocial concerns, not merely the more obvious physical effects of their illness. Some of these effects develop during active treatment and linger or persist over time, including fatigue, body-image disturbance, altered social and interpersonal relationships, changes in work capacity, and diminished quality of life. This population is also at risk for problems that manifest months or years after treatment ends and are secondary to cancer or its treatment. The most worrisome of these is recurrence or a second cancer, whose events bring a whole new cascade of psychosocial challenges. But long-term adaptation may also require managing fear of recurrence, depression/suicide, infertility, and altered life trajectories (15).

Finishing treatment itself can be stressful. In addition to worry that the cancer will come back when therapy stops, there are concerns about how to cope with the continued effects of the illness. Survivors may find themselves feeling sicker than when they started treatment and uncertain as to what is 'normal' or how to resume life as before. There can be accompanying anxiety about leaving a treatment setting and team where they felt their needs were understood and met. Separation from fellow travellers on their journey—others who shared the treatment experience—can increase a sense of isolation. Who will understand what they have been through at home or be willing to talk with them about their experience? Cancer may even be a taboo topic in the regions where they live. Questions arise about who will provide their ongoing care or what this should look like when they return home. At the same time, family and friends may expect their loved one to come home and be the person they knew before cancer arrived in their lives. All these factors can contribute to making the transition to recovery rocky at best.

At a minimum, receipt of education about what to expect when treatment ends is key. In several high-income countries, one approach to this has been to recommend the development and communication of a survivorship care plan (SCP) (16). The SCP has two main parts: first, treatment summary with details of the tumour characteristics, treatments received, and major complications experienced, and second, a plan for follow-up care that outlines actions needed to monitor for a recurrence/new cancer (surveillance), identification and care for persistent effects of the cancer or its treatment, prevention of adverse late effects including an emphasis on health promotion, and information concerning who will be responsible for, or who to contact regarding, all of the above (Box 20.1) (17). Ideally, the SCP is generated and discussed as part of a transition meeting with the cancer survivor and treating staff. While the document itself is useful for cancer survivors to have as part of their medical record and to share with future healthcare providers responsible for their care, more important is the conversation that accompanies its completion.

Participants in the 5th Breast Health Global Initiative Global Summit outlined a set of recommendations for delivery of supportive care after curative treatment for breast cancer that might be reasonable to provide, depending on the resources available in a

---

Box 20.1 Survivorship Care Plan (SCP) contents per the Institute of Medicine

1. Surveillance for recurrence or new cancer
2. Assessment and treatment or referral for persistent effects (e.g. pain, fatigue, sexual dysfunction, functional impairment, depression, employment issues)
3. Evaluation of risk for and prevention of late effects (e.g. second cancers, cardiac problems, osteoporosis); health promotion
4. Coordination of care (e.g. including frequency of visits, tests and who is performing these)

Source: based on Hewitt ME et al. *From Cancer Patient to Cancer Survivor: Lost in Transition*, Washington DC: The National Academies Press; 2006 (17).

---

certain country. These use breast cancer care as the model, but the content of the re-commendations is readily generalizable to survivorship care for cancer more broadly (see Tables 20.1 and 20.2) (18).

Assisting Health Practitioners to Provide Psychosocial Care—The Role of Guidelines

Evidence presented in this chapter represents a small fraction of the available psy-chosocial research. It is enormously challenging for busy clinicians to keep abreast of emerging research, so clinical practice guidelines can be a helpful aide. Clinical practice guidelines are sets of non-mandatory rules, principles or recommendations for prac-tice based on systematic reviews and critical appraisal of evidence. Guidelines should be developed by a multidisciplinary panel of experts and key stakeholders, and they consider subgroups and patient preferences as necessary. The quality of evidence pre-sented should be rated, and the process for their development should be clearly de-scribed to exclude distortions, biases, and conflicts of interest. In addition, they should be revised as new evidence emerges (see Chapter 9).

Although guidelines in clinical medicine have existed for some decades, they are relatively new in psycho-oncology. The National Comprehensive Cancer Network (NCCN) first launched Distress Management Guidelines in 1997 with the introduction of a Distress Thermometer in which patients rate their distress on a scale from 0 to 10. This was designed to be less stigmatizing than asking about issues such as depression or anxiety. Inclusion of a problem list assists health professionals to recognize and be responsive to the core concerns of the individual.

The first clinical practice guidelines specifically for the psychosocial care of women with breast cancer were launched in Australia in 2000 by the National Breast Cancer Centre, and these were later broadened to encompass the psychosocial concerns of adults with cancer. The guidelines were innovative in that they were designed for use by all members of the treatment team and incorporated recommendations about

Table 20.1 Healthcare delivery issues: health education, community adaptation, and patient support following curative treatment

	Basic	Limited	Enhanced	Maximal
Health professional education[a]	BC recurrence, second primary cancer Long-term TX complications Women's health Psychosocial (survivorship) consideration[c] Lifestyle modifications	Psychosocial risk assessments Psychosocial complications of survivorship Sexual health	Psychosocial screening methods	
Patient and family education[b]	BC recurrence or new cancers; symptoms to report Long-term and late TX complications Appropriate use of CAM Women's health issues Psychosocial issues (survivorship) Lifestyle modifications	Follow-up schedules Adherence to endocrine therapy Sexual health		
Community awareness	Community awareness of BC survivorship issues			
Psychosocial (survivorship)	Patient and family education[b] Psychosocial (survivorship) consideration[c] Peer support by trained BC survivors	Psychosocial assessments, including depression Emotional and social support by health professionals	Screening and referral for depression/distress by mental health specialist Psychosocial counselling by mental health specialists Availability of pharmacotherapy Social service counselling for financial, employment and legal issues	Psychiatrist-, psychologist-, or social worker- coordinated care

The table stratification scheme implies incrementally increasing resource allocation at the basic, limited, and enhanced levels. Maximal level resources should not be targeted for implementation in low- and middle-income countries (LMICs), even though they may be used in some higher-resource settings.

BC, breast cancer; CAM, complementary and alternative medicine; TX, treatment.

[a]The term 'health professional' is used to acknowledge the range in medical and other professionals who provide supportive care services in LMICs. When specialists are identified as a required resource, it is assumed that a specialist has a certification for their area of expertise.

[b]Patient, family and/or partner education may be the primary intervention for some supportive care services.

[c]'Consideration' is a term used in this table to refer to basic patient evaluation through patient–provider interactions, including dialogue, observations, and other appropriate means of evaluation.

Reproduced with permission from Ganz PA et al. 'Supportive care after curative treatment for breast cancer (survivorship care): resource allocations in low- and middle-income countries. A Breast Health Global Initiative 2013 consensus statement.' *Breast.* Volume 22, Issue 5, pp. 606–15. Copyright © 2013 Elsevier Inc. DOI: https://doi.org/10.1016/j.breast.2013.07.049 (18).

Table 20.2 Survivorship issues: long-term complications, lifestyle modifications, monitoring and documentation following curative treatment

	Basic	Limited	Enhanced	Maximal
Long-term treatment-related complications	Patient and family education[b] on long-term TX complications Antibiotics for cellulitis or lymphangitis Basic lymphoedema supplies	PT, OT, CDT for lymphoedema management Fatigue, insomnia management, Pain management	Coordinated care by oncology-trained personnel/nursing staff Custom compression garments	Pneumatic pump Perometer
Women's health[a]	Patient and family education[b] on early menopause, body image	Patient and family education[b] on sexual health Treatment of menopausal symptoms: topical agents and simple behavioural strategies	Pharmacotherapy for menopausal symptoms Breast reconstruction for asymmetry Bone-modifying agents	Clinical assessment and tailored intervention for menopausal symptoms and sexual health
Lifestyle modification	Patient education[b] on diet and exercise	Weight management and daily exercise counselling	Exercise programme Individualized education by nutritionist	Weight management programme
Monitoring	Monitor for BC recurrence, secondary primary cancers Monitor for long-term TX complications	Monitor for endocrine medication adherence		Genetic testing and counselling Screening for high-risk cancers
Documentation	Patient care record (e.g. discharge summary)	Patient treatment summary	Survivorship care plan	

The table stratification scheme implies incrementally increasing resource allocation at the basic, limited, and enhanced levels. Maximal level resources should not be targeted for implementation in low- and middle-income countries, even though they may be used in some higher-resource settings.

BC, breast cancer; CDT, comprehensive decongestive therapy; PT, physiotherapy; OT, occupational therapy; TX, treatment.

[a]Women's health issues for breast cancer patients include menopause, reproductive health, fertility, body image, and sexual health; educational efforts should include partners, as appropriate.

[b]Patient, family and/or partner education may be the primary intervention for some supportive care services.

Reproduced with permission from Ganz PA et al. 'Supportive care after curative treatment for breast cancer (survivorship care): resource allocations in low- and middle-income countries. A Breast Health Global Initiative 2013 consensus statement'. *Breast*. Volume 22, Issue 5, pp. 606–15. Copyright © 2013 Elsevier Inc. DOI: https://doi.org/10.1016/j.breast.2013.07.049 (18).

communication techniques and strategies for non-psychosocial clinicians to explore and respond to anxiety and depression. Since then, many guidelines have been produced including Canadian guidelines providing recommendations about development of psychosocial services and best practice in delivery of supportive care.

The American Society of Clinical Oncology (ASCO) has established a repository of guidelines, many of which represent adaptation or refinement of existing guidelines. The most recent publication relates to patient–clinician communication (19). Although not specific to breast cancer, this guideline was rigorously developed by a multidisciplinary panel and provides recommendations about clinical interactions across all phases of the cancer trajectory. There are clear recommendations about core communication skills and their application in discussions about goals of care and prognosis, treatment options, clinical trials, and engaging family members in care. A major strength of this ASCO guideline is its inclusion of recommendations about training for all those engaged in clinical care of the patient with cancer. It is advocated that training in communication skills should include skills practice and experiential learning with opportunities for role-play and direct observation of patient encounters. Perhaps more critically, the training should foster practitioner self-awareness and include reflection on personal attitudes and beliefs which may affect communication or lead to bias in decision-making. The latest version of the NCCN Distress Management Guidelines provides clear algorithms to assist in evaluation and guide treatment in relation to a range of problems ranging from adjustment disorder, depression, and anxiety, and continues through to delirium, psychosis, and substance-related disorders. These guidelines promote the importance of care by social workers and chaplaincy and provide descriptions of the evidence supporting specific psychotherapeutic interventions such as cognitive behaviour therapy and supportive psychotherapy.

However, the proliferation of guidelines now poses a dilemma for health professionals. As of November 2016, the Guidelines International Network database contained more than 6,000 guidelines, evidence reports, and related documents. Determining which are relevant to clinical practice requires access to databases and the ability to search topics of clinical relevance. For psycho-oncology, these searches are not straightforward. The discipline of psycho-oncology is broader than mental health per se; it is more focused than public health and must incorporate the context of cancer. Accessing relevant reports is thus a complex task.

The nature of the guidelines relevant for psycho-oncology is also different from other guidelines. For example, a guideline about handwashing before and after patient contact targets a specific behaviour/practice by defined practitioners who are likely to readily identify this guideline as relevant to their clinical role. Psycho-oncology advocates a tiered model of care in which only those with higher distress are referred for specialized psychosocial treatment. However, in this model all patients, including those with low or minimal distress, are considered to benefit from good communication of treating health professionals. This includes *all* who have contact with patients (nurses, oncologists, surgeons, etc.). Hence implementation of this recommendation mandates skills development and/or behaviour change in those who may not see this as their 'core business'.

As patient need and distress increase, the tiered model of care recommends more specialized interventions, delivered by psychologist, social worker, or psychiatrist depending on the specific problem, and evidence has been presented in this chapter about the effectiveness of such interventions. However, this requires referral to psycho-social professionals whose role may be unfamiliar, or expertise unclear, to the treating practitioner. Implementation of psychosocial guidelines is thus more complex than recommendation of specific discrete behaviours (such as handwashing) for which the clinician is solely responsible.

Production of guidelines alone does not change practice, and there is an emerging body of research describing the complexity of translating evidence into practice. Implementation strategies need to be tailored across stakeholder groups and to address identified barriers. Changes in mindset are fundamental for systems reform, and local opinion leaders are likely to play an important role in promoting evidence-based practice (20). We still have insufficient understanding of the complex factors affecting clinical decision-making. It is self-evident that familiarity with clinical practice guidelines and professional confidence are likely to lead to enhanced implementation of guideline recommendations. Qualitative research with nurses affirms that implementation should not be regarded as a single-step intervention, and this highlights the importance of ongoing engagement, follow-up, and feedback for all staff who are seen as active participants in the implementation process (21). It is also important to consider the dynamic nature of practice change, and the inherent tension between maintaining what is known and familiar and developing new ways of responding. Clinicians who have participated in communication skills training are likely to be keenly aware that it is not only the acquisition of new knowledge or skills that is necessary, but sometimes it is the 'unlearning' of accustomed habits (22). 'Knowledge tools' that are short, flexible, and focused on the clinical problem raised by the patient may be valuable in assisting clinicians in implementing evidence-based care. However, implementation cannot focus exclusively on individual practitioners and must incorporate awareness of enablers and barriers related to systems, policy-makers, and health care managers.

An area that is currently largely neglected in psycho-oncology is the importance of more robust engagement of patients to advocate for psychosocial care. The National Institute for Health and Care Excellence guidance on overcoming barriers to change notes the importance of engagement with patients as advocates. We have compelling evidence about unmet needs of patients with cancer and their family members across many domains, and there is no doubt that patient expectations and political voice can lead to change. NCCN has launched guidelines for patients on distress, and this represents an important step towards more active patient education and engagement (23). The indispensable role of patient advocates and progress in initiatives to change policy and attitudes towards psychosocial care are described in more detail in the following section.

Progress to Date—Delivery of Psychosocial Care in Europe and Around the World

Translation of evidence into clinical practice requires not just research evidence but also changes in policy and attitudes towards clinical care. At the beginning of the millennium, international initiatives attempted to address this. In 2000, The Charter of Paris promoted awareness of cancer epidemiology (incidence, mortality, and survival) gaps in care and the need to improve these by making use of best science to translate it into better-targeted policies. In February 2000, more than 100 international leaders of government, patient advocacy leaders, cancer research organizations, and corporations met in Paris at the first World Summit Against Cancer. Participants reaffirmed their commitment to the global eradication of cancer, namely to 'prevent and cure cancer, and to maintain the highest quality of life for those living with and dying from this disease', by signing The Charter of Paris Against Cancer (24). As an international initiative, in its ten points, this Charter intended to mobilize efforts and investments to empower those affected by cancer, guarantee their human rights, and improve treatment worldwide. The Charter of Paris is a landmark in the world response to cancer and has set the stage for further actions. February 4th was thus designated 'World Cancer Day.'

This activity led to further initiatives. One was the creation, in 2003, of the European Cancer Patients' Coalition, a federation of cancer patients' organizations across Europe under the motto 'Nothing about us without us!' (http://www.ecpc-online.org). This Coalition began strategic lobbying with the Members of European Parliament and set up an informal all-party forum, Members of European Parliament Against Cancer (the MAC group), as an initiative inside the European Parliament committed to promoting action on cancer as an EU priority. This initiative was supported by the Portuguese and Slovenian EU Presidencies and presented as a priority in the EU health agenda. An important outcome of these joint efforts was the EU Resolution document, *Council Conclusions on Reducing the Burden of Cancer in Europe*, which was signed by the 27 Member States in Luxembourg in June 2008. This document included recognition of the important role of psychosocial oncology in cancer care and led to the launch of the European Partnership for Action Against Cancer (EPAAC) by the President of the European Commission (EC) in 2009. This joint action was co-financed by the EC, Member States, and stakeholders to support Member States and stakeholders in their efforts to respond to cancer more efficiently by providing a framework for identifying and sharing information, best practices, capacity, and expertise in cancer prevention, control, and care (http://www.epaac.eu/).

In Europe, EPAAC has provided an umbrella for the recognition and development of psychosocial oncology care. A Psychosocial Oncology Action integrated in the Healthcare work package mapped the resources of psychosocial care in Europe and piloted a training strategy to improve psychosocial care and communication skills among health care providers in Europe, which was delivered and successfully tested in Romania. An additional deliverable of EPAAC was the *European Guide for Quality National Cancer Control Programmes* (NCCPs), which includes a chapter on Psychosocial Oncology Care, as part of the main components of effective and high-quality NCCPs (4). This chapter discusses the necessary programme elements for quality psycho-oncological care delivery, such as:

- training of health care professionals in the psychosocial aspects of cancer;
- inclusion of routine screening for distress, the 6th vital sign of cancer patients;
- employing evidence-based treatments for symptoms and psychosocial needs identified through screening for distress;
- development of minimum practice standards in psycho-oncology services;
- implementation and integration of psycho-oncology programmes into cancer multidisciplinary teams;
- allocation of funds at the national health system level to ensure that comprehensive cancer care includes psychosocial care as standard.

A set of indicators for psychosocial cancer care was also proposed, to best monitor the services and its resources (Table 20.3) (25):

Table 20.3 Indicators for psychosocial oncology care

Indicators	Core	Additional/ supplementary
Structural	Inclusion of the psychosocial care services for cancer patients in the National Cancer Control Plan. Existence of the psychosocial care services/units in the national healthcare system. Number of psychosocial care professionals working in cancer care services. Continuity in participation of psychosocial care specialists in the multidisciplinary team meetings per service and per hospital treating cancer patients. Inclusion of communication skills training (CST) in curricula and continued professional development programmes for medical doctors and nurses: - undergraduate curricula; - postgraduate curricula; - continued professional development programmes. Inclusion of psychosocial care in curricula and continued professional development programmes for medical doctors and nurses: - undergraduate curricula; - postgraduate curricula; - continued professional development programmes. Having a budget for psychosocial care services.	Number of cancer care facilities with psychosocial care services per number of cancer care facilities in the country. Availability of postgraduate courses and/or MSc courses in psycho-oncology provided by universities.
Process	Proportion of cancer patients that are screened—routinely and on a regular basis—for distress against the number of cases of cancer per year. Proportion of cancer patients that receive psychosocial care.	Cost-offset analyses to clarify benefits.
Outcome	Patient satisfaction. Quality of life.	General wellbeing.

Despite these advances, psychosocial concerns of patients with cancer have been, and still are, too often dismissed or underestimated, and psycho-oncology services are still not yet offered on a regular basis as part of the treatment of cancer patients. This constitutes a major gap in cancer care and the rehabilitation of cancer patients. A recently published study on the psychosocial care resources available in Europe, conducted under the EPAAC, showed that although many European countries include psychosocial oncology care in their NCCPs ($n = 21/27$; 78%), only one-third of those ($n = 10$; 37%) reported having a specific budget for it (25). Moreover, provision of psychosocial care was still found, in many cases, to be under local/hospital or charities/non-governmental organization's budgets and responsibility, mainly available in general or university hospitals and cancer centres, and seldom available in other facilities. The authors concluded that although many countries have referred to psychosocial oncology care in their NCCP, there is still much to do in terms of allocating resources and delivering the care equitably among European countries. Furthermore, they reported that there is a need to promote training and certification in this area as well as to have a national cancer policy that includes a recommendation for the use of existing psychosocial cancer care clinical guidelines.

Likewise, a report conducted by the EC Initiative on Breast Cancer, which focused on the development of a voluntary European quality assurance scheme for breast cancer, identified an irregular landscape regarding the provision of psycho-oncological support for women treated for breast cancer in European Breast Units (26). The report noted that the identified gaps in care could be overcome by making provision of psycho-oncological care a requirement for the accreditation of Breast Units, a goal which the working group plans to pursue.

In early 2017, the Cancer Control in Europe initiative, the last Joint Action co-financed by the EC, EU Member States, and stakeholders, with its many experts in the field, delivered the *European Guide for Quality Improvement in Comprehensive Cancer Control*. A chapter on 'Survivorship and Rehabilitation' refers to the lack of attention and resources in most of the European countries and states that 'the most impeding factors for the quality of cancer follow-up care were poor coordination of care, lack of communication among health care providers, uncertainties about 'who is responsible' for the follow-up care, and occurrence of many psychosocial unmet needs'. The chapter provides a full set of recommendations and guidance on how to provide and implement quality rehabilitation and survivorship care.

A survey conducted worldwide by the IPOS Federation of National Psycho-Oncology Societies reported that about 50% of the countries that already have a National Psycho-Oncology Society do not have psychosocial care integrated into mainstream cancer services. The biggest challenges faced Africa, South America, and South-East Asia concerning non-existing resources or isolated care provision. The better-resourced regions were North America and Australia. Europe is quite diverse, and has a total of 16 IPOS-federated psycho-oncology societies among 44 countries, which is just a little more than one-third of the European countries that have psycho-oncology organized in their country. Even when services do exist, they face funding and workforce shortfalls.

The European and world landscape surveys on psycho-oncology resources report unequivocally that there is a lack of widespread availability of professional psychosocial care, and what is offered varies greatly between regions and countries as well as across continents. Services are linked mostly to the country's income and health budget, and the organization of cancer care, namely, the existence of an effective NCCP as well as accreditation of clinical centres. We have learned that it requires political will to bring about change and improvement in cancer policies, including specialized psychosocial cancer care in treatment plans, treatment guidelines, and its provision in routine cancer care. This may be achieved through joint efforts of public demand and lobbying by psycho-oncology and advocacy organizations.

Key Messages

- A significant number of women diagnosed with breast cancer have a high level of cancer-related distress: as many as 32% of women with early breast cancer and 60% of those with advanced disease.
- High levels of distress have negative consequences for clinical outcomes, quality of life, and wellbeing.
- It is recommended that patients' distress and psychosocial needs be regularly assessed as the 6th Vital Sign and that psychosocial oncology care services be delivered by specialized professionals.
- Psychosocial interventions can have an important benefit in effectively reducing distress and psychological morbidity, and in improving patients' wellbeing and quality of life across all phases of disease and survivorship.
- Psychosocial oncology care guidelines assist clinicians in delivering care and promote standardization of clinical practice through the best available science translated into evidence-based recommendations tailored to patients' needs.
- Psychosocial oncology care is considered one of the main components of effective and high-quality cancer care and of the accreditation of breast cancer units.
- Whereas the quality standard cancer care requires psychosocial care access and availability to cancer patients, there is still a lot to be done to implement it.

References

1. Carlson L et al. High levels of untreated distress and fatigue in cancer patients. *Br J Cancer* 2004;90(12):2297–2304.
2. Mitchell AJ et al. Depression and anxiety in long-term cancer survivors compared with spouses and healthy controls: a systematic review and meta-analysis. *Lancet Oncol* 2013;14(8):721–732.
3. Grassi L and Travado L. The role of psychosocial oncology in cancer care. In Coleman MP et al., editors. *Responding to the Challenge of Cancer in Europe*. Ljubljana: Institute of Public Health; 2008. p. 209–229.

4. Travado L and Dalmas M. Psychosocial oncology care. In Albreht T et al., editors. *European Guide for Quality National Cancer Control Programmes*. National Institute of Public Health, Ljubljana: Slovenia; 2015. p. 35–39.

5. Mosher CE and DuHamel KN. An examination of distress, sleep, and fatigue in metastatic breast cancer patients. *Psychooncology* 2012;21(1):100–107.

6. Holland J et al. The IPOS new International Standard of Quality Cancer Care: integrating the psychosocial domain into routine care. *Psychooncology* 2011;20:677–678.

7. Bultz BD and Carlson LE. Emotional distress: the sixth vital sign in cancer care. *J Clin Oncol* 2005;23(26):6440–6441.

8. Mitchell AJ et al. Identification of patient-reported distress by clinical nurse specialists in routine oncology practice: a multicentre UK study. *Psychooncology* 2011;20:1076–1083.

9. Bultz BD et al. Implementing Screening for Distress, the 6th Vital Sign: a Canadian strategy for changing practice. *Psychooncology* 2011;20(5):463–469.

10. Bruera E et al. The Edmonton Symptom Assessment System (ESAS): a simple method for the assessment of palliative care patients. *J Palliat Care* 1991;7:6–9.

11. Gil F et al. Use of distress and depression thermometers to measure psychosocial morbidity among southern European cancer patients. *Supp Care Cancer* 2005;13(8):600–606.

12. Faller H et al. Effects of psycho-oncologic interventions on emotional distress and quality of life in adult patients with cancer: systematic review and meta-analysis. *J Clin Oncol* 2013;31:782–793.

13. Duijts SFA et al. Effectiveness of behavioral techniques and physical exercise on psychosocial functioning and health-related quality of life in breast cancer patients and survivors—a meta-analysis. *Psychooncology* 2011;20:115–126.

14. Matthews H et al. The efficacy of interventions to improve psychosocial outcomes following surgical treatment for breast cancer: a systematic review and meta-analysis. *Psychooncology* 2017;26:593–607.

15. Andersen BL et al. Screening, assessment, and care of anxiety and depressive symptoms in adults with cancer: an American Society of Clinical Oncology Guideline Adaptation. *J Clin Oncol* 2014;32:1605–1619.

16. Mayer DK et al. Summit it up: an integrative review of studies of cancer survivorship care plans (2006–2013). *Cancer* 2015;121(7):978–996.

17. Hewitt ME et al., editors. *From Cancer Patient to Cancer Survivor: Lost in Transition*. Washington DC: National Academies Press; 2006.

18. Ganz PA et al. Supportive care after curative treatment for breast cancer (survivorship care): resource allocations in low- and middle-income countries. A Breast Health Global Initiative 2013 consensus statement. *Breast* 2013;22(5):606–615.

19. Gilligan T et al. Patient-clinician communication: American Society of Clinical Oncology consensus guideline; *J Clin Oncol* 2017;35(31):3618–3632.

20. Bohmer RMJ. The hard work of health care transformation. *N Engl J Med* 2016;375:709–711.

21. Bahtsevani C et al. Experiences of the implementation of clinical practice guidelines—interviews with nurse managers and nurses in hospital care. *Scand J Caring Sci* 2010;24;514–522.

22. Gupta DM et al. The physician's experience of changing clinical practice: a struggle to unlearn. *Implement Sci* 2017;12:28.

23. National Comprehensive Cancer Network Guidelines for patients. Distress. Available at: https://www.nccn.org/patients/guidelines/distress/files/assets/common/downloads/files/distress.pdf

24. Kerr D. World Summit Against Cancer for the New Millennium: The Charter of Paris. *Ann Oncol* 2000;11:253–254.

25. Travado L et al. Psychosocial oncology care resources in Europe: a study under the European Partnership for Action Against Cancer (EPAAC). *Psychooncology* 2015;26:523–530.

26. Neamțiu L et al. Psycho-oncological support for breast cancer patients: a brief overview of breast cancer services certification schemes and national health policies in Europe. *Breast* 2016;29:178–180.

21

Genetics

Marjanka K. Schmidt, Alexandra J. van den Broek, Mark E. Robson,
Ornella Campanella, and Soo Hwang Teo

Acknowledging: Irene L. Andrulis, Eveline M. Bleiker,
and Fred H. Menko

Genetic Landscape of Breast Cancer

Breast Cancer is Partly a Heritable Disease

The accumulation of somatic mutations in breast tissue leading to the development of breast cancer occurs largely by chance. However, well-established breast cancer risk factors including lifestyle factors, hormonal factors, and germline genetics place women at higher risk of developing breast cancer. About 10–30% of breast cancers are estimated to be explained by known (mostly modifiable) lifestyle and environmental factors such as body mass index and use of hormones; this is population dependent. Based on monozygotic twin studies, it has been estimated that another 20–30% of breast cancers can be explained by germline genetics caused by the specific genetic make-up passed from parents to child (Box 21.1). The remaining risk might be due to rare variants, yet unknown environmental or lifestyle factors, as well as interactions between lifestyle and germline genetic variants.

Genetic Variants
Genetic variants, often called mutations, that a child inherits within the genetic make-up from its parents are called *germline* mutations. Because such a mutation was present in the egg or sperm cell, it is present in all cells throughout the body of the offspring. These mutations define the heritable risk for a disease. Gene mutations that are not inherited from a parent but acquired throughout life are called *somatic* mutations. These mutations can be acquired in any type of cell and can also cause various diseases, cancer being the most common. Another type of somatic mutation acquired early in embryonic development, called *mosaic* mutations, can also cause predisposition for a disease similar to germline mutations but limited to the specific tissues that originated from the embryonic stem cell.

The influence of germline genetics on breast cancer risk is reflected by the strong relationship observed between family history of breast cancer and risk of breast cancer for an unaffected female relative. The incidence of breast cancer in males is low (approximately 1% of all breast cancer cases), but, based on limited data, a larger proportion

---

Box 21.1 Heritable Risk

Genetic *inheritance* is defined as the passing on of the genetic make-up from parents to child. This inherited genetic make-up of persons is also referred to as *germline genetics*. The proportion of variation in a particular disease that is attributable to *germline genetics* is called the *heritability* or *heritable risk* of a disease. For breast cancer, two heritable forms are defined, specifically *familial breast cancer*, which is breast cancer in a family with more (breast) cancers than statistically expected, but no specific pattern of genetic inheritance, and *hereditary breast cancer*, which is breast cancer with an apparent autosomal dominant inheritance. Breast cancer that is likely not due to germline genetics is called *sporadic breast cancer*. Gradually, this concept of a separation between heritable breast cancer and sporadic breast cancer is shifting with the realization that *all* breast cancers have a heritable and a sporadic component.

---

of male breast cancers compared to female breast cancers is thought to be heritable. In Figure 21.1, an example of a breast cancer family pedigree is shown including inheritance through the male line in the middle generation. Although the entire heritable component of breast cancer risk (20–30% of total risk) cannot yet be explained, an increasing number of genetic variants have been identified that account for approximately 40% of this heritable risk (Figure 21.2).

High-Risk BRreast CAncer Genes

The first breast cancer risk genes discovered were BReast CAncer1 and 2. These genes, abbreviated *BRCA1* and *BRCA2* and which harbour pathogenic germline mutations, were discovered in 1990 and 1994 using linkage analysis of a large group of families with cases of early-onset breast cancer. About 3–5% of all breast cancer cases are related to pathogenic germline mutations in the *BRCA1* or *BRCA2* genes, and

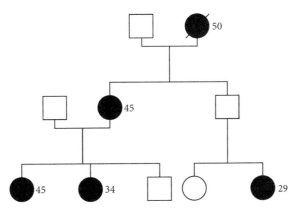

Figure 21.1 Pedigree of a family with familial/hereditary breast cancer. ○: female without breast cancer; ●: female with breast cancer; ◕: female deceased with breast cancer; □: male without breast cancer. Ages at diagnoses of the breast cancer are indicated.

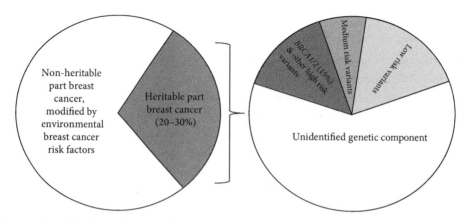

Figure 21.2 The heritable part of breast cancer. Currently, the genetic variants that are identified can explain around 40% of the heritable part of breast cancer by BRCA1/2 and moderate- and low-risk variants. The remaining part is still unexplained.

Reproduced from A. Rudolph et al. 'Gene-environment interaction and risk of breast cancer'. *British Journal of Cancer*, Volume 114, Issue 2, pp. 125–33. Copyright © 2016 Springer Nature Publishing. DOI: 10.1038/bjc.2015.439.

these are estimated to explain around 15% of the total heritable risk of breast cancer (Figure 21.2). In several populations, founder *BRCA1* and *BRCA2* mutations with a higher prevalence have been described. The best-known are founder mutations in the Ashkenazi Jewish population (prevalence approximately 2.5% and accounting for approximately 85% of carriers). However, specific founder mutations in *BRCA1* have also been identified in other populations (accounting for approximately <20% of carriers in those populations), for example the Dutch and Polish populations, and the existence of founder mutations in the Chinese population has also been suggested.

Lifetime risk of developing breast cancer differs among countries (1); for example, the lifetime risk for the general White female population to develop breast cancer in the USA is estimated to be around 12% (2). Carrying a pathogenic germline mutation in the *BRCA1* or *BRCA2* gene leads to a much higher risk for breast cancer. The risk is estimated to be between 27% and 80% by age 70 years with *BRCA2* mutation carriers on the lower end of the range and *BRCA1* mutation carriers on the higher end (3). Relative risks for *BRCA1* and *BRCA2* mutation carriers compared to non-carriers are similar globally, although the absolute risks differ according to differences in population baseline risks. The risk for ovarian cancer is also substantially increased in *BRCA1* (about 44%) and *BRCA2* (about 17%) mutation carriers compared to women not carrying a *BRCA1* or *BRCA2* germline mutation (4). Clinicians should be aware that BRCA pathogenic mutations, specifically *BRCA2*, also predispose to other cancers such as pancreatic and prostate. Specific regions and mutations in *BRCA1* and *BRCA2* may determine a differential relative breast compared to ovarian cancer risk. Moreover, the large inter-individual variability in the risks of breast and ovarian cancer for *BRCA1* and *BRCA2* mutation carriers is also determined by environmental factors and other genetic elements.

Breast Cancer Risk Variants in Other Genes

Through whole-exome analysis of thousands of breast cancer patients from multiplex families, it seems unlikely that there are other high-risk breast cancer genes comparable to *BRCA1* and *BRCA2* with mutations that are relatively frequent (though still rare) in the population. Only a few other, very rare, high-risk genes implicated in multiple cancer syndromes have been identified that also lead to a largely increased breast cancer risk, for example, PTEN and TP53. The remaining part of the heritable risk is more likely explained by variants in genes associated with lower risks (or with high risks but being very rare). Large collaborative efforts using case–control study designs have discovered moderate-risk variants, such as CHEK2 c.1100delC and pathogenic (truncating) variants in PALB2, and low-risk variants, which are predominantly single nucleotide polymorphisms (SNPs) in non-coding regions (Figures 21.2 and 21.3). These SNPs are, in most instances, markers of risk rather than causal factors in themselves. Due to technological developments and increasing availability of large genome-wide association studies, the list of low- and moderate-risk gene variants is still growing. Estimation of the exact associated risks of these variants, and in some instances whether a gene (e.g. *BRIP1*) is truly associated with breast cancer, is also an ongoing effort.

Variants of Unknown Significance

Pathogenic germline mutations in high-risk genes are mostly truncating variants, resulting in aberration or even loss of function of the transcribed protein. Although it is generally accepted that different pathogenic mutations in the same gene may lead to different increases in risk, risks are currently estimated for all such pathogenic mutations together per gene. This is largely because individually BRCA1 and BRCA2 variants are rare, making it very difficult to derive variant-specific prospective risk estimates. In addition, for a large number of variants that do not appear to cause protein truncation, the effect on protein function is unknown or unsure, making it difficult to predict the consequences on cancer risk. Such variants are called 'variants of unknown significance' (VUS). In the *BRCA1* and *BRCA2* genes many VUS have been reported; up to 20% of the BRCA1/2 genetic tests will report VUS. While the majority of studies show that when VUS are classified only a small percentage (<10%) of VUS are upgraded to being potentially pathogenic, these remain reported as VUS, because the misinterpretation of VUS can lead to clinical harm for women and their families (5).

Breast Cancer Risk Prediction

As discussed above in this chapter, mutations in the *BRCA1* and *BRCA2* genes lead to a high-risk of breast cancer, and the mutation status of unaffected family members can be used for breast cancer risk prediction in healthy individuals. However, for families

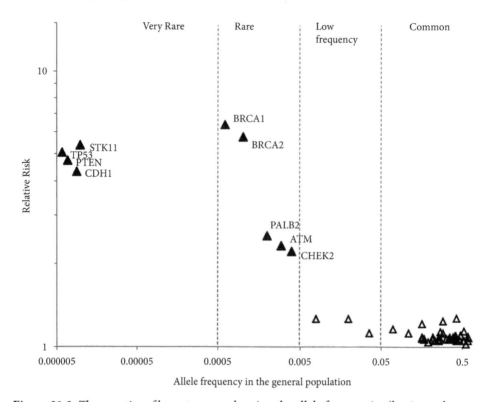

Figure 21.3 The genetics of breast cancer showing the allele frequencies (horizontal axis) and risk distributions (vertical axis) for breast cancer risk variants, for which risk estimation has been established. Allele frequencies: very rare (<0.05%); rare (0.05–0.5%); low frequency (0.5–5%); common (>5%). The variants mentioned here refer to pathogenic variants (mostly truncating) in those genes.

Source: This figure is a moving target; at time of publication the most recent list of common variants was available from Michailidou et al. 'Association analysis identifies 65 new breast cancer risk loci.' Nature. Volume 551: pp. 92–94. Copyright © 2017, Springer Nature Publishing. DOI: 10.1038/nature24284.

with (multiple) cases of cancer, even when no pathogenic variant in these genes is detected, persons can still be at increased risk of breast cancer due to a mutation in a gene that was not tested, or, more likely, a polygenic heritable component that is not (yet) known. There are many families (60–80% depending on referral setting) in which multiple relatives are affected by breast cancer but no known high-penetrance mutation is found. In these families, the number of relatives with breast cancer in a family and the age at diagnosis of the cancers (cancers with a heritable component more often occur at younger ages) are the main components used to estimate the breast cancer risk for healthy woman.

To estimate a person's breast cancer risk, risk prediction models have been developed. Depending on the model and the population, these models include germline genetic status, family history, and possibly lifestyle and environmental factors as well as mammographic density. Although generally applicable to all women, the models have mostly been developed for healthy women who have relatives with breast cancer and who are BRCA1 and BRCA2 mutation negative or not tested. The most important component of all these risk prediction models is examining the pedigree of a woman (Figure 21.1), as family history of cancer remains the most significant predictor of breast cancer risk. Such use of family history information is important, particularly in low- and middle-income countries, where genetic testing might not be as widely available. Also, without genetic testing information, by using among others the family history of a person, an adequate prediction may be made using risk prediction models (6).

There is a large diversity in breast cancer risk prediction models; some are published as software packages or online tools. Examples include the Tyrer–Cuzick model, Gail model (7), and the BOADICEA model (8). Validation studies have shown that the (referred) Tyrer–Cuzick model as well as the BOADICEA model perform well, although improvements continue to be made. Performance of each model depends on whether appropriate calibration has been conducted in the population, and, clearly, choosing the right risk model is important, since the output of the different models could vary even for an identical pedigree. Unfortunately, most of these models are not yet suitable for populations from non-European descent. In Europe, the BOADICEA model is the most widely used and best validated for the clinical genetics setting. BOADICEA also includes risk estimates for other genes such as CHEK2 and ATM (8). Future challenges include being able to provide better dynamic models, which show changing risks with increasing age and changing lifestyle risk factors and, then, keeping these models up to date. For the western population, it is likely that the two factors most likely to affect the performance of the model are the increasing population age-specific incidence of breast cancer and the decreasing sizes of families.

Genetic Counselling and Testing

A woman who is at increased risk of breast cancer, determined by an (extensive) family history of cancer or young age at breast cancer diagnosis, should be referred for genetic counselling. Referral can be done by any treating physician. Although referral guidelines for genetic counselling differ among countries throughout the world, they are all based on family history and age with minor differences in the details (9). Other indications are strongly associated with being a BRCA1 and BRCA2 carrier and are also used for referral for genetic counselling. These include being a member of a population with a high incidence of BRCA1 founder mutations such as Ashkenazi Jewish, having bilateral breast cancer or both breast and ovarian cancer, having a triple-negative breast cancer (oestrogen receptor and progesterone receptor and HER2/NEU negative), and having male breast cancer. In the USA all male breast cancer patients are candidates for referral to the Clinical Genetic Centre.

At Clinical Genetic Centres, specialized physicians (clinical geneticists) and genetic counsellors estimate the a-priori probability of a woman carrying a breast cancer-causing or -associated mutation, and they provide counselling on whether genetic testing is appropriate. In most countries, testing is criteria-based, i.e. a threshold for genetic testing of ≥10% a-priori probability of carrying a BRCA1 or BRCA2 mutation. Several breast cancer risk prediction models, such as the BOADICEA or BCRCAPRO, can also assess the a-priori probability of being carrier of a BRCA1 or BRCA2 mutation.

Although genetic testing has previously only included the *BRCA1* and *BRCA2* genes, increasingly, other genes such as *PALB2, TP53* have been included. In some countries, testing for specific founder mutations such as the medium risk CHEK2 c.1100delC mutation have already been introduced. With the advent of less expensive genetic testing methods, gene panel testing is now being implemented, and these often include genes for which the association with breast or other cancer risk may not be well defined. It is best practice that clinical genetic centres are appropriately supported by a certified laboratory with either the automated pipelines or the appropriately trained laboratory clinical genetic specialists to assure the appropriate selection of genes to be tested and the right classification of the detected germline variants. For the classification of variants (see 'Variants of Unknown Significance'), a resource was built to gather all information on variants, and several decision-support software programmes exist (10). The result should be communicated in an unequivocal letter to the counsellor, who should discuss the outcome with the counselee. Counselees should discuss the outcome of the testing with their family, but, for example in the Netherlands, the counsellors are increasingly proactive in approaching family members with the consent of the counselee with the test result. Notably, genetic counselling and testing services are currently underdeveloped in low- and middle-income countries, including in many parts of South America, Africa, and Asia (11).

When to Test?

The timing of genetic counselling and testing of healthy women is of course dependent on the manifestation of a family history of breast cancer and a woman's age. Hereditary breast cancer rarely manifests before age 20–30 years, so counselling will not change screening and follow-up recommendations before then. Some countries have introduced preimplantation genetic testing for BRCA1/2 mutations to give BRCA1/2 mutation carriers the opportunity to conceive children without passing on the BRCA1/2 mutation. However, there is still limited consensus with respect to preimplantation or prenatal genetic testing for BRCA1/2 mutations.

For BRCA1 or BRCA2 carriers who have developed breast or ovarian cancer, having the genetic testing results could help determine treatment choices including choice of surgery or chemotherapy for breast cancer or the choice of chemotherapy or targeted therapy for ovarian cancer. Since it is possible to generate DNA test results quickly after diagnosis, this has led to the concept of 'rapid genetic testing', or 'treatment-focused genetic testing'. Rapid genetic testing provides a window of opportunity for the counselling and genetic test results to guide the choice of surgery and systemic treatment. Moreover, given that there is currently insufficient capacity for genetic counselling services to meet future demands of genetic testing in the current infrastructure, it has become critical to review the mode of delivery of genetic counselling and genetic testing from conventional clinical genetics services to surgical and oncological departments. A new trend for providing genetic testing is called mainstreaming. Only when a genetic test is 'positive' will the patient be referred for counselling by a genetic specialist. Although mainstreaming can lead to increasing access to genetic testing and other advantages of this approach have been identified, there are also several challenges. Among others, the education of non-geneticists to ensure appropriate information and support is provided when offering a genetic test, plus a solid infrastructure to ensure all patients with a 'positive' test or complex case are referred. The first implementation programmes are currently underway, with pioneering programmes in the UK (http://www.mcgprogramme.com/), Australia, and Malaysia (12).

Advice Based on the Testing Result

The results of a genetic test, positive or negative, are used to inform the assessment of breast cancer risk of the referred person and her family, preferably using up-to-date breast cancer risk prediction models (see 'Breast cancer risk prediction'). Based on this assessment of risk, further counselling will be provided. Advice will be provided regarding preventive measures to decrease the breast cancer risk, such as intensified surveillance (screening) or prophylactic risk-reducing surgery of the breasts (and/or ovaries and tubes to reduce the risk of ovarian cancer). The counsellor also discusses and recommends that all family members of a high-risk family, who might also be at increased breast cancer risk, are informed. In the future, with more personalized risk estimations on their way, each family member may receive their own risk estimates including other personal genetic and lifestyle factors.

The advice given to women is based on the estimated risk, the woman's age, and taking the woman's preferences into account. The process of counselling, but also the guidelines on how to deal with different estimated risks, differ among countries (National Institute of Health and Care Excellence guidelines in the UK, https://www.nice.org.uk/; Dutch guidelines, http://www.oncoline.nl/). In Table 21.1 a simplified example is given of the Dutch guidelines.

Women with a very high estimated lifetime risk for breast cancer, such as BRCA1 and BRCA2 mutation carriers, can, instead of intensified surveillance, also choose prophylactic risk-reducing bilateral breast mastectomy as an option to manage their breast cancer risk. After a risk-reducing mastectomy the risk for breast cancer falls to less than 1% (13). Uptake of prophylactic mastectomy is high among high-risk women, certainly when carrying a BRCA1 and BRCA2 mutation, but differs between countries. These differences may in part be explained by differences in attitudes towards

Table 21.1 Simplified version of the Dutch recommendations of surveillance for familiar breast cancer and hereditary breast cancer (Breast Cancer Guideline, NABON 2012: http://www.oncoline. nl/; revision 2017)

Risk category	Estimated lifetime risk	Starting age screening (years)	Interval (years)	Surveillance method
Familial breast cancer—slightly increased risk	<20%	50–75	2	Mammogram[a]
Familial breast cancer—moderately increased risk	20–30%	40–50	1	Mammogram
		50–75	2	Mammogram[a]
Familial breast cancer—strongly increased risk	>30%	35–60	1	Clinical breast examination and mammogram
		60–75	2	Mammogram[a]
Hereditary breast cancer—BRCA1 or those with 50% probability of carrying a mutation	>40%	25–40	1	Clinical breast examination and MRI
		40–60	1	Clinical breast examination and MRI and mammogram (every 2 years)
		60–75	1	Clinical breast examination and mammogram
Hereditary breast cancer—BRCA2 or those with 50% probability of carrying a mutation; PTEN; STK11; ATM c.7271T→G	>40%	25–30	1	Clinical breast examination and MRI
		30–60	1	Clinical breast examination and MRI and mammogram
		60–75	1	Clinical breast examination and mammogram
Hereditary breast cancer—CHEK2, without additional family history	20–30%	40–50	1	Mammogram
		50–75	2	Mammogram[a]
Hereditary breast cancer—CHEK2, with additional family history	>30%	35–60	1	Clinical breast examination and mammogram
		60–75	2	Mammogram[a]

[a]Dutch population screening programme; available for all Dutch women.

risk-reducing surgery between physicians in different countries. When considering prophylactic risk-reducing surgery many factors should be considered such as the estimated breast cancer risk, options for surveillance and thereby early detection, the advantages but also disadvantages of the surgery and possible breast reconstruction, and psychosocial aspects (such as negative body image and problems with sexual functioning) (14). Specifically, for BRCA1 and BRCA2 mutation carriers, salpingo-oophorectomy to reduce ovarian cancer risk should be part of the risk management strategy.

Challenges to Deal with Findings in Genes Other than *BRCA1* and *BRCA2*

With all of the technical advances of sequencing in recent years, gene panel testing has been developed, which enables simultaneous testing for mutations in a set of multiple genes. There are several commercially available multigene testing panels for breast cancer. These multigene panels include not only genes for which the clinical impact has been established (e.g. BRCA1, BRCA2, TP53, and CHEK2; see Figure 21.2), but also many genes for which the clinical significance is not yet established. One such gene, included in many of the multigene breast cancer panels, is *BRIP1*. *BRIP1* was previously considered to be a gene related to breast cancer risk; however, recent studies showed it to be unlikely that mutations in this gene lead to an increased overall breast cancer risk. Due to the decreasing costs of sequencing, it is expected that the use of these multigene panels will soon become widespread. Multigene panels have already started entering the care system, though ideally this should only be done when all essential questions regarding the interpretation of the results have been answered. Moreover, high rates of VUS (see 'Variants of Unknown Significance') up to 30% have been reported using multigene panels.

Notably, there is currently no evidence on the impact of increased screening or prophylactic risk-reducing surgery on carriers of other genes, and the evidence is largely based on BRCA-negative carriers with strong family history of breast cancer. Moreover, there is evidence that risk-reducing mastectomy only appears to reduce cancer risk with no apparent difference in (short-term) mortality in BRCA1 and BRCA2 carriers. In this context, advice regarding prophylactic risk-reducing surgeries is increasingly complicated because of a lack hitherto of accurate information regarding absolute risk of cancer, the impact of family history of cancer on cancer risk, and the lack of robust methods for characterization of variants in these genes. For example, without a family history of breast cancer, the lifetime risk of breast cancer for CHEK2 c.1100delC mutation carriers is estimated to be around 20%, whereas this is higher in the context of a family with a history of breast cancer in which other genetic components add up to the risk of around 35–55%. In addition, novel variants in CHEK2 or, for example, ATM have not yet been evaluated for their clinical significance. This is similar to the VUS in the *BRCA1* and *BRCA2* genes; those VUS are identified during genetic testing, but the clinical implications of such a variant are often largely unknown as there are no robust functional assays for these genes. Even more so, specifically age-dependent risk estimates are important, because those are needed to tailor advice regarding screening and preventive measures. These estimates are lacking even more for many of the newly discovered risk genes.

Nevertheless, multigene panel testing could eventually make a useful contribution to predict woman's risk of breast cancer, but robust evidence and clinical validation are first needed for all the genes included in such a panel. Currently, end-users should be aware of the limitations that still exist with many of these panels.

Risk Communication

Appropriate communication of breast cancer risks to women and their relatives will ensure informed decision-making about possible intensified follow-up and/or prophylactic surgeries. How to communicate and make risks interpretable for women is a challenge and consequently an evolving field of research (15,16). In general, patients tend to forget or incorrectly recall medical information. The support of written information, including pictograms to visualize risks, will lead to better recall than spoken information alone. However, it is not so much the recall of actual risk that is related to the impact on the experienced distress and risk-reducing behaviour, but more the interpretation of these risks, i.e. the perceived risk. These risk perceptions are heavily influenced by personal experience with breast cancer as well as the experiences of first- and second-degree relatives who succumbed to the disease. Thus, the perceived risk may be the motivator in risk-reducing surgery, more than the actual risk estimates themselves. Therefore, counsellors should be aware of the individual interpretation of the cancer risk more than the correct recall of the actual risk.

Germline Genetics *and* Breast Cancer Treatment Decisions

Next to having implications for the lifetime breast cancer risk, counselling and genetic testing results might also have implications for treatment options for patients diagnosed with breast cancer. Since rapid genetic testing has been available in many countries, treatment decisions can be made from the genetic test results. For example, patients who carry BRCA1 and BRCA2 pathogenic mutations have a 10–20% 10-year risk of developing a second breast cancer in the other breast, i.e. contralateral breast cancer, compared to a 4% risk for non-carriers. Because of this increased risk, some women opt for direct preventive surgery in addition to their breast cancer treatment. Patients with BRCA1 often have breast cancers with aggressive biological features that are less commonly seen in tumours arising in patients without the mutations, making them prone to a worse survival (17). It has also been suggested that mutations in BRCA1 or BRCA2 make tumours more sensitive to adjuvant chemotherapy. Novel chemotherapeutic agents, the poly(ADP-ribose) polymerase (PARP) inhibitors, are a promising treatment strategy that has been approved for the treatment of ovarian cancer in BRCA1 and BRCA2 mutation carriers, and results in breast cancer are encouraging. Because of the expanding role of germline genetics in treatment decisions for patients, including a clinical geneticist in the multidisciplinary breast team is of great importance and will become even more relevant in the future with the evolving developments in this field.

The Role of Patient Organizations; Empowering Patient Decision-Making

One of the main goals of patient organizations is to raise awareness on familial and/ or hereditary breast and ovarian cancer among patients and their relatives, doctors, nurses, and other professionals, but also among the general population. Patient organizations have traditionally provided a supporting role for patients, but their activities are constantly developing and evolving.

The ABRCAdaBRA Story

ABRCADABRA was born on Facebook in 2015. A 'closed group' with specific criteria to be accepted as a member was set up. The criteria to become a member included carrying a BRCA1/2 germline mutation, carrying a VUS in a BRCA gene, having a high prevalence of breast and/or ovarian cancer within the family, and cases of male breast cancer waiting for their genetic test result. Italian women met during a conference on breast cancer in young women. Experiences were shared about critical issues on Italian management of high-risk patients, and it was pointed out that Italy did not yet have advocacy activity in the 'BRCA' field. Then, the 'closed group' on Facebook was opened and named: 'BRCA1–BRCA2 NAZIONALE ITALIANO'. It is now a very active group counting more than 850 members, mostly women and a few men. The group is very interactive and creates a wonderful connection among women from every part of Italy, from the North to the South. They share experiences and emotions and ask questions and investigate any personal and sometimes intimate aspects that are not so easy to discuss even with physicians.

Being a BRCA mutation carrier has multiple aspects that need to be investigated and explained to each woman. It has many effects on a relationship, and sometimes it can influence the desire for motherhood (for the fear of passing on the mutation to children). Being a BRCA mutation carrier very often means that you need to live with the 'Syndrome of the Sword of Damocles', living with the constant fear of getting breast or ovarian cancer, who knows if or when. After Angelina Jolie came out for being a BRCA mutation carrier, many authors, journalists, and physicians gave their 'personal opinion' about her decisions which influence the choice of women and the general opinion and the common sense on this delicate topic. A BRCA mutation carrier needs to be strictly followed and accompanied by a team of experts such as breast surgeons, psychologists, and geneticists, before doing the test and after the results are obtained.

The possibility of undergoing prophylactic surgery to reduce the risk of breast and ovarian cancer significantly during one's lifetime needs to be well explained and discussed with women and their family (for example, the husband). It is an irreversible type of surgery, and bilateral mastectomy is not a 'cosmetic surgery': it changes the breast forever and it impacts the perception of the body. Women need to know that they will lose body sensation in the breast and the nipple, and that the breast remains cold and hard to the touch, especially in case of breast implants. If a woman and her partner are not well informed, this could create negative outcomes in the quality of life. And what about bilateral oophorectomy? It reduces the risk of ovarian cancer significantly, but, especially for younger women, it means entering early menopause with all the well-known side-effects: vaginal dryness, loss of libido, hot flushes, and rejection of maternity. So, reducing breast and ovarian cancer risk with prophylactic surgery has many objective side-effects that need to be well explained to allow a conscious choice by women.

From the virtual world with the group on Facebook, BRCA1-BRCA2 NAZIONALE ITALIANO moved into the real world and founded the first national patient advocacy association focused on BRCA mutation carriers called 'aBRCAdaBRA'. The most important goal of this association is to work closely with clinical experts focused on high-risk women and men and their families, thereby improving the management of this special patient population and giving voice to the needs of BRCA mutation carriers. In less than one year, aBRCAdaBRA met with women, citizens, and the press to explain the real meaning of BRCA mutation and about not placing too much trust in a lot of false statements about the role of risk-reducing surgery, health care professionals, geneticists, breast surgeons, oncologists, gynaecologists, and psychologists to increase the culture of knowledge by giving all women the chance to discover whether they are BRCA mutation carriers. aBRCAdaBRA worked with other relevant organizations such as Europa Donna. Well-informed women will choose the better solution for them: risk-reducing surgery or surveillance. aBRCAdaBRA hopes that in the future nobody will choose for women; rather, let women decide for themselves. aBRCAdaBRA advocates that knowledge is power!

The Future of Breast Cancer Genetics

A part of heritable breast cancer risk has been explained (Figure 21.2). More genes and variants are discovered every year, and these explain an increasing part of the heritable risk. The variants that have been discovered over the last decade have mostly led to only a small increase in risk (Figure 21.3, lower right corner). However, combining information from many low-risk variants can be of clinical significance. 'Polygenic Risk Scores' (PRS) have been developed for breast cancer that stratify breast cancer risk in women, both in those with and without a family history of breast cancer. For example, a study by the Breast Cancer Association Consortium indicated that the lifetime risk of breast cancer for women in the lowest and highest quintiles of the 77-SNP PRS are 5.2% and 16.6% for a woman without family history, and are 8.6% and 24.4% for a woman with a first-degree relative with breast cancer. Including this information in risk prediction models can be very valuable for cancer risk prediction. It should be noted that in research many more genes and variants, in addition to those discussed above, are identified and being tested for an association with breast cancer risk. Although of great interest, these variants are not yet applicable for clinical use, though they may be in the future.

Population-Based Genetic Testing

Currently, genetic testing and breast cancer risk prediction is mainly done for high-risk individuals and families in the clinical genetic setting. Population-based genetic testing for cancer susceptibility, independent of family history, has currently only been done for BRCA1 and BRCA2 germline mutations in defined population subgroups with a high incidence of founder mutations. Extending population-based genetic testing to non-founder populations creates considerable financial and infrastructural challenges, but is already being considered (18). As more information for more accurate breast cancer risk prediction becomes available and testing methods become cheaper, it might be of interest to use broader genetic information for breast cancer risk prediction in the general population. Risk stratification based on genetic information could, for example, inform population-based screening programmes. The first risk-based screening programmes are already being tested in the research setting: women who elect to participate will receive a comprehensive risk assessment (including, for example, the standard non-genetic risk factor assessment and genetic testing of low-risk variants). Their risk profiles will then be used to personalize screening frequency: very low-risk women will be offered less frequent screening schedules whereas women at high risk would receive enhanced surveillance and prevention options (19).

When developing infrastructures for population-based genetic testing for (breast) cancer susceptibility, the question arises: why not exploit the powerful genetic testing techniques now available and examine the whole genome instead of (a set of) selected genes? Single gene testing implemented in clinical practice is currently moving to multiple gene panel testing; a subsequent move to whole exome or genome testing is expected. Breast cancer susceptibility genes will then be embedded in a more comprehensive programme of population-based genetic testing for many genes/variants related to different diseases. The costs of whole exome/genome sequencing are falling, and discussions are ongoing about all aspects of implementing whole exome/genome genetic testing in screening of newborns (20), who then might benefit from personalized prevention and treatment during their lifetimes. One of the larger criticisms is that information relevant later in life would be revealed early. Storage of data and release of parcels of information during life would be preferable, but this generates the need for storage and protection of large amounts of sensitive data and appropriate infrastructures. Important limitations also include our current ability to integrate comprehensive genetic information into clinical care. For example, not all data generated can or should be used; filtering will need to make sure that only results will be generated for genes/variants for which risk interpretations are stable and clinical applicability is clear. Even more so, the knowledge base continues to grow with the discovery of new genes/variants and updated risk information, showing the need for a pipeline which is regularly updated. Moreover, the number of incidental findings, which generates discussions about the 'right not to know' and the amount of information becoming available, substantially surpasses our current experience. The limitations discussed regarding genetic testing in high-risk families apply far more to population-based genetic testing. Risks will be smaller, risk differences will be subtler, and decisions that need to be made based on that information become even more complicated. Several other points should be considered; the cost-effectiveness, the need for well-trained professionals and infrastructures for counselling and communication of the results, and the burden for healthy persons to receive and comprehend all of this information.

Direct-to-Consumer Genetic Testing

Even though there are still many considerations and challenges related to population-based genetic testing, direct-to-consumer genetic testing is already available. Traditionally, genetic tests have only been available through healthcare providers. However, in the last decade, direct-to-consumer genetic testing has also been made available through commercial companies. These genetic tests are marketed directly to consumers and allow any person to have part or their full genome sequenced without consultation with, and supervision by, a health care professional. All the limitations discussed regarding genetic testing are also applicable to this situation, and a consumer is vulnerable to being misled by the results of unproven or invalid tests. They may receive incomplete, incorrect, and unclear information about their health. Genetic testing provides only one piece of information about a person's health, but many other factors affect a person's risk. These factors are discussed during a consultation with a healthcare professional, but are potentially not addressed with direct-to-consumer testing.

Because of the potential hazards related to direct-to-consumer genetic testing, the US Food and Drug Administration (FDA) restricts commercial companies from offering direct-to-consumer genetic tests that function as diagnostic/health tests, until they have been analytically or clinically validated. In 2017, the FDA allowed marketing of the first direct-to-consumer genetic test that provided diagnostic information, but only for certain conditions (https://www.fda.gov/NewsEvents/Newsroom/PressAnnouncements/ucm551185.htm; date: 6 April 2017). Soon after in 2018, the FDA authorized the first direct-to-consumer test that reports three mutations in the BRCA genes, related to an increased breast cancer risk, therefore with significant medical consequences (https://www.fda.gov/NewsEvents/Newsroom/PressAnnouncements/ucm599560.htm; date: 6 March 2018). In contrast to the situation in the USA, the regulatory framework in Europe is fragmented due to lack of

European Union or national legislation, and substantial differences exist among individual countries. Efforts are being made for harmonization of the regulation in Europe in a new version of the European Commission's In Vitro Diagnostics directive (which will come into force in 2022), but it is not likely that this will include mandatory medical supervision, rather it will only regulate the performance and safety (21). Even so, whereas in many countries commercial companies are not allowed to offer diagnostic tests directly to the consumer without medical supervision, companies still can provide persons their genetic information by including simple authorization by any physician (but market the test to consumers), or may provide customers with the raw genotyping data (without clinical interpretation). Interpretation of the raw data can be requested through third-party companies, but this has been shown to be highly sensitive for false positives and misinterpretation of variants in genes with potential clinical impact. Due to these potential hazards, there is an ongoing debate about the balance between medical paternalism, protecting people from the hazards of direct-to-consumer genetic testing, and individuals' right to obtain information about themselves.

Key Messages

- Around 20–30% of breast cancers are explained by genetic inheritance.
- Genetic variants now identified explain around 40% of this heritable component.
- Variants in the high-risk genes *BRCA1* and *BRCA2* explain around 15% of breast cancers; the remaining 25% are explained by more recently identified variants in medium- and low-risk genes.
- Clinical implications of most variants, certainly those in medium- and low-risk genes, are largely unknown.
- Even in known breast cancer risk genes, VUS remain.
- Women at high-risk of developing breast cancer, who are currently still identified mainly through a family history of cancer or who are young at diagnosis, should be referred for genetic counselling and testing.
- Online risk prediction tools are available for prediction of breast cancer risk.
- Advice about risk-reducing strategies, such as intensified surveillance or prophylactic risk-reducing surgery of the breasts, should be given to patients based on the estimated breast cancer risk and taking patient preferences into account.
- Multigene panels are upcoming and should be critically viewed for content and use.
- Infrastructures for implementation of population-based genetic testing are under development.
- Direct-to-consumer genetic testing by commercial companies fuels the debate about medical paternalism and protecting people from the hazards of this direct-to-consumer genetic testing versus individuals' right to obtain information about themselves.

References

1. Ferlay J et al. GLOBOCAN 2012 VI .0, Cancer incidence and mortality worldwide: IARC CancerBase No. I. Lyon, France: International Agency for Research on Cancer; 2013. Available from: http://globocan.iarc.fr/Pages/fact_sheets_cancer.aspx

2. Howlader N et al. SEER Cancer Statistics Review (CSR), 1975–2013. Available from: http://seer.cancer.gov/csr/1975_2013/sections.html

3. IBIS software (Tyrer–Cuzick model). Available from: http://www.ems-trials.org/riskevaluator/

4. Kuchenbaecker KB et al. Risks of breast, ovarian, and contralateral breast cancer for BRCA1 and BRCA2 mutation carriers. *JAMA* 2017;317:2402–2416.

5. Eccles DM et al. BRCA1 and BRCA2 genetic testing-pitfalls and recommendations for managing variants of uncertain clinical significance. *Ann Oncol* 2015;26:2057–2065.

6. Garcia-Closas M et al. Combined associations of genetic and environmental risk factors: implications for prevention of breast cancer. *J Nat Cancer Inst* 2014;106(11):pii: dju305.

7. Breast Cancer Risk Assessment Tool. Available from: https://bcrisktool.cancer.gov/

8. BOADICEA—Centre for Cancer Genetic Epidemiology. Available from: http://ccge.medschl.cam.ac.uk/boadicea/

9. Lee AJ et al. Incorporating truncating variants in PALB2, CHEK2, and ATM into the BOADICEA breast cancer risk model. *Genet Med* 2016;18:1190–1198.

10. Hampel H et al. A practice guideline from the American College of Medical Genetics and Genomics and the National Society of Genetic Counselors: referral indications for cancer predisposition assessment. *Genet Med* 2015;17:70–87.

11. Rehm HL et al. ClinGen—the clinical genome resource. *N Eng J Med* 2015;372:2235–2242.

12. Mainstreaming Cancer Genetics. Available from: http://www.mcgprogramme.com/

13. Ormond KE et al. Genetic counseling globally: where are we now? *Am J Med Genet* 2018;178:98–107.

14. Hartmann LC and Lindor NM. The role of risk-reducing surgery in hereditary breast and ovarian cancer. *N Engl J Med* 2016;374:454–468.

15. Mendes A et al. How communication of genetic information within the family is addressed in genetic counselling: a systematic review of research evidence. *Eur J Hum Genet* 2016;24:315–325.

16. Stellamanns J et al. Visualizing risks in cancer communication: a systematic review of computer-supported visual aids. *Patient Educ Couns* 2017;100(8):1421–1431.

17. Schmidt MK et al. Breast cancer survival of BRCA1/BRCA2 mutation carriers in a hospital-based cohort of young women. *J Natl Cancer Inst* 2017;109(8):329.

18. Manchanda R et al. Cost-effectiveness of population-based BRCA1, BRCA2, RAD51C, RAD51D, BRIP1, PALB2 mutation testing in unselected general population women. *J Natl Cancer Inst* 2018;110(7):714–725.

19. Shieh Y et al. Breast cancer screening in the precision medicine era: risk-based screening in a population-based trial. *J Natl Cancer Inst* 2017;109(5):djw290.

20. Howard HC et al. Whole-genome sequencing in newborn screening? A statement on the continued importance of targeted approaches in newborn screening programmes. *Eur J Hum Genet* 2015;23:1593–1600.

21. Kalokairinou L et al. Legislation of direct-to-consumer genetic testing in Europe: a fragmented regulatory landscape. *J Commun Genet* 2018;9:117–132.

PART 6

HEALTH INFORMATION
TECHNOLOGY

22

Improving Treatment Value Using Health Information Technology

Roma Maguire, Antonio Ponti, and Fernando Suarez

Introduction

Advances in diagnostics and treatment in addition to a rapidly ageing population are putting an unprecedented strain on care services across the globe. There is an urgent need to transform and modernize the way care is delivered in order to meet the needs of our society now and in the future. The triple aims of care (better health, better care, lower cost) still prevail; however, we need to think about how we can deliver care more intelligently and, importantly, at a pace to meet these increasing demands.

Advances in information and communication technology offer a means of providing solutions to the significant challenges that we face and crucially act as a mechanism to enable and sustain much-needed system transformations. Technologies are constantly developing, advancing, and becoming smarter. Devices such as smart phones and sensor technologies are growing in availability and reducing in price. Increasingly large and diverse data-systems are integrated, from DNA sequencing to electronic health records and the linkage of large medical or non-medical databases built for other, often administrative, purposes (1,2).

Connected Health

The field of 'connected health' has emerged in response to this significant demand and pervasiveness of information and communication technology within all aspects of our society. Connected health is defined by Richardson as 'patient-centred care resulting from process-driven health care delivery undertaken by healthcare professionals, patients and/or carers who are supported by the use of technology (software and/or hardware)' (3). It is a virtual ecosystem of care that extends beyond the confines of physical health-care establishments and which uses deepening technology integration, information exchange, data analytics, and advances in genomics to intelligently support citizens and patients to stay well within their communities for as long as possible and, importantly, quickly access services in times of need.

While the vision of 'connected health' has significant potential to transform and revolutionize the ways in which healthcare is delivered now and in the future, we need to be cognizant of preventing information overload and, importantly, identifying what information we need, and in what format, to optimize and enable the delivery of this model of care.

For example, in the field of breast cancer in 2017 there were more than 20,000 papers published on this subject alone, and 250 of those papers were on breast cancer clinical trials. Furthermore, the number of publications on genomics and breast cancer grew from one thousand between 2005 and 2010 to more than two thousand between 2011 and 2016. While this explosion in the amount of research has led to advancements in our understanding of cancer and by extension to better treatments, it has also created the problem of cognitive overload for clinicians.

In the field of genomics, the advancements and clinical adoption of DNA sequencing technologies have had an impact on the cost of sequencing. The cost of a complete human exome has fallen below US$1,000 and will most likely fall below US$100 in the near future (Figure 22.1) (4–6). As the field of cancer moves from genomics to 'panomics', the amount of data is only going to grow, so making sense of and visualizing the data will be a challenge in coming years. The positive impact that this will have on patient treatment and care, however, will be unprecedented. Today there are more than 200 drugs with pharmacogenomics information on their label, and about a third of those are for oncology (6). Moreover, 73% of drugs currently in development have the potential to become personalized treatments (8).

All these advancements in the field of oncology are being enhanced by significant developments in the field of information and communications technology and data

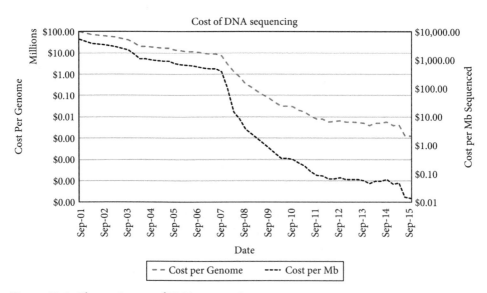

Figure 22.1 Change in cost of DNA sequencing.

Source: Data from: National Human Genome Research Institute. DNA Sequencing Costs: Data. Available from: https://www.genome.gov/sequencingcostsdata/; Lyman GH et al. Impact of a 21-gene RT-PCR assay on treatment decisions in early-stage breast cancer. An economic analysis. *Cancer* 2007;109(6):1011–1018; Nooman MA et al. Cognitive computing and the future of health care. *IEEE Pulse.* Available from: https://pulse.embs.org/may-2017/cognitive-computing-and-the-future-of-health-care/

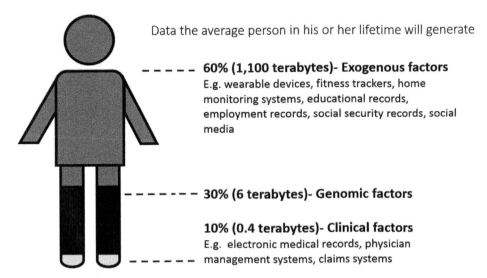

Data the average person in his or her lifetime will generate

60% (1,100 terabytes)- Exogenous factors
E.g. wearable devices, fitness trackers, home
monitoring systems, educational records,
employment records, social security records, social
media

30% (6 terabytes)- Genomic factors

10% (0.4 terabytes)- Clinical factors
E.g. electronic medical records, physician
management systems, claims systems

Figure 22.2 The quantified self.

Source: data from Mohamed Nooman Ahmed et al. 'Cognitive Computing and the Future of Healthcare: The Cognitive Power of IBM Watson Has the Potential to Transform Global Personalized Medicine'. *IEEE Pulse.* Volume 8, Issue 3, pp.4-9. Copyright © 2017 IEEE. DOI: 10.1109/MPUL.2017.2678098.

analytics. Patients will potentially generate close to 1.2 petabytes of information in their lifetime. Around 60% of these data will consist of non-traditional sources: structured, e.g. wearable devices and home monitoring systems; and non-structured, e.g. educational records, employment records, and social media. Thirty per cent will consist of genomic and other molecular tests and the last 10% will be stored in their electronic medical record (Figure 22.2). These data, at present, are often disorganized, redundant, and in many cases not available to the clinician or the patient. The human mind cannot process such large amounts of data and, importantly, deem what is and what is not useful. The optimal utility of such data will rely on the use of cognitive technologies and artificial intelligence. Such systems can deal not only with the volume of data but also with the velocity, variety, and veracity required to provide the clinician, in general, and the oncologist, in particular, with a complete view of the 'quantified self'.

It is currently impossible for a single doctor to keep up to date with all these developments in a traditional way, and only with the assistance of information and communications technology will patients and clinicians benefit from this revolution. The promise of truly personalized medicine can only be reached by our ability to bring these three spheres together: patient records, new research, and genomics. Generation of insights using artificial intelligence and machine learning will be the driving force of healthcare now and in the future (Figure 22.3) (9). Nevertheless, data quality problems and the human input remain a major issue, making intelligent data platforms, for the moment, the best alternative for breast cancer specialists.

Along with all these developments the issue of cybersecurity is always a concern.

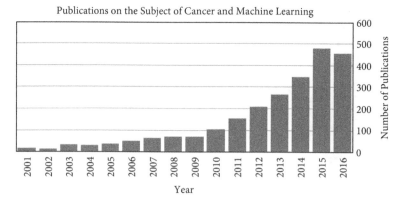

Publications on the Subject of Cancer and Machine Learning

Figure 22.3 Trends in machine learning and cancer research.
Pubmed query 'cancer[sb] machine learning' on 13 January 2017.

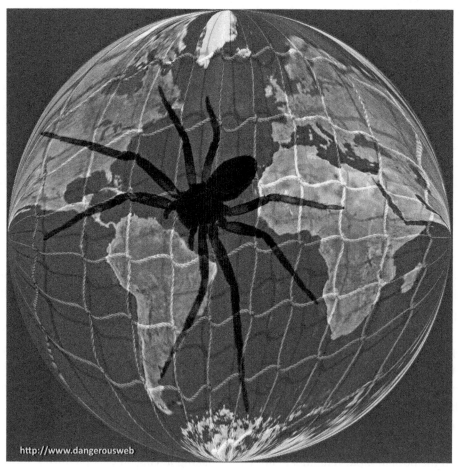

Figure 22.4
www.maybehazardous, Robert Paridaens (with permission).

Just as these data can be used by doctors to positively influence patient care, they may also be misused if not protected. The consequences of such a breach could affect the patient's capacity to maintain insurance or employment as well as impact their financial wellbeing. Our inability to protect such data can also have a negative impact on the public's trust in the system, and, therefore, affect access to the very data that are necessary to drive the advancements into the future. The responsibility of keeping the patient's data secure should be shared between patients, providers, and legislation. The protection of mobile devices, education of the workforce, and the proper maintenance and updates of the technological infrastructure along with advancements in the prevention, detection, and response to data breaches are central to progressing the genomic and digital revolution and the significant advances that these will bring to the field of oncology.

Another caveat of big data research is that it is not sufficient that large data-systems are integrated; sound study designs and analytical methods as well as transparency should be applied as well. As Khoury puts it, 'Big Error can plague Big Data', including selection bias, confounding, and 'false alarms' (casual associations or ecological fallacies leading to false positive) (10). Furthermore, in data-driven research the principles of causality should always be appropriately considered (9) (Figure 22.4).

Key Messages

- Increasingly large data-systems are integrating data from DNA sequencing into large medical databases.
- Generation of insights using artificial intelligence is challenging and remains a work in progress.
- Public discussion about benefits and challenges of big data in breast cancer will continue in the coming years.
- It is important to use big data to improve treatment value while maintaining transparency and giving attention to sound study design.

References

1. Meyer AM and Basch E. Big data infrastructure for cancer outcomes research: implications for the practicing oncologist. *J Oncol Pract* 2015;11(3):207–208.
2. Enright KA et al. Setting quality improvement priorities for women receiving systemic therapy for early-stage breast cancer by using population-level administrative data. *J Clin Oncol* 2017;35:3207–3214.
3. Richardson I. Connected Health: People, Technology and Processes. Lero-TR-2015-03. Lero Technical Report Series. University of Limerick; 2015.
4. National Human Genome Research Institute. DNA Sequencing Costs: Data. Available from: https://www.genome.gov/sequencingcostsdata/
5. Lyman GH et al. Impact of a 21-gene RT-PCR assay on treatment decisions in early-stage breast cancer. An economic analysis. *Cancer* 2007;109(6):1011–1018.

6. Nooman MA et al. Cognitive computing and the future of health care. *IEEE Pulse*. Available from: https://pulse.embs.org/may-2017/cognitive-computing-and-the-future-of-health-care/
7. US Food and Drug Administration. Table of Pharmacogenomic Biomarkers in Drug Labeling. Available from: https://www.fda.gov/Drugs/ScienceResearch/ucm572698.htm
8. Pharmaceutical Research and Manufacturers of America. Value of Personalized Medicine. Available from: http://phrma-docs.phrma.org/sites/default/files/pdf/chart_pack-value_of_personalized_medicine.pdf
9. Obermeyer Z and Emanuel EJ. Predicting the future—big data, machine learning and clinical medicine. *N Engl J Med* 2016;375(13):1216–1219.
10. Khoury MJ and Ioannidis JPA. Big data meets public health: human well-being could benefit from large-scale data if large-scale noise is minimized. *Science* 2014;346(6213):1054–1055.

23

Teleoncology

Groesbeck Parham, Hans Junkermann, Gert G.G.M. Van den Eynden,
and Paul van Diest

Introduction

E-health can be defined as the application of information and communications technologies (ICTs) across the whole range of functions that affect the health sector. As a constantly evolving science that incorporates new technological advances and adaptations to the ever-changing health needs of different global settings, it can be further divided into the domains of telehealth, e-learning, and health informatics. Telehealth involves the use of ICTs to deliver health services, expertise and information over distance. E-learning is concerned with the delivery of individualized, comprehensive, dynamic learning content in real-time. Health informatics deals with storage, retrieval, and optimal use of biomedical data, information, and knowledge for problem-solving and decision-making. One of telehealth's newly evolved disciplines is teleoncology, defined as the delivery of clinical oncology services from a distance for diagnosis, treatment, and patient follow-up using ICT (1). Its fundamental aim is the reduction of inequities in cancer care and the development of health professionals. Teleoncology may use mobile devices or fixed communication systems and can be classified in two main groups: (a) synchronous (real-time), based on interactive communication such as videoconferencing, and (b) asynchronous, or store-and-forward method by non-real-time interaction (Chapter 10). The technology is applicable to medical establishments located in different nations (internationally) and within the same country. Areas where teleoncology has been most successfully applied are surgery, radiology, and pathology.

To reach its full transformational potential, teleoncology must become applicable in areas where its impact is most needed—the developing world and underserved areas in the developed world. To do so, future platforms will need to focus on health system strengthening by taking into consideration the people (healthcare providers and patients) that are to be served, local healthcare needs, and what actually makes a difference. Qualitative studies of provider and patient acceptability are needed. Costs analyses are required to document the economic benefits of teleoncology (2) (Table 23.1).

Table 23.1 Major challenges related to teleoncology in sub-Saharan Africa

- Local technical expertise remains essential even to process specimens
- Resources to train personnel and establish and maintain equipment and servers
- Strong commitments by participating pathologists, clinicians, and IT collaborators
- Minimum computing and image capture technologies
- Stable source of funding to maintain and replace equipment over time as required
- Insufficient bandwidth for smooth communication and timely loading of scanned slides
- Unpredictable Internet service provider outages
- High cost of Internet service

Telesurgery

Worldwide, more than 80% of people with cancer will require surgery during their disease course, but less than 25% have access to safe, affordable, and timely surgery (3). Among the barriers to increasing surgical capacity are the time and costs required to train novices. Oncologic surgical care in many low- and middle-income countries (LMICs), when available at all, is often provided by non-physician medical officers, general physicians, and surgeons without formal oncologic training or certification. Subspecialty training in oncology in the western hemisphere is expensive, and many trainees from LMICs do not return home after becoming qualified (Chapter 8). In-country surgical oncology training would most likely require one to two years of instruction combined with on-site clinical mentoring by an expert (4). Most foreign experts are not available for such lengthy periods. However, recent advances in tele-communications, distance education, and surgical education have made it feasible to develop forms of surgical training based on a blended approach of computer-based (telementoring) and on-site tutoring. Telementoring and remote teleconsultation in surgery are widely available in developed countries, and their use in developing countries is beginning. While telementoring in high-income countries (HICs) is based on minimally invasive surgical platforms (laparoscopic and robotic surgery), in most LMICs it will need to be adopted to open surgery, which remains the most commonly used approach. Indeed, computer-based learning and telementoring have been shown to be highly effective in enhancing surgical skills among surgical trainees in low-resource settings, where faculty time is limited and access to visiting faculty is sporadic (5). These novel approaches to teaching and learning surgical procedures offer the advantage of standardized teaching, so that trainees can receive high-quality examples upon which to base their skills, regardless of their location or setting.

Teleradiology

Teleradiology makes the evaluation of medical images independent of the location of the image acquisition. It thus enables the reading of every image by an expert within an acceptable timeframe without travelling time or laborious handling of images.

Mammography screening is the situation most amenable to teleradiology in the subfield of breast imaging. A physician is not required at the location of the acquisition of the mammograms. Clinical information is of minor importance for the interpretation of the images and can be given easily on an accompanying proforma. Double reading by two independent experts enhances the sensitivity of the screening. Reading of the images must not be immediate. If there are divergent results of the double reading, then a conference and/or arbitration are recommended in order to keep the specificity at an acceptable level before the women are invited for assessment of the detected lesions. All these steps can be supported by teleradiology, which makes participation of distantly located experts possible and efficient, thereby improving the quality of the screening programme.

Recent results from magnetic resonance imaging breast cancer screening programmes for high-risk women support the idea that double reading is just as advantageous in this situation. Since the number of cases is much smaller than in mammography screening programmes, it is even more difficult for the local radiologist to acquire the necessary experience to provide a high-quality evaluation of the images.

In symptomatic breast disease, the advantage of teleradiology is less obvious. In this situation, the clinical examination leads to symptom-guided ultrasound examination, which is complemented by mammography except in well-defined situations. The ultrasound examination is performed with a handheld ultrasound probe. The documented images are very much dependent on the operator's technique and are thus not suited to an independent second opinion. The mammography in this situation has to be assessed in the context of the clinical and ultrasound examination. Furthermore, the decision on further assessment by needle biopsy is usually rendered immediately after the examination, and it is impractical to include the result of a second opinion by teleradiology into this primary decision-making. For less experienced readers, however, a second reading could be beneficial, because auditing supervision by an expert can enhance the quality of the mammography reading (the European guidelines suggest double reading for readers reading fewer than 3000 cases per year). Teleradiology could make this feasible, especially in multisite breast centres, where an expert is not always present at the mammogram-acquiring sites. The second reader, of course, must have access to all the results of the clinical and ultrasound examination of patients for evaluating the mammogram in light of all symptoms and findings.

Technical Requirements

To use teleradiology effectively, it must be assured that the reader at the distant site receives the images of the same quality as the reader on site. This means that a workstation equipped with (expensive) high-resolution monitors required for mammography reading must be available. General purpose monitors are not sufficient. The software should be able to display and exchange annotations made by any of the readers. The results of the ancillary examinations and patient history should be displayed to the second reader. The working place should meet the same requirements regarding ambient light and exclusion of distraction as a typical mammography reading place. The distant reading workplace must be totally included in the technical quality management of the mammography unit. The distant reader should also take responsibility for, and be involved in, the quality management of the technical aspects of mammography acquisition (positioning of the breast and handling of the machine) if the reader on site is less experienced.

Data transfer requires a stable, fast, and encryption-protected data connection. In screening cases, the data transfer of the daily batch of images, including priors, should be accomplished at least overnight. For clinical cases, an even faster transfer for the usually smaller number of cases would be necessary, if the result is to be integrated into the clinical decision. Compression without loss should only be used to improve the transfer speed of the image files.

In cases where teleradiology is used in multidisciplinary or consensus conferences, it must be assured that the lesions pointed out during the discussion of the images can be identified by all participants.

It may be anticipated that because of the decreasing cost, increasing transfer speeds, and improved handling by smarter software, teleradiology will be increasingly used in breast imaging with the aspects of knowledge-sharing, auditing, quality management, and education. This will potentially allow a higher and more evenly distributed quality of breast imaging in all parts of the world.

Telepathology and New Opportunities for Pathology Networking

Pathology remains the keystone in cancer diagnostics, even in the era of molecular biology. In fact, rapidly increasing insights in tumour biology challenge the pathologist to translate this knowledge to the bedside. Exhaustive subtyping, the assessment of increasingly complex tumour parameters, and innovative pharmacodiagnostic markers require subspecialization of pathologists (e.g. haematopathology, neuropathology, breast pathology). In small institutions and low-resource settings such pathology manpower needs are largely unavailable.

In general, there are four basic telepathology platforms: (a) static images, (b) whole-slide scanning, (c) dynamic non-robotic telemicroscopy, and (d) dynamic robotic telemicroscopy (6). These approaches vary widely in terms of technology costs, ICT support, and the need for local pathology expertise. For instance, static images require only limited technical infrastructure (a microscope, digital camera, and Internet connection), but they depend on appropriate selection of diagnostic fields. All require local technical expertise for purposes of specimen processing, and some degree of financial support and local pathology expertise. The major determinant of each of these variables is the complexity of the technology.

Major improvements of whole-slide image scanning hardware and software and the necessary ICT infrastructure (storage capacity and network speed), have catalysed the transition of pathology from analogue (glass slides and microscope) to digital (reading of slides on a computer screen) in routine practice. This will completely change pathology logistics over the next 5 to 10 years. The use of digital pathology in routine practice has many advantages, one of the most important of which is knowledge-sharing within (long-distance) networks of (expert) pathologists.

The implementation of telepathology platforms, assisted by networks of expert pathologists, can offer support to laboratories and/or hospitals with limited pathology resources, regardless of whether the cause is due to small institutional size, limited pathology manpower, lack of availability of pathology subspecialist knowledge, remote location, or a combination of factors. Telepathology support in such situations can serve multiple needs. For instance, easy access to a colleague's expertise for a second opinion in challenging cases, and/or assistance during difficult intraoperative examinations, can prevent bottlenecks in treatment. On the other hand, primary reading of cases in situations of pathology manpower shortages enables hospital/laboratory management to ensure short turnaround times and continuity of care. Telepathology can also facilitate certain aspects of the laboratories' quality management system, such as continuous auditing of cases, third-line/external quality control, and continuous education of pathologists.

Although it opens new opportunities, telepathology also leads to new challenges. Besides the logistical challenges associated with integrating images in the lab flow, validation is necessary before telepathology can be used in primary diagnosis. International 'virtual' collaboration of medical professionals and the exchange of sensitive (patient) data demands an ethical and legal framework, something that is not yet fully established in many countries. Telepathology also requires powerful yet user-friendly ICT applications, which must be adapted to local needs and contexts. High-cost technologies must be avoided in LMICs because they are economically unsustainable. Organizations such as the International Telepathology Foundation (http://www.itpf.eu) can assist (groups of) pathologists in overcoming these hurdles.

Another concern raised by telepathology and the growth of artificial intelligence technology is its potential to make pathologists in developing countries redundant. Despite these concerns, the role of the local pathologist as the 'expert guardian of the patient's tissue' remains essential. Displacement of crucial disciplines such as pathology can diminish local knowledge and decision-making. Furthermore, the lack of local pathologists can hinder the implementation of telepathology initiatives. As diagnostic procedures become less invasive, biopsies and surgical resections progressively smaller, and as information expected from resected material increases, the pathologist is the expert needed to perform, supervise, and guarantee optimal tissue handling. Using telepathology to embed local pathologists within a larger (international) community of experts actually strengthens, rather than threatens, their position. In addition, easy access to automated image analysis tools will assist the pathologist to perform semiquantitative analyses. Digital pathology opens doors to connect to the rest of the world by facilitating easy access to remote specialists, enabling education and training, and creating opportunities to study very rare and valuable cases, all while saving time and money previously used to physically travel with or ship slides.

An example of the use of telepathology in an HIC is the Dutch Pathology Image Exchange Platform which has been supported by the nationwide network and registry of histo- and cytopathology in the Netherlands (Pathologisch-Anatomisch Landelijk Geautomatiseerd Archief, PALGA) and developed by Sectra (7). Launched in April 2018, this national platform was built to digitally exchange whole-slide images between pathology laboratories. The three circumstances in which it is used are reassessment of pathology material in the event of patient transfer to another hospital ('revision'), consultation for difficult cases, and digital expert panels. Using a digital technology platform, the Pathology Image Exchange Platform obviates the need for sending slides using traditional mail, thereby improving the turnaround time of revisions, consultations, and expert panels. This improves quality of diagnostics by engaging suitable experts independent of geography. The exchange of relevant patient data associated with the images is done through the highly secured network of PALGA, which ensures complete anonymized exchange of images by international standards.

By contrast, one example of a successful telepathology programme in an LMIC is the University of North Carolina Project Malawi Telepathology Program (8). In 2013 at Kamuzu Central Hospital in Lilongwe, Malawi, a telepathology programme using whole-slide imaging on the Aperio Digital Pathology System (Leica Biosystems, Buffalo Grove, IL, USA) was initiated. Its purpose was to support local pathologists, clinical care, and research efforts. At Kamuzu Central Hospital, biopsies and cytology specimens are submitted to the pathology laboratory (directed by a Malawian pathologist) that provides basic cytology, histology processing, and a limited panel of manual immunohistochemical stains. Cases are initially reviewed by local pathologists, who generally communicate an initial impression to clinicians. In difficult cases, slides are scanned and loaded to a secure server, which collaborating USA pathologists access via a virtual private network connection. Once each week, Malawi-based clinicians and pathologists present these patients at a telepathology conference, which is attended by local providers and their counterparts in the USA. After discussion, a consensus diagnosis is rendered by the pathologist in Malawi. More recently, the group has begun to experiment with alternative teleconferencing solutions using the online Zoom Video Conferencing system (ZoomVideo Communications, San Jose, CA, USA). When coupled to a microscope-mounted digital camera, this system allows dynamic telemicroscopy driven not by the USA-based collaborating pathologist (as would be the case in robotic telemicroscopy) but by local pathologists in Malawi.

Key Messages

- Although teleoncology experiences in developing countries are promising, human resource and technological barriers must be addressed to realize its full impact on cancer care.

- Best practices must be identified for each local setting in LMICs.
- Telementoring and teleconsultation can be highly effective in enhancing surgical skills among surgical trainees in low-resource settings.
- Mammography screening is the situation most amenable to teleradiology in breast imaging.
- The role of the local pathologist as the guardian of the patient's tissue remains essential.

References

1. Hazin R, Qaddoumi I. Teleoncology: current and future applications for improving cancer care globally. *Lancet Oncol* 2010;11(2):204–210.
2. Ferrari R et al. Tele-oncology in sub-Saharan Africa: a literature review. *J Cancer Policy* 2018;17:9–14.
3. Sullivan R et al. Delivering safe and affordable cancer surgery to all. *The Lancet* Oncology Commission on Global Cancer Surgery. *Lancet Oncol* 2015;16(11):1193–224.
4. Chinula LA et al. A tailored approach to building specialized surgical oncology capacity: early experiences and outcomes in Malawi. *Gynecol Oncol Rep* 26;2018:60–65.
5. Autry AM. Teaching surgical skills using video internet communication in a resource-limited setting. *Obstet Gynecol* 2013;122(1):127–131.
6. Pantanowitz L. Digital images and the future of digital pathology. *J Pathol Inform* 2010;1:pii:15.
7. van Diest PJ et al. Pathology Image Exchange (PIE): the Dutch national digital pathology platform for exchange of whole slide images for efficient teleconsultation, telerevision and virtual expert panels. *JCO Clin Cancer Inform* 2019;3:1–7.
8. Gopal S et al. Early experience after developing a pathology laboratory in Malawi, with emphasis on cancer diagnoses. *PLoS One* 2013;8(8):e70361.

PART 7

BREAST CANCER RESEARCH

24

The Changing Clinical Research Pathway

Didier Verhoeven, Evandro de Azambuja, Wim Demey, Luis Teixeira,
Gilberto Schwartsmann, Etienne Brain, Fatima Cardoso, and Ahmad Awada

Introduction

Cancer research is one of the fastest-growing research areas of medicine. *Breast Cancer Research* is the highest-ranking breast cancer-specific title in the top oncology journals worldwide. Certainly, the efforts of breast cancer research become apparent when these directly benefit patients. In order to develop innovative approaches, a good understanding of the molecular bases of tumour growth, invasion and metastasis, causality, risk reduction, detection, and early diagnosis is necessary. Understanding biological mechanisms allows us to first understand the core of the disease, and this understanding makes it possible to develop new treatments for our patients. Fundamental research gives us the ideas and knowledge to achieve new insights and new treatment options (1).

In 2013, the 35 members of the Organisation for Economic Co-operation and Development devoted, on average, 22% of their research budget to basic research. Early in 1960, the first conclusive evidence between DNA damage and cancer was reported, and this marked a turning point for cancer research (2). After that, big discoveries were made. A good illustration of the bench-to-bedside strategy was the discovery in 1987 of a mutated gene, Her2, which stimulates the excessive growth of a group of breast cancer cells. Some years later, the team of Dennis Slamon found the correlation between high levels of this protein and poor patient outcomes, i.e. a poor prognosis. The next step was the identification of a monoclonal antibody to block this pathway of cell proliferation, and personalized breast cancer treatment with monoclonal antibodies became possible for the first time. In practice, much research follows such bench-to-bedside strategies.

Although surgery and radiation therapy are also key for breast cancer treatment, systemic treatment is most prominent. It is driven by the desire for improved outcome and quality of life and directly applies laboratory research to develop new ways to treat patients more effectively. Surgery, radiation therapy, and research concerning supportive and palliative issues are less common, and this is partly because financial support from Pharma is less available. 'Comprehensive cancer centres' were created to stress the need for multidisciplinary care and to secure the connection between basic, translational, and clinical research as well as the provision of services directly to our patients.

Historically speaking, research was once more focused on public health questions. Much effort was placed on basic research at the academic level, and a lot of preclinical drug discoveries were supported by universities and funded by public money. The most economically risky stages of fundamental research were done mostly at our research institutions, and when a compound was promising, clinical trials were performed mostly with the financial support of pharmaceutical companies. The potential for profit and return on investment were the main incentives for further research by industry. Clinical trial methodology has changed, however, and results are needed more quickly. Drug-oriented clinical research has evolved from chemotherapy and endocrine treatments to molecular-targeted therapies and, more recently, new immunotherapeutic approaches.

From Preclinical to Late-Stage Clinical Research

Preclinical research using in-vitro, animal, and, more recently, xenograft models are needed to test drugs before they can be offered to our patients with cancer. This is a daunting task, because less than 10% of investigational new drugs proceed beyond early development, and the approval rate for new oncology drugs is, at best, 5%. Here, preclinical animal models play a central role in identifying pharmacological toxicities (3). These models, although imperfect, remain an important means to predict safety and efficacy prior to first use in humans. In accordance with the Nuremberg Code of 1947, experiments must be done with minimal risk for the patients (4). The current animal models for breast cancer drugs are xenografts of breast cancer cell lines growing in immunodeficient mice or chemically, virally, or genetically manipulated mouse models. The use of the right model remains an important step in introducing successful new molecules into the clinic. One of the problems is the heterogeneity of human breast cancer and the more homogeneous nature of animal models. Great care is needed in designing preclinical models. An accurate preclinical animal model screening can reduce cost and increase the successful introduction of new drugs for treating breast cancer.

Traditionally, clinical cancer research can be separated in phase I, II, III, and IV studies. The later phase studies concern late side-effects and efficacy during longer-term follow-up.

Phase I trials: the first experiment of a new drug in humans. The a-priori benefit after inclusion is minimal. The aim of these trials is not to improve survival or quality of life, but rather to determine the dose and document side-effects. Careful selection of the participating patients is mandatory with a reduced 90-day mortality. If this mortality rate is too high (>20%) or if there are toxic deaths, it means that either patients are included without adequate evaluation of their health condition at the screening phase of the study, or that the drug is too toxic to pursue its further development (5).

Phase II–III trials: phase II trials concern evaluation of safety and efficacy of a new treatment. A higher number of patients are enrolled in these studies than in a phase I study, and the patient population is more homogeneous. Although few data are available, an improvement in the patient's health is possible, certainly because more trials are now considered as being between phase II and III. The aim of phase III trials is to compare new treatments with the standard treatment. These new treatments may also be less effective, more toxic, or more expensive than the current standard. The HERA trial, for example, showed that a longer treatment with trastuzumab for two years was more costly, toxic, and no more efficacious than treatment for one year. The ALTTO trial showed that the lapatinib-only arm was less effective than trastuzumab, and this led to premature discontinuation of this arm. The BETH trial showed that the combination of trastuzumab and bevacizumab was more toxic and more expensive without better outcome (6).

A clear evolution in the methodology of drug development has been observed in the past few years. Previously, the time between the start of the phase I and phase III studies was nearly ten years; nowadays, however, a period of less than five years is the goal. Phase I studies are started with an expansion phase of selected groups of patients or tumours by clinical, pathological, or molecular criteria. Many phase II studies end with a randomized phase II study, a nearly phase III study, and some drugs are now approved with these phase II results while waiting for confirmation from large phase III trials. Another more recent concept is the I-SPY2 trials to predict the therapeutic response with imaging and molecular analysis. The framework here is an adaptive phase II trial in the neoadjuvant setting of locally advanced breast cancer to provide a model for more rapid assessment of novel phase II drugs and to determine which subtypes will benefit from treatment. It allows new agents to enter and leave the study without having to stop enrolment or resubmit the entire protocol for regulatory review (https://www.ispytrials.org) (7).

Competing interests are present at the intersection of academic medicine and clinical research. Advancement for academic physicians requires publications and productive research. In the case of clinical trials, this means enrolling patients and proposing investigator-initiated trials. The non-financial conflicts of interest in clinical research are unavoidable, but these must be handled with respect to bedside care and bioethical concerns (8). Caution is also required with respect to financial rewards.

The improvement in survival for breast cancer patients has changed the disease to that of a manageable condition. Still, better care and support after treatment are crucial, and additional research on long-term follow-up and toxicities is required in registration studies or so-called phase IV studies. For this reason, the European Organisation for Research and Treatment of Cancer (EORTC) recently started the EORTC YOU umbrella protocol to follow long-term outcome and toxicity (9).

Important ethical considerations must be taken into account during clinical research. Middle-income countries are a fast-growing market for pharmaceutical companies as well as for clinical trials. The number of trials registered with clinicaltrials.gov has increased rapidly since 2005 on the Asian continent, especially in China and India. A reason for this could be that rules about patient rights might be less restrictive, and that participation in a clinical trial could be a way to obtain a new drug or treatment at no cost.

Another issue is the ethics committees examining protocols and informed consents. There is a significant difference globally regarding their function and independence.

Additionally, there is a continuously increasing administrative burden associated with the conduct of a clinical trial. Several legal regulations hinder clinical research, some of which appear to accommodate pharmaceutical companies' needs. In essence, regulations should guarantee patients' rights and facilitate research. A single Health Research Agency should replace the variety of regulatory bodies in order to facilitate this.

The Use of Observational 'Big Data'

The use of (retrospective) observational data, such as data gathered by cancer registries, could be considered in situations where a randomized trial is no longer considered ethical, because both treatment options are already implemented in daily practice or in case of a low event rate and a very long follow-up period. The latter implies that the final results of the trial will be available only after 10–15 years, which prevents patients from benefiting from the treatment only at a very late stage. Moreover, observational studies do not exclude, for example, elderly patients, who are often an excluded group in randomized clinical trials. Although confounding by indication can be a problem in studying observational data, the results can support certain hypotheses for a broad patient group. Furthermore, the main reason for gathering the data should be kept in mind before using it to answer a research question. The ability to develop 'big data' comprising structured and unstructured data as well as statistical methods such as machine learning techniques may be of help, but these techniques should always be interpreted with caution (10) (Chapter 22).

Evolving Therapeutic Approach

The therapeutic approach in breast cancer has changed towards molecular biology-driven research. We have moved from empirical oncology with chemotherapy (recently also with antibody–drug conjugates) to a molecular-targeted and immunological approach (Table 24.1).

The types of clinical trials in advanced breast cancer during 2007–2011 were approximately 21% cytotoxic, 72% targeted therapies, and 7% immunotherapies (11). The evolution towards these targeted therapies brought some new insights and lessons to our researchers in different tumour types:

1. Treatment of unselected populations should be discouraged.
2. Tumour dependency should be defined to stress the use of uni-targeted versus multi-targeted tyrosine kinase inhibitors.
3. The identifications of a driver genetic abnormality are key as well as the discovery of a selective targeted agent (e.g. Her-2 alteration).
4. Rare tumours are 'good' niches for selected targeted agents (e.g. BRCA mutated).

Table 24.1 Targets involved in carcinogenesis and inhibitors/pathway

Target	Agent	Marker of sensitivity / resistance	Indication
ER	Tamoxifen, aromatase inhibitor, fulvestrant	ER mutation (resistance)	Early and M+
Her-2	Trastuzumab, pertuzumab, lapatinib, Neratinib, T-DM1	Her-2 amplification or overexpression	Early and M+
VEGF	Bevacuzimab	Neovascular density?	M+?
m-TOR	Everolimus	NA	M+
CDK 4/6	Palbociclib, ribociclib, abemaciclib	NA	M+
Rank 1	Denosumab	NA	M+ (bone)
PARP	Olaparib, rucaparib	BRCA mutation	M+
PI3K	Alpelisib	PIK3CA mutations	M+
PD-L1	Atezolizumab	Expression on immune cells	M+

ER, oestrogen receptor; M+, metastatic; adj, adjuvant; NA, not available.

5. One gene may predict resistance, but no single gene, protein, or pathway can predict full efficacy (Her-2, receptor status).
6. Discovery of the resistance mechanisms are a high priority (e.g. endocrine therapy, anti-Her-2 therapies).
7. Patients and tumour characteristics remain important (tumour size, lymph node status, menopausal status).
8. The emergence of pharmacogenetics has been difficult (e.g. Cytochrome CYP 2D6 and tamoxifen).
9. Expected and unexpected side-effects have arisen from targeted therapies.
10. Chemotherapy, but also radiotherapy, remain important, especially for the synergy with targeted agents (e.g. chemotherapy with anti-Her-2 agents).

One sign of potential success for targeted therapy is that the target is a driver of carcinogenesis (not only abnormal) and preferably associated with poor outcome for a selected population. A tumour dependent on a single-gene abnormality with a rational and selective drug will result in a smart trial.

The clinical research landscape has shown a remarkable evolution in the adjuvant as well as the metastatic settings. In the past, large randomized controlled trials were performed in the adjuvant setting, and thousands of unselected patients received modest benefits (taxane trials, anthracycline trials, etc.). Now and in the future, more selected groups of patients will be included. Large benefits are sought and will hopefully be obtained by using biomarkers for selection and surrogate markers for efficacy.

Previously in the metastatic setting, trials were small and used response rate as the endpoint. Later, randomized trials were performed with hundreds (or thousands) of unselected patients. Progression-free survival was mainly used as surrogate endpoint, and only rarely was overall survival used. Nowadays, randomized controlled trials or single-arm trials aim to demonstrate a larger effect on outcome. Selected groups of patients and high-quality databases are needed by clinical, pathological, or molecular criteria. This research requires fewer patients to be enrolled in the study, but a rather large number of patients to be screened. This has given birth to basket (one qualifying group of alterations, tumour agnostic) and umbrella (multiple qualifying alterations, single histology) studies. ESMO provided a comprehensive view for the interpretation of oncological studies with its Magnitude of Clinical Benefit Scale that has been adopted by pharmaceutical companies as well as by regulatory bodies (12).

Clinical breast cancer research is divided between industry-sponsored (70%), academic partnership with the Pharma industry (20%), and pure academic research (10%).

Pharmaceutical industry-sponsored clinical research comprises mostly phase I–II studies. An important pressure of regulatory bodies is observed with business-oriented focus and an increase in the costs. The trials are designed and controlled by drug companies and their medical advisors, and some concerns have been raised about the control and reporting of data. Recently, more action was taken to report all data of all studies. The World Health Organization created the International Clinical Trials Registry Platform to ensure that a complete view of research (phase I through phase IV) is accessible to all those involved in health care decisions. The registration was seen as a scientific, ethical, and moral responsibility (13).

Clinical research in 'partnership' with the pharma are initiated by investigators or co-operative groups. These trials are designed and mostly controlled by academic centres, cooperative groups, or networks and result in fewer concerns about the reporting of the data.

Finally, pure academic research has produced a wide range of clinical trials in mainly randomized phase II studies or translational research. They are supported mainly by research grants or foundations, and minimally by governments. They focus on public health questions or treatment strategies (e.g. Finnish SOLD Trial about short duration of adjuvant trastuzumab with a result only slightly inferior than one year of trastuzumab (14). Such findings could give opportunities for developing countries with more cost-effective strategies. These important academic studies, unfortunately, are less frequent and require considerable logistics.

Key Messages

- Preclinical studies remain necessary for further understanding of tumour biology.
- Breast cancer research has exhibited an evolution towards molecularly targeted drug therapy.
- Ethical considerations are of utmost importance to protect patients' rights.

- Bureaucratic regulatory considerations limit cancer research and should be thoughtfully reconsidered.
- A smart trial is defined by a tumour dependent on one gene/protein abnormality and a rational and selective drug.
- A risky trial is defined by a tumour (different genes/proteins/pathways involved in carcinogenesis) and a less selective drug.
- Clinical research shows an evolution towards selected groups of patients, but with a high number of patients screened and an increase in benefit.
- 'Pharma only' clinical research raises concerns about control and the reporting of all data. Models of collaboration should continue to be developed.

References

1. Institute of Cancer Research, London. The Drug Discoverer—Why 'basic research' is critical for understanding and treating cancer. 2018. Available from: https://www.icr.ac.uk/blogs/the-drug-discoverer/page-details/why-basic-research-is-critical-for-understanding-and-treating-cancer.
2. Brookes P and Lawley PD. Evidence for the binding of polynuclear aromatic hydrocarbons to the nucleic acids of mouse skin: relation between carcinogenic power of hydrocarbons and their binding to deoxyribonucleic acid. *Nature* 1964;202:781–784.
3. Clarke R. The role of preclinical animal models in breast cancer drug development. *Breast Cancer Res* 2009;11(Suppl 3):S22.
4. The Nuremberg Code. Available from: http://www.cirp.org/library/ethics/nuremberg/
5. Chau NG et al. Early mortality and overall survival in oncology phase I trial participants: can we improve patient selection? *BMC Cancer* 2011;11:426–436.
6. Pritchard K. Optimizing the delivery of targeted research: an opportunity for comparative effectiveness research. *J Clin Oncol* 2010;28(7):1089–1091.
7. Barker AD et al. I-SPY 2: An adaptive breast cancer trial design in the setting of neoadjuvant chemotherapy. *Clin Pharmacol Therapeut* 2009;86(1):97–100.
8. Rosenberg A. 'Get the consent' Nonfinancial conflict of interest in academic clinical research. *J Clin Oncol* 2017;35(1):11–13.
9. Liu L et al. A unique research infrastructure from the European Organisation for Research and Treatment of Cancer (EORTC) to optimise long-term follow up of patients. The YOU (Your Outcome Update) protocol: Rationale, scope, design and research opportunities. *J Cancer Policy* 2018;15:118–121.
10. Shah ND et al. Big data and predictive analytics: recalibrating expectations. *JAMA* 2018;320(1):27–28.
11. Dogan S et al. Issues in clinical research for metastatic breast cancer. *Curr Opin Oncol* 25(6):625–9.
12. European Society of Medical Oncology Clinical Trial Resources | OncologyPRO. Available from: https://oncologypro.esmo.org/Education-Library/Clinical-Trial-Resources
13. World Health Organization | Welcome to the WHO ICTRP. 2018. Available from: http://www.who.int/ictrp/en/
14. Joensuu H et al. Effects of adjuvant trastuzumab for a duration of 9 weeks vs 1 year with concomitant chemotherapy for early human epidermal growth factor receptor 2-positive breast cancer. The Sold Randomized Clinical Trial. *JAMA Oncol* 2018;4(9):1199–1206.

25

A Global Perspective on Cooperation

Fatima Cardoso, Evandro de Azambuja, Gilberto Schwartsmann, Nuria Kotecki,
Wim Demey, Luis Teixeira, Didier Verhoeven, Etienne Brain, and Ahmad Awada

The Need for a New Model for Clinical
Research Collaboration

Breast cancer research is highly demanding in terms of resources, researchers, and patients. Because of these demands, the creation of a breast cancer research network was necessary for the growth of global research. The aim was to obtain the best results, avoid duplication of trials, and especially to avoid conducting trials which would ultimately not answer a specific question. The US National Cancer Institute (NCI) is the world's largest funder of breast cancer research. In 2016, NCI invested more than US$500 million in breast cancer research (one-tenth of its total budget) (1).

This sort of collaboration is now applied to most tumour types, and this is mainly due to progress in understanding the molecular biology of cancer. Due to the increased costs of new therapies, a model that renders systemic targeted therapies affordable in all countries is a high priority (2). The keys for the success of clinical research networks are summarized below (Figure 25.1).

- High degree of professionalism and motivation of the team is required.
- High degree of dedication of all to clinical and translational research with improving access to clinical material and support of large data bases.
- Sufficient human resources at all levels: increased funding will enhance our knowledge and broaden our talent pool.
- Close collaboration of the team with the other partners (pharmaceutical industry, clinical research organizations, laboratories, fundamental researchers, etc.) in the interest of the network.
- Open new studies quickly and successfully recruit and retain patients.
- Include academic questions in the methodology (not focus on financial results).
- Global high-quality standards with a culture of competence.
- A visionary strategy with cross-discipline collaboration between physicians, technologists, engineers, and all interested parties.
- Creation of a network of satellite centres around the academic centres (essential for patients/tumours screening).
- Democratic and pragmatic governance and functioning.
- Breaking with the 'power, business, and fashion' strategy of current clinical research!

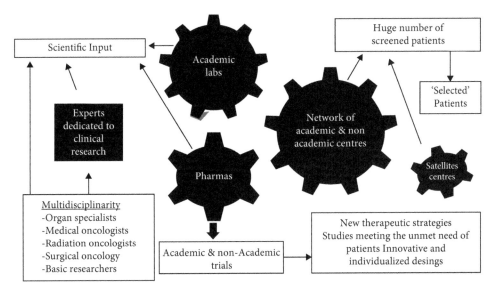

Figure 25.1 A new model of clinical research collaboration (Oncodistinct Network).

Adapted with permission from Kotecki, N. et al. 'How to emerge from the conservatism in clinical research methodology?' *Current Opinion in Oncology*. Volume 29, Issue 5, pp. 400–4. Copyright © 2017 Wolters Kluwer Health, Inc. DOI: 10.1097/CCO.0000000000000399

International Breast Cancer Networks

There are many breast cancer-specific networking groups in Europe, the USA, and worldwide. Some of the most important are mentioned in this chapter; however, some groups are not listed, although they are active in different regions of the world.

BIG (https://www.bigagainstbreastcancer.org/). The Breast International Group was created in 1996 as an international non-profit organization for academic breast cancer research from around the world. The mission of BIG is to facilitate breast cancer research by stimulation of cooperation between its 59 member groups and academic networks collaborating with, but independent of, pharmaceutical companies. BIG is convinced that global research and collaboration are needed to find a cure for breast cancer. BIG functions in more than 50 countries, more than 3,000 hospitals, and more than 10,000 breast cancer experts. So far, more than 70,000 patients have taken part in BIG trials worldwide.

NABCG. The North American Breast Cancer Groups comprise a network of major US- and Canadian-based research groups supported by the US National Cancer Institute and working in topic-specific working groups (such as breast cancer) since 2005. Together NABCG and BIG strive to improve the care and cure rates of patients with breast cancer through international collaboration.

EORTC Breast Cancer Group (https://www.eortc.org/research_field/breast). The European Organisation for Research and Treatment of Cancer was founded in 1962 by leaders in cancer medicine, who realized that patient management could not advance without a solid understanding of the disease and its biology, vigorous testing of novel treatments, and cross-disciplinary collaboration beyond state borders. The Breast Cancer Group, as part of the EORTC, challenges, redefines, and develops standards of care in all areas of breast cancer diagnosis and therapy. The group's research area is broad and goes beyond systemic treatment (radiotherapy, surgery, male breast cancer, management of ductal carcinoma in situ, understanding of molecular biology, etc.). More than 50,000 breast cancer patients have already participated in EORTC trials. One of the largest trials was the landmark study conducted in the 1980s which showed similar overall survival between mastectomy and breast conservation with a follow-up of 20 years (3).

NSABP (http://www.nsabp.org). The National Surgical Adjuvant Breast and Bowel Project was founded 50 years ago in Pittsburgh, PA, USA. It designs and conducts practice-changing cancer research. With more than 700 research sites, it conducts clinical trials and laboratory studies in the medical, surgical, and prevention settings to improve outcome and quality of life of patients with breast and colorectal cancer. Its aim is to benefit the worldwide community. It has published follow-up studies of more than 20 years, which lend the data a robust character.

EBCTCG (http://www.ctsu.ox.ac.uk). The Early Breast Cancer Trialists' Collaborative Group established in 1983, based in Oxford, UK, includes researchers from every important randomized trial worldwide. The EBCTCG involves all trials worldwide that have done relevant randomized trials on the treatment of women with breast cancer. Since 1985, the world's trials have shared their data every 5 years so as not to miss any moderate difference in long-term survival. In 2011, 620 names of their collaborators in local and systemic therapy trials were published in *The Lancet*. Several hundred research groups have shared patient data on more than 450,000 women in 400 randomized trials for meta-analyses. The treatments include surgery, radiotherapy, chemotherapy, endocrine treatment, other forms of systemic treatment, and screening.

IBCSG (http://www.ibcsg.org). The International Breast Cancer Study Group (previously named the Ludwig Breast Cancer Study Group) was created in 1978 and has been conducting large phase III clinical trials since then. The IBCSG has been a leader of tailored approaches for specific subpopulations of breast cancer patients.

In addition to the above-named groups, there are other interesting, international, mainly breast cancer-specific research groups, which are introduced below.

LACOG (http://www.lacog.org.br). The Latin American Cooperative Group is a non-profit organization founded in 2008 by a group of Latin American medical oncologists interested in the development of clinical research. It was the first multinational cooperative group in Latin America exclusively dedicated to clinical and translational research.

ANZBCTG (http://www.bcia.org.au). The Australia–New Zealand Breast Cancer Trials Group has for more than 35 years been the largest independent clinical trial research group in Australia and New Zealand. More than 14,000 women have participated already in more than 75 clinical trials.

ENBDC (http://www.enbcd.org). The goal of the European Network of Breast Development and Cancer is to foster interactions between laboratories working on mammary gland development and cancer worldwide.

IBIS (http://www.ibis-trials.org). The International Breast Cancer Intervention Studies are designed to investigate the use of endocrine treatment, zoledronic acid, and other products in preventing breast cancer and its recurrence in women. IBIS-I ended in 2001 having recruited 7,154 women in nine countries.

JBCRG (http://www.jbcrg.jp/en). The Japan Breast Cancer Research Group was founded to activate breast cancer clinical trials and to disseminate information from Japan to the world. Their mission is to become a global opinion leader, acting as a united Japanese team. Currently more than 260 institutes are registered as members. Basic as well as clinical research are performed.

Oncodistinct Network (http://www.oncodistinct.net). This international network was recently created to perform innovative and academic clinical trials in solid tumours including breast cancer. Oncodistinct is a pragmatic network taking into consideration the recent understanding of cancer biology and the need for a complete shift in clinical research.

In addition, many very important, mainly national groups are performing outstanding clinical breast cancer research. They can be found on the BIG (59 members in 2018) and NABCG websites.

The Changing Pattern of Global Clinical Trials

On the website http://www.clinicalTrials.gov, all worldwide registered cancer studies, including those in breast cancer, can be found, with the record going back many years. Since 2000, 284,374 studies in 204 countries were posted up to 2018 based on the year when these data were first made available. Since 2005, a considerable rise was observed in registered studies. In 2018, 8,465 breast cancer studies were registered worldwide: 4,782 in North America (4,445 in the USA), 2302 in Europe, 1,416 in Asia (561 in China), 192 in Russia, 278 in South America, 295 in the Middle East, 231 in Oceania, and 146 in Africa (see Figure 25.2).

When looking at the evolution of research in different countries, clinical trials in breast cancer are becoming more frequent in Asia. Availability of a vast patient pool, high-quality infrastructure, comparable quality, and lower costs in comparison to the USA and Europe have been the driving force for pharmaceutical companies to outsource trials to Asia.

A large treatment-naive patient pool is available as well as numerous trial centres with advanced technology. One analysis of article output found that the worldwide growth has been driven by an upsurge in China (more than 19% growth per year). Fudan University in Shanghai is China's most active centre, forming collaborations with many centres in the USA, the UK, and Germany (1). In addition, the low healthcare

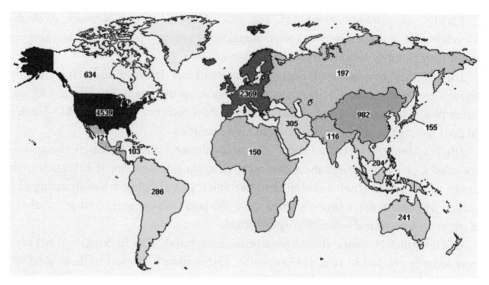

Figure 25.2 World map with the number of performed clinical breast cancer studies.
Source: www.ClinicalTrials.gov

expenditures by many governments in Asia make clinical trials an attractive way for patients to access innovative therapies.

Data from Asia are mostly of high quality, with even lower critical findings from the US Food and Drug Administration (FDA) and European Medicines Agency than in the USA indicating a high international standard. Opinion leaders in Asia are often members of international expert groups, and their international reputations via citations are growing rapidly (4). However, the Asian population might differ from the rest of the world, and results of trials conducted there may not be generalized as such, due to the different metabolism of some drugs in Asian compared to Caucasian populations.

The cost:effectiveness ratio of their trial organization is favourable. The cost for all procedures and visits is 25–40% lower than in western countries.

Specialized trial centres have a high-quality infrastructure. In addition, some of them are enhancing information technology systems and are at the forefront of innovation.

India is the most important source of generic drugs and is, for example, the largest producer (76%) of generic antiretroviral drugs (anti-HIV) used in impoverished countries (5). Although India is a country with fewer regulations and quality control, the FDA and World Health Organization are working on standards and pre-qualifications.

On the contrary, clinical trials are underdeveloped in Latin America, although expertise and infrastructure are present and increasing. Cancer has overtaken infectious disease as the principal cause of mortality in middle-income countries such as Brazil. The logistics and difficulties of introducing high standards of translational research, data handling, and monitoring of clinical trials in developing countries, e.g. Brazil, are evident. In the mid-1990s, some Brazilian basic and clinical investigators created a drug development initiative that was responsible for the identification of some new compounds from the region. They were helping preclinical and early clinical evaluation as well as the education of a new generation of scientists interested in the field. As part of an extramural US NCI-sponsored drug discovery programme, a large-scale project of acquisition and testing of compounds isolated from South American medicinal plants was implemented. Under the framework of the South-American Anticancer Drug development office, the first phase I trial and pharmacokinetic study of a new anticancer drug was performed in Latin America in 2006 (6). Over the years, Brazilian medical oncologists have markedly increased their participation in clinical trials and consensus papers in the management of breast cancer. This has resulted in improvements of the infrastructure for drug development in the country with the creation of several clinical trial units at academic and non-academic institutions as well as the formal recognition of ethics and scientific committees by the government. The creation of LACOG enabled coordination and performance of multicentre clinical trials in the region. Furthermore, considering that several of the newly approved targeted agents and biologicals are not available for the majority of the patients in routine practice, patient inclusion in clinical trials has become a means to gain access to novel therapies.

Key Messages

- A new model of clinical breast cancer research is needed based on molecular biology and the new understanding of cancer biology and ensuring that all countries can participate in the new discoveries.
- Close international collaboration with many different partners is required.
- A lot of international as well as national network groups are active and performing outstanding academic research.
- Asia is becoming an important destination for future solid cancer research including breast cancer. China is taking the lead in breast cancer research, while India is highly involved in the production of drugs.
- Success in the future will depend on a new strategy of pragmatic governance and high-quality standards.
- New regulations in clinical trials should improve research quality without being too much of a burden on academic research.

References

1. Elsevier Research Intelligence. Whitepaper: Working Toward a Cure. Examining the State of Global Breast Cancer Research. October 2011. Available at: https://www.elsevier.com/__data/assets/pdf_file/0017/53225/4108-SciVal-Breast-Cancer-Whitepaper-v3-LO-singles.pdf
2. Eccles A et al. Critical research gaps and translational priorities for the successful prevention and treatment of breast cancer. *Breast Cancer Res* 2013;15:R92.
3. Litière S et al. Breast conserving therapy versus mastectomy for stage I–II breast cancer: 20 year follow-up of the EORTC 10801 phase 3 randomised trial. *Lancet Oncol* 2012;13(4):412–419.

4. Wong L. Cancer research in Asia: challenges and opportunities. Clinical Cancer Research 2010
5. Waning B et al. A lifeline to treatment: the role of Indian generic manufacturers in supplying anti-retroviral medicines to developing countries. *J Int AIDS Soc* 2010;13(1):35.
6. Schwartsmann G et al. A phase 1 trial of the bombesin/gastrin-releasing peptide (BN/GRP) antagonist RC3095 in patients with advanced solid malignancies. *Invest New Drugs* 2006;24(5):403–412.

26

Challenges and Threats

Evandro de Azambuja, Fatima Cardoso, Gilberto Schwartsmann, Didier Verhoeven, Wim Demey, Luis Teixeira, Philippe Aftimos, Etienne Brain, and Ahmad Awada

Do Clinical Trial Designs Currently Meet the Needs of Our Breast Cancer Patients?

Although much has already been done to better organize breast cancer research, a gap remains between actual clinical trial designs and the needs of patients.

Although several new anticancer agents have reached clinical practice faster than in the past, a redundancy remains in their development. Improvements in progression-free survival and disease-free survival are often observed, but rarely is a clear improvement in overall survival seen in early stage disease or in metastatic patients. The designs are mostly inappropriate, and the dose-limiting toxicities are unclear. The commonly used endpoints are, for example, not relevant for immunotherapy. Therefore competitive trials by different companies are performed in similar settings, but comparative studies between drugs of competing companies are rare. Few studies try to look at the best 'therapeutic strategy', or the studies are performed in unmet-needs clinical settings and focus on rare forms of breast cancer (e.g. male breast cancer). More biomarkers are studied, but their validation for clinical use is limited.

Patients play an integral and active part in the clinical trial process. They have the right to more innovative approaches of drug development. Without patients, there would be no trials and no drugs on the market. The involvement of patient advocates is required in the design of new trials. For example, collecting additional biopsies can help researchers predict tumour response, but this can be uncomfortable for the patients. So, their support and compliance are needed (1).

We also need a more individual research with close collaboration between the pharmaceutical industry, investigators, and patient representatives coupled with an academic network in line with the revolution on drugs development and supported by quality control of clinical research sites. High-performing sites are essential for effective and efficient conduct of the clinical trial. True standards for research centres must be developed. Independence, transparency, and effectiveness are important aspects of research units (2). The key to global recognition of accreditation as a 'Clinical Research site' will be the acceptance of its value by trial sponsors, contract research organizations, patients, regulators, and researchers. An emphasis on a culture of competence and high performance is most relevant for robust accreditation (3).

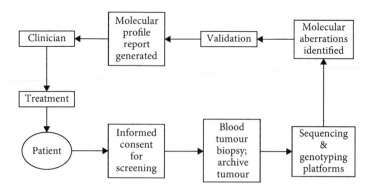

Figure 26.1 Dream or future reality? The circuit of matching patient/tumour/test platform/drug.

Challenges of Clinical Research and Precision Medicine

In the era of targeted therapy and precision medicine, there is an urgent need for an improved drug development methodology. New anticancer agents need optimization of their development, and unmet needs such as the optimization of immunotherapy trials must be addressed. Most of all, the desperate hunt for biomarkers is a priority. Although more biomarkers have been studied (a recent PubMed search identified 42,636 biomarker studies!), very few are validated for clinical use. Therefore new trials must integrate a high level of translational research with a clear potential for clinical practice. Validation must be done by a proper statistical strategy and with reproducible high-quality datasets. Although precision medicine is highly promoted among clinicians as well as patients, only a limited number of actionable/targetable mutations have been found. In addition, relevant trials have limited access. The MOSCATO-01 trial included 1,100 patients from 2011 to 2016, found 411 targetable mutations, but only 119 were treated (4). Although this search for molecular profiles of breast cancer patients is a priority, next generation sequencing is not recommended for clinical practice and remains wishful thinking. Nevertheless, Figure 26.1 proposes a model of matching patient/tumour/test-platform/drugs as a research issue, but it is uncertain for future use and has many limitations and challenges.

Bridging the Gap between Innovation and Clinical Practice

Cancer clinical trials are mostly dedicated to therapeutic innovation leading to regulatory approval. The gap between innovation and clinical practice and between regulatory approval and real-world use of anticancer drugs must be narrowed. Each country determines its real-world use based on its own criteria such as pricing, reimbursement, and clinical indications. Reforming this system from an 'innovation-centred' to a truly 'patient-centred' system with involvement of all stakeholders in the care delivery system requires an independent research infrastructure (Figure 26.2) (5). Regulatory approval by the US Food and Drug Administration or the European Medicines Agency does not

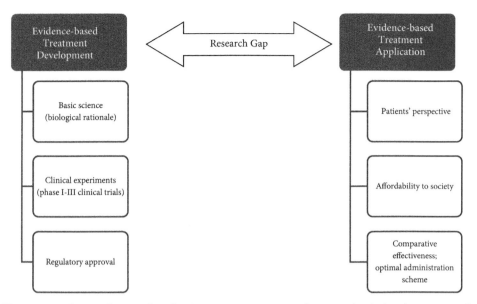

Figure 26.2 Research gap related to innovative treatments between both development and application in real-world clinical practice.

Reproduced with permission from Kempf et al. 'Mind the gap' between the development of the therapeutic innovations and the clinical practice in oncology: A proposal of the European Organisation for Research and Treatment of Cancer (EORTC) to optimize cancer clinical trial research'. *European Journal of Cancer.* Volume 86, pp. 143–149. Copyright © 2017 Elsevier Inc.

guarantee patients' access to innovative treatments. Patients, health professionals, academia, pharmaceutical industry, regulators, payers, and policymakers have the task of collaborating as team players. Too many times in the past, each of these players has defined their own priorities and, thereby, looked differently at innovative treatments: for their own profit, for development of medical possibilities, for advancement of an academic career, for therapeutic efficacy, and for cost to society.

Another important concern is the number of patients who inadequately understand many elements of the presented informed consent. Obtaining this consent from the patient remains essentially the responsibility of the treating physician, but this task should be shared more with other qualified professionals in order to promote a high-quality informed consent through teamwork (6).

Threats and Challenges of Breast Cancer Research

The current strategy of breast cancer research is dominated by business, fashion, and power. Too many 'market- and regulatory-oriented' trials are running compared to patient-directed ones based on real patient needs. The performance of pivotal trials for regulatory purposes remains important. But we also need trials with more individualized research that makes use of well-designed biomarkers and a biological rationale. Unresolved scientific questions in the context of nosological fragmentation of diseases must be highly promoted. To be successful, we need a new and pragmatic model for clinical research networks between investigators, cooperative groups, and the pharmaceutical industry. Improvement in trial design should encompass endpoints that more accurately reflect patient needs (7). Together, all stakeholders must determine the best approach, ensure accountability, and make the best use of resources.

An important point is to realize that clinical research provides us with about the best data we can obtain in a highly selected population. Inclusion and exclusion criteria form an important bias, and, consequently, the participating patients should not be seen as a window to the real-world. The data in cancer registries, on the contrary, provide real-life data about limited variables covering the whole population. This makes benchmarking possible, but it also presents opportunities for population-based research. In the future, further expansion of research to 'big data' has the potential to give us a lot of additional information about many missing variables of the whole population (see Chapter 22).

Key Messages

- There is lack of funding at all levels of breast cancer research.
- Too many business-oriented and too few patient-directed trials are performed.
- Power, business, and fashion dominate clinical research projects.
- There are not many clinical research trials conducted to study surgery, radiation therapy, epidemiological, and causality aspects of breast cancer.
- Clear endpoints must be defined and be understandable for all stakeholders, and these must take patient needs into account, including patient-reported outcomes.
- Patients are the risk-takers in the clinical trials and must be represented in the design of the trials, especially in case of additional biopsies. The informed consent has to be understandable for the patients.

References

1. Batten L et al. Patient advocate involvement in the design and conduct of breast cancer clinical trials requiring the collection of multiple biopsies. *Res Involv Engagem* 2018;4:22.
2. Johnston S et al. Voluntary site accreditation—improving the execution of multicenter clinical trials *N Engl J Med* 2017;377:1414–1415.
3. Koski G et al. Accreditation of clinical research sites—moving forward. *N Engl J Med* 2018;379(5):405–407.
4. Massart M et al. Better outcomes with precision medicine. *Cancer Discov* 2016;6(12):1296–1297.
5. Kempf E et al. 'Mind the gap' between the development of the therapeutic innovations and the clinical practice in oncology: a proposal of the European Organisation for Research and Treatment of Cancer (EORTC) to optimize cancer clinical trial research. *Eur J Cancer* 2017;86:143–149.
6. Fernandez-Lynch H et al. Informed consent and the role of the treating physician. *N Engl J Med* 2018;378:2433–2438.
7. Wilson M. Outcomes and endpoints in cancer trials: bridging the divide. *Lancet Oncol* 2015;16(1):PE43–E52.

PART 8

THE ECONOMICS OF BREAST CANCER CARE

27

Assessing Costs and Value for Money

Manuela Joore, Xavier Pouwels, and Bram Ramaekers

Introduction

Worldwide, health care expenses have increased substantially over the last decades, even when taking the increasing welfare over time into account (Figure 27.1). In the European Union (EU), the costs of cancer care were estimated to be €51 billion (2009), which comprises 4% of the total health care expenses. When including productivity losses and informal care costs, the total economic burden of cancer was estimated to be €126 billion in the EU, representing 1% of the gross domestic product (GDP) (1). Breast cancer accounted for the highest health care expenses (€7 billion; 13% of the total cancer-related costs) in the EU. Medication costs accounted for approximately 50% of the health care costs relating to breast cancer treatment (approximately €3 billion out of the €7 billion), which represents 20% of the total economic burden of breast cancer in the EU. Similarly, productivity losses due to mortality and informal care are both associated with high costs (both exceeding €3 billion). The total economic burden of breast cancer was estimated to be €15 billion, representing on average €13 per capita in the EU (1).

These increasing health care expenses are not sustainable. Different initiatives aim at containing these increasing expenses by preventing overdiagnosis and overtreatment (http://www.choosingwisely.org/). Precision oncology may also be promising for containing health care expenses by improving breast cancer treatment efficiency. However, opinions on the potential of precision oncology in decreasing health care expenses are divided. Only future and broader implementation of precision oncology will determine whether it can contribute to a more efficient use of limited health care resources.

Decision-makers resort to health economics to inform reimbursement decisions on new breast cancer interventions. A fundamental objective of health economics is to determine the optimal use of the limited funds that are available. The underlying principle is that a decision-maker will allocate the funds available such that health is maximized. In reality, this means that priorities are set: some interventions are reimbursed, whereas others are not or only partially reimbursed (Box 27.1). In order to make these priority-setting decisions, decision-makers can rely on the results of cost of illness studies and budget impact analysis (to assess affordability) as well as economic evaluations (to assess efficiency) of new interventions. The following sections contain an explanation of these techniques as well as examples of applications to breast cancer care. In addition, the use of these techniques in health care policy decision-making is described.

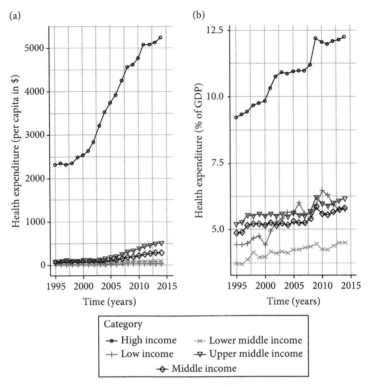

Figure 27.1 Health expenditure over time per capita in dollars and as percentage of gross domestic product (GDP).

Source: World Bank Open Data (obtained June 15, 2017 from http://data.worldbank.org/). Reproduced under the Creative Commons Attribution 4.0 International License https://creativecommons.org/licenses/by/4.0/.

Assessing the Costs of Breast Cancer Care

Cost-of-illness (COI) studies estimate the costs associated with a specific condition. A COI study starts with determining the target population, which is a subset of the population with the disease (for instance patients with HER2-positive breast cancer). The population with the disease is a subset of the total population; this is particularly relevant to consider if a preventive intervention (such as breast cancer screening) is considered, because this will impact the incidence of the condition. Once the target population is defined, the resources used by patients in this population are estimated. Depending on the perspective, this might include only health care resources, or be broadened to include costs in other sectors (productivity for instance) and patient and family costs (such as out-of-pocket expenses, travel costs, and informal care costs). A distinction can be made between a prevalence-based and an incidence-based approach. In the prevalence-based approach, resource use of all patients affected in a certain time-period is considered. In the incidence-based approach, the resource use over the remaining lifetime of incident patients in a specific period of time is considered. A budget impact analysis (BIA) can be used to inform budget planning. In a BIA, the expected expenditures associated with the adoption of a new health care intervention are assessed. This means that the COI in the current environment is compared to the COI in the new environment after adoption of the new intervention (Figure 27.2).

BIAs are used by budget holders, and these differ between jurisdictions. The budget holders may include administrators of national health care programmes or private insurance plans, employees of health care delivery organizations, and employers who pay for health care of their employees. It is important to tailor the perspective of the BIA to the budget holder. The International Society of Pharmacoeconomics and Outcomes Research (ISPOR, https://www.ispor.org/budget-impact-health-study-guideline.asp) has published principles of good practice for BIA. In these publications, an analytical framework containing all important aspects in the design of a BIA is described.

Assessing Value for Money of Breast Cancer Care: Economic Evaluation

Economic evaluations compare the costs and effects of at least two interventions. The difference in costs is divided by the difference in effects between the new and old interventions to obtain an incremental cost-effectiveness ratio (ICER) (Figure 27.3).

Economic evaluations of breast cancer care are mostly cost-effectiveness analysis (CEA) and cost-utility analysis (CUA). These two types of economic evaluation differ in the way effects are measured and valued. In a CEA, the effects are expressed in natural

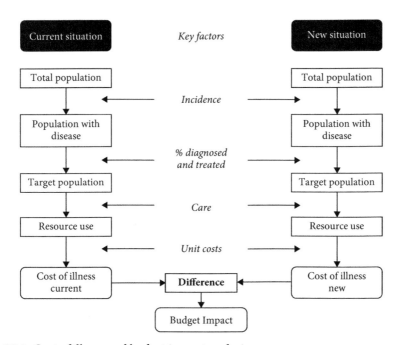

Figure 27.2 Cost of illness and budget impact analysis.

Adapted with permission from Sullivan et al. 'Budget Impact Analysis-Principles of Good Practice: Report of the ISPOR 2012 Budget Impact Analysis Good Practice II task force'. *Value in Health,* Volume 17, Issue 1, pp. 5–14. Copyright © 2014 Elsevier Inc. DOI: https://doi.org/10.1016/j.jval.2013.08.2291 (2)

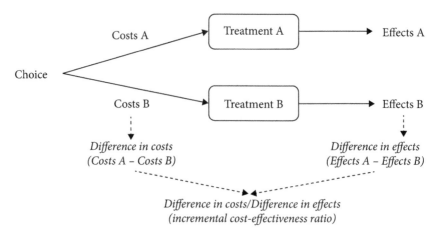

Figure 27.3 Cost-effectiveness and cost-utility analysis.
In cost-utility analysis the effects are expressed in quality-adjusted life-years.

units, such as number of life-years gained or proportion of patients with serious toxicity avoided. In a CUA, the effects are expressed in quality-adjusted life-years (QALYs). QALYs are a combined measure of survival and health-related quality of life, with one QALY representing one year in perfect health. The health-related quality-of-life valuation used to calculate QALYs is often referred to as *utility*, and is mostly obtained using instruments such as the EuroQol 5 dimensions (EQ-5D) (http://www.Euroqol.org) or the 36-Item Short Form Survey (SF-36) (https://www.rand.org/health/surveys_tools/mos/36-item-short-form.html). These instruments (so-called multi-attribute utility instruments) combine a descriptive part containing questions regarding health that is completed by patients and a tariff that can be used to turn these scores into a utility. This utility presents the value of a health state, from the perspective of the general public. Alternatively, patient's preferences for health and health care can be used as outcomes in economic evaluations (see Chapter 29). The advantage of CEA is that it has a very clear link to the outcomes in clinical trials. The advantage of CUA is that the results of CUAs can be easily compared across all populations and for all types of interventions, because the measure of effect (the QALY) is generic. Several handbooks and good practice guidelines (e.g. ISPOR, https://www.ispor.org/workpaper/Modeling-Good-Research-Practices-Overview.asp) exist on the methods for economic evaluations in health care, and measuring and valuing health effects for economic evaluations (3,4).

There are two approaches to conducting an economic evaluation: trial-based and model-based (3). Trial-based economic evaluations are conducted alongside clinical trials, in which resource use is collected besides clinical outcomes and if a cost-utility analysis is planned, multi-attribute utility instruments are used to collect utility data. These economic evaluations serve primarily the purpose of information gathering. Model-based economic evaluations consist of a model (a series of mathematical and statistical relationships) that describes a situation based on all available knowledge. Model-based economic evaluations are evidence synthesis tools to estimate the performance of an intervention in the real-world context for which a decision has to be made. This context often is or cannot be observed in a trial. For instance, the trial follow-up may be too short to capture all consequences, the patient population is not representative for the real-world situation, and often not all relevant comparator interventions are observed in a single trial (4).

It is considered good practice to address uncertainty surrounding the (incremental) costs, effects, and cost-effectiveness ratio. Because costs are often skewed, bootstrapping is recommended to construct confidence intervals. The costs and effects are calculated from each bootstrap sample, and these bootstrap estimates are then used to build up an empirical distribution of costs and effects. The number of bootstrap samples required depends on the sample data, but typically should be at least 1,000. The bootstrap results are often plotted on a cost-effectiveness plane, with the incremental costs on the y-axis and the incremental effects on the x-axis (Figure 27.4A).

To show the probability of an ICER being acceptable to decision-makers, the value of the unit of effect (in CUA the QALY) has to be known. This value is established in some jurisdictions. An intervention is considered cost-effective if the ICER is below this value. The National Institute of Health and Care Excellence in the United Kingdom (https://www.nice.org.uk), for instance, uses a threshold of £20,000 for most types of intervention. In situations where the threshold is uncertain, a cost-effectiveness acceptability curve can be drawn, based on the results of the bootstrapping, by calculating the proportion of bootstrap replicates below the threshold for a range of thresholds (Figure 27.4B) (5).

Priority Setting and Managed Entry Agreements in Health Care

Since health maximization with available resources is often one major objective of health systems, it is increasingly recognized that merely effectiveness of a new intervention is not a persuasive factor for inclusion in public insurance plans (Box 27.1). To illustrate this, Dakin et al. (6) estimated that cost-effectiveness alone correctly predicted 82% of reimbursement decisions in the UK. Nevertheless, other factors are often considered next to cost-effectiveness when making these decisions. In the UK, the willingness to pay is higher for end-of-life treatments (https://www.nice.org.uk/guidance/gid-tag387/documents/appraising-life-extending-end-of-life-treatments-paper2), whereas in the Netherlands, the willingness to pay is higher for diseases with a higher burden (https://english.zorginstituutnederland.nl/publications/reports/2015/06/16/cost-effectiveness-in-practice).

Based on the cost-effectiveness evidence and other relevant criteria, decision-makers might decide whether to reimburse a (new) intervention. However, these decisions are often made under considerable uncertainty, making the trade-off between these different criteria difficult. In response to this uncertainty and growing financial risks (due to the increasing costs of medical technology), decision-makers increasingly opt for

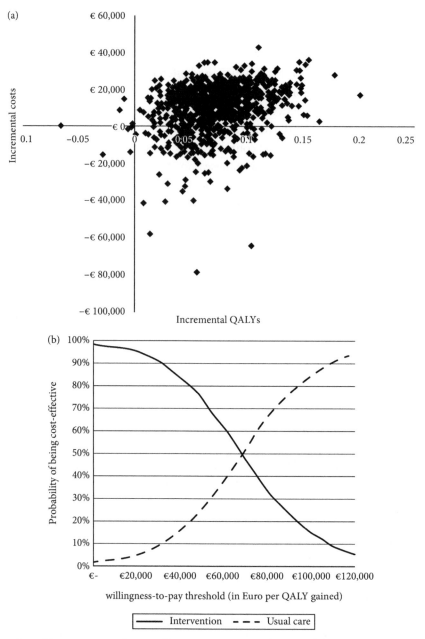

Figure 27.4 The incremental cost-effectiveness plane and cost-effectiveness acceptability curve.

QALYs, quality-adjusted life-years.

(a) Incremental cost-effectiveness plane showing the bootstrapped incremental costs and effects (in QALYs) of an intervention versus usual care.

(b) Cost-effectiveness acceptability curve. The curve indicates the probability (*y*-axis) of an intervention being cost-effective compared to usual care with different threshold values (*x*-axis).

Box 27.1 Priority setting using cost-effectiveness to maximize health

To use cost-effectiveness analyses for reimbursement decision-making, it is necessary to specify a willingness to pay threshold, i.e. the amount society should be willing to pay per additional unit of effect, often specified as quality-adjusted life-years. Setting this willingness to pay threshold incorrectly (e.g. too high or too low) will lead to opportunity costs and health benefits forgone (2). This is illustrated in Figure 27.5 using hypothetical health systems (I–IV), wherein each bar represents an intervention with a certain height (representing the health benefit per $1,000), and a certain width (representing the total costs of this intervention). The vertical line represents the budget limit. All interventions to the left of this line are reimbursed in the hypothetical health system, whereas the others are excluded given the constrained budget. In health system I, the interventions are prioritized based on cost-effectiveness; consequently interventions A–H are reimbursed whereas interventions I–L are not. In health system II, interventions are prioritized based on criteria other than cost-effectiveness; consequently interventions A and B, which generated a relatively large amount of health benefit per $1,000, are displaced by intervention L which generated a relatively low amount of health benefit per $1,000. Thus, with the same budget, health system II produces less health (i.e. health benefits forgone) compared with health system I due to prioritization based on criteria other than cost-effectiveness.

I: prioritized based on cost-effectiveness

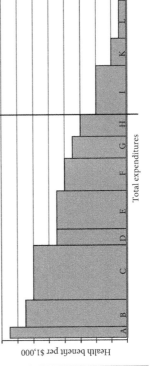

II: prioritized based on criteria other than cost-effectiveness

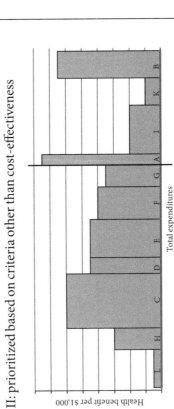

Health system III is confronted with the question whether to adopt interventions X–Z. From a cost-effectiveness perspective, it should be questioned whether these new interventions produce more health benefit per $1,000 than the interventions that have already been adopted (A–H). Since the health benefit per $1,000 for intervention Z is above this 'threshold'; this intervention should be adopted, as shown in health system IV. Here it also becomes clear that this threshold is inherently dependent on the health care budget; for instance if the health care budget increases, then the 'threshold' should be altered to include interventions producing less health benefit per $1,000 (e.g. readopting intervention H again in health system IV).

III: adopting new interventions (X–Z) in health system A

IV: intervention H is displaced by intervention Z

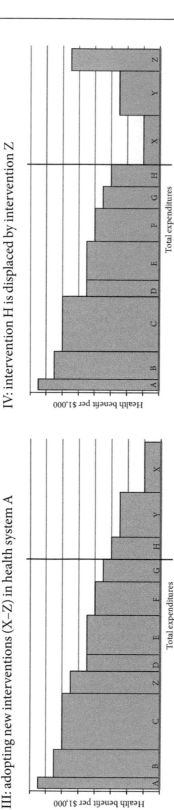

Figure 27.5 Based on Culyer et al. 'Cost-effectiveness thresholds in health care: a bookshelf guide to their meaning and use.' *Health Economics, Policy and Law.* Volume 11, Issue 4. pp. 415–432. Copyright © 2016, CUP. DOI: https://doi.org/10.1017/S1744133116000049

managed entry agreements (MEAs; also termed risk-sharing agreements) instead of a simple yes/no recommendation (https://www.ispor.org/risk-sharing-health-program-guideline.asp). MEAs are arrangements, typically between payers and manufacturers of an intervention and might involve (1) effective price changes/discounts (either dependent or independent on outcome) and (2) the collection of evidence while the technology is temporarily adopted within a health system. In case MEA schemes are well designed and used appropriately, these arrangements can help decision-makers to optimize recommendations regarding the adoption of interventions in a predictable, transparent, and rational manner (http://nicedsu.org.uk/methods-development/managed-entry-agreements-mea/).

Key Messages

- Societal health care expenditures, of which a considerable part is due to breast cancer care, are rising to levels that may not be sustainable.
- Health economics can assist decision-makers to adopt and reimburse care that is affordable and efficient.
- Results from economic evaluations inform the allocation of available budgets in order to maximize health and patients' outcomes.

References

1. Luengo-Fernandez R et al. Economic burden of cancer across the European Union: a population-based cost analysis. *Lancet Oncol* 2013;14(12):1165–1174.
2. Sullivan SD et al. Budget impact analysis—principles of good practice: report of the ISPOR 2012 Budget Impact Analysis Good Practice II task force. Value in Health 2014;17:5–14.
3. Drummond MF et al. *Methods for the Economic Evaluation of Health Care Programmes.* Oxford University Press; 2015.
4. Ratcliffe J et al. *Measuring and Valuing Health Benefits for Economic Evaluation.* Oxford University Press; 2016.
5. Aarts MJ et al. Cost effectiveness of primary pegfilgrastim prophylaxis in patients with breast cancer at risk of febrile neutropenia. *J Clin Oncol* 2013;31(34):4283–4289.
6. Dakin H et al. The influence of cost-effectiveness and other factors on NICE decisions. *Health Econ* 2014;24(10):1256–1271.

28

The Economic Impact of Breast Cancer in the South-East Asian Region

Merel Kimman, Sanne Peters, Stephen Jan, Nirmala Bhoo-Pathy, Cheng-Har Yip, Manuela Joore, and Mark Woodward

Introduction

The economic burden of cancer treatments to health systems across the world will grow since the population is ageing and the availability of medical technologies and treatments expands. The economic burden falls not only on the health systems, but also on patients, families, and societies as a whole. Most patients and families incur costs as a result of a cancer diagnosis. These can include direct medical costs such as those associated with seeing general practitioners, medical specialists, allied health professionals, receiving treatment (e.g. surgery, radiotherapy, chemotherapy), and those associated with buying medications to help alleviate the symptoms of cancer and the side-effects of treatment. The majority of patients also have out-of-pocket expenses in relation to travelling to hospital appointments. Furthermore, patients may be unable to continue working due to the burden of their symptoms, treatment, or side-effects, and this leads to decreases in household income as well as costs to society in terms of lost productivity.

Health insurance generally reduces the out-of-pocket costs of treatment. The extent of financial protection, however, is highly health system specific and varies in services covered and the level to which expenses are reimbursed. When financial protection is limited and social safety nets are not present, patients diagnosed with cancer face the prospect of financial ruin. The financial burden of a cancer diagnosis is felt most strongly in socioeconomically disadvantaged groups, and particularly those in low- and middle-income countries where out-of-pocket payments are the principal means of financing health care.

Financial burden is commonly defined in terms of the incidence of *financial catastrophe*, where out-of-pocket expenditure for health care exceeds a defined threshold proportion of annual income, usually 30% of annual household income or 40% of non-food expenditure or income. Another important indicator of financial burden is *economic hardship*, which can be defined as a household's inability to pay living or medical expenses or the use of financial coping strategies (e.g. drew on accumulated savings or sought financial assistance) in order to pay a living expense (1). In this chapter, the economic impact of a breast cancer diagnosis is illustrated using data from the Asean CosTs In ONcology (ACTION) study (2).

The Economic Impact of Breast Cancer in Low- and Middle-Income Countries

The ACTION study was a unique observational study of the household burden of cancer conducted in eight low- and middle-income countries in South-East Asia (Cambodia, Indonesia, Laos, Malaysia, Myanmar, Philippines, Thailand, and Vietnam) (3) (Box 28.1). Patients diagnosed with a first-time cancer were consecutively recruited (within 12 weeks from initial date of diagnosis) from 47 sites, including public and private hospitals and cancer centres, and followed through their first year following diagnosis. The main outcomes of interest of the ACTION study comprised incidence of financial catastrophe, economic hardship, and all-cause mortality at one year following cancer diagnosis. Mortality is an important competing outcome of financial burden, since patients may avoid incurring high out-of-pocket costs due to (early) death or because data on out-of-pocket costs are not captured due to death. Financial catastrophe was defined as out-of-pocket costs at 12 months equal to or exceeding 30% of annual household income. Costs included medical costs (inpatient/outpatient care, purchase of drugs, medical supplies and equipment, traditional medicine) and non-medical costs due to illness (transportation, accommodation, etc.), which were directly incurred by patients at point of delivery and not reimbursed by insurance.

Between March 2012 and September 2013, 9,513 patients were recruited into the ACTION study, of whom 2435 were female patients with a breast cancer diagnosis. The mean age of these breast cancer patients was 50 years, with the majority diagnosed with stage II or III cancer. Most patients (62%) were from lower middle-income countries (Indonesia, Laos, Philippines, or Vietnam), 28% from upper middle-income countries (Thailand or Malaysia), and 10% of patients were from low-income countries (Myanmar or Cambodia). Half of the patients had some form of health insurance. See Table 28.1 for key characteristics of the breast cancer sample. It must be noted that patients with advanced cancer stages or those who are very poor may have been underrepresented in the study population, since they may not have presented to the health system for care.

Financial Catastrophe

One year after diagnosis, data on financial catastrophe and death were available for 1667 (69%) of the study sample; of these, almost two-thirds (61%, $n = 1027$) experienced financial catastrophe, 13% ($n = 217$) died, and just 26% ($n = 432$) had a favourable outcome one year after diagnosis, i.e. alive and no financial catastrophe (Figure 28.1B). Figure 28.1C illustrates that around 10% of the financial catastrophe cases were driven by excessive non-medical expenditures. Factors such as high age (aged >54 years), being unmarried, having below-average income, not having health insurance, and not having paid work were associated with a higher odds of experiencing financial catastrophe. In relation to the outcome mortality at one year, an older age, low

Box 28.1 Patients' experiences with breast cancer diagnosis and treatment in Malaysia and Indonesia

I. Patient Experience: Malaysia

Mei[a] is a very busy 32-year-old mother of three from Kuala Lumpur, Malaysia. She first noticed a lump when she was breast feeding with her second child. Worried, she was unsure who to consult or where to seek help. She went to her gynaecologist several times and was told repeatedly that nothing was wrong. It wasn't until she was heavily pregnant with her third child that her symptoms were taken seriously and she was referred to a breast surgeon. A biopsy revealed, to her shock, that she had breast cancer. Because the diagnosis was delayed, by that stage, it had also spread to her lymph nodes. She was angry and scared.

To make matters worse, Mei had a long and anxious wait until her baby was born until she could be treated. Two weeks after the birth and still in postnatal recovery, Mei started chemotherapy to shrink the tumour. She later underwent surgery and then radiotherapy for six weeks alongside targeted therapy.

Mei's journey continues to be a struggle, but despite this she considers herself one of the lucky ones; first, because her pregnancy made her a priority case for doctors; second, because insurance covered the costs of her expensive treatment. Despite this, Mei still sees an impact on her household income from health supplements and other out-of-pocket expenses, which were burdensome especially with three small children.

'I used to be a caretaker, now I am the patient too.'

II. Patient Experience: Indonesia

Melati[a] is aged 52 years and lives in Jakarta, Indonesia. From when she first noticed symptoms, a lump in the breast, it took two years and five check-ups with five different doctors until a biopsy confirmed that she had stage 2 breast cancer.

Frustrated the cancer was not caught earlier, Melati underwent surgery and several courses of chemotherapy at one of the main hospitals in Jakarta. Conditions in the wards were crowded and, consequently, patients have to wait long periods of time. The oncologist had limited time to converse about her diagnosis and outlook. Given the situation, Melati understood that the doctor would not have enough time to explain more about her disease. For this reason, she decided to ask her doctor questions proactively to get a better understanding of her condition.

Now in remission, Melati has been able to get back to a relatively normal life taking care of the family home and her husband. She feels very fortunate that cancer treatment was covered by insurance, but despite this, her children, who are in their 20s, still needed to support with some out-of-pocket expenses.

[a]The patient names have been changed.

Table 28.1 Baseline characteristics of 2,435 female breast cancer patients

Characteristic	N	%
Age group (years)		
<45	765	31
45–54	899	37
55–64	552	23
≥65	218	9
Missing	1	<1
Marital status		
Married	1,829	75
Not married	606	25
Level of education		
0–6 years (primary)	824	34
6–12 years (secondary)	972	40
>12 years (tertiary)	638	26
Missing	1	<1
Country income type		
Low-income (Myanmar, Cambodia)	244	10
Lower middle-income (Indonesia, Laos, Philippines, Vietnam)	1,503	62
Upper middle-income (Thailand, Malaysia)	688	28
Household income		
Low	838	34
Medium	436	18
High	747	31
Don't know	414	17
Health insurance		
No	1,236	51
Yes	1,198	49
Missing	1	<1
Cancer TNM stage		
I	198	8
II	864	36
III	614	25
IV	157	7
Unknown/missing	602	24

Reproduced with permission from The ACTION Study Group. 'Policy and priorities for national cancer control planning in low- and middle-income countries: Lessons from the Association of Southeast Asian Nations (ASEAN) Costs in Oncology prospective cohort study.' *European Journal of Cancer*. Volume 74, pp. 26–37. Copyright © 2017 Elsevier Inc. DOI: https://doi.org/10.1016/j.ejca.2016.12.014

income, not having paid work, lower levels of education, as well as a more advanced cancer stage were associated with higher odds of death (Table 28.2). The mortality rate may be underestimated, because severely ill and terminal patients were not recruited into the study for ethical reasons. Also, the lost to follow-up group (*n* = 768) may include a relatively high proportion of patients who could not be contacted due to death and thus could not be coded as such.

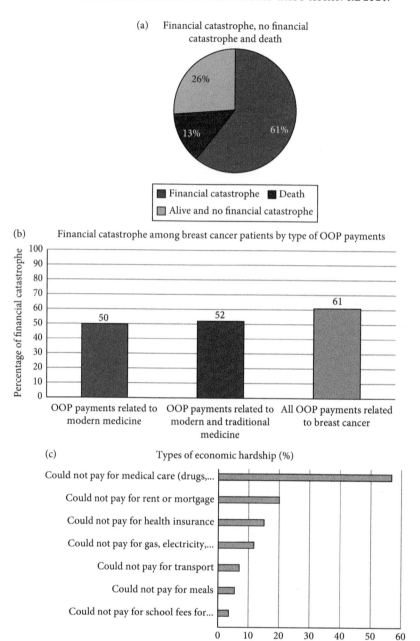

Figure 28.1 Financial catastrophe, economic hardship, and death at 12 months after diagnosis among breast cancer patients. OOP, out-of-pocket.

(a) Study outcomes 12 months after diagnosis among breast cancer patients ($N = 1,667$). (b) Financial catastrophe at 12 months after diagnosis, by type of out-of-pocket payments ($N = 1,667$). (c) Types of economic hardship ($n = 393$). (d) Types of coping strategies used ($n = 393$).

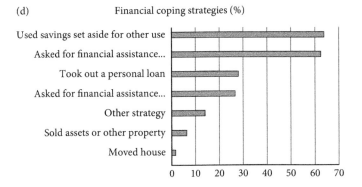

Figure 28.1 Continued

Economic Hardship

A year after diagnosis, of patients who were financially solvent at baseline, economic hardship was reported by a quarter of families. Around 56% of these families, for example, could not pay for their cancer medicines, medical tests, or consultations, 20% were unable to pay their rent or mortgage, and 12% could not pay their utility bills (not mutually exclusive) (Figure 28.1A). To cope with economic hardship, 64% of affected families used their savings that were set aside for other use, 28% resorted to taking personal loans, and 14% had sold their assets or property (not mutually exclusive) (Figure 28.1D).

Breast Cancer in Relation to Other Cancer Types

Across all other cancers represented in the ACTION study sample (i.e. excluding breast cancer), financial catastrophe was experienced by 44% of the population, and by one year after diagnosis 35% of the population had died. Across other cancers, financial catastrophe was most frequent in participants with gastrointestinal cancers (51%) and gynaecological cancers (51%). The finding that financial catastrophe was thus most frequent in breast cancer (61%) is not surprising, because breast cancer is generally amenable to chemotherapy, radiotherapy, hormone therapy, and targeted therapy, all inducing potential costs to patients. Furthermore, breast cancer is less fatal than other cancers, and patients who live longer incur more costs. Other risk factors for financial catastrophe and death, such as higher age or a low income, were similar across breast and other cancers.

Table 28.2 Odds ratios (and 95% confidence intervals) for financial catastrophe and death, relative to no financial catastrophe (reference) in breast cancer patients with complete outcome data (n = 1,667), adjusted for age, sex, cancer stage, and geographic region

Characteristic		Financial catastrophe	Death
Age (in years)	<45	Reference	Reference
	45–54	1.22 (0.85; 1.73)	1.01 (0.60; 1.72)
	55–64	1.64 (1.10; 2.88)	1.28 (0.53; 3.09)
	65	1.74 (1.06; 2.88)	1.28 (0.53; 3.09)
Highest level of education	Tertiary	Reference	Reference
	Secondary	1.39 (0.97; 1.99)	1.76 (1.00; 3.11)
	Primary	1.19 (0.81; 1.75)	2.52 (1.41; 4.50)
Marital status	Married	Reference	Reference
	Unmarried	1.35 (0.96; 1.89)	1.01 (0.59; 1.73)
Health insurance	Yes	Reference	Reference
	No	1.12 (0.84; 1.49)	1.36 (0.87; 2.13)
Income level	High	Reference	Reference
	Med	2.06 (1.40; 3.01)	2.17 (1.06; 4.41)
	Low	4.88 (3.39; 7.02)	8.87 (4.83; 16.29)
Paid Work	Yes	Reference	Reference
	No	1.57 (1.17; 2.11)	1.91 (1.22; 2.98)
Cancer TNM stage	1	Reference	Reference
	2	1.32 (0.86; 2.01)	1.63 (0.53; 4.96)
	3	0.98 (0.62; 1.54)	4.61 (1.53; 13.91)
	4	0.89 (0.47; 1.67)	11.45 (3.45; 37.99)

Reproduced with permission from Jan S et al. 'Financial catastrophe, treatment discontinuation and death associated with surgically operable cancer in South-East Asia: Results from the ACTION Study.' *Surgery*. Volume 157, Issue 6, pp. 971–982. Copyright © 2015 Elsevier Inc. DOI: https://doi.org/10.1016/j.surg.2015.02.012

Policy Implications

Breast cancer can lead to major financial burden, especially in low- and middle-income countries, because treatments are costly and out-of-pocket expenses are high. This was illustrated by the ACTION study conducted in South-East Asia: among the study's breast cancer population, almost two-thirds of families faced catastrophic expenditures for treatment, and one in four families experienced economic hardship within one year after diagnosis. Older patients and patients with greater levels of disadvantage (e.g. low income or education) tended to have higher risk of financial burden. Findings in the breast cancer population differed from results obtained for other types of cancer, in that financial catastrophe was higher and mortality lower (3–5). There is a clear need for governments to re-examine their health financing systems and extend financial protection through social health insurance and publicly supported cancer care to better protect citizens from the costs associated with cancer treatment. Health insurance alone, however, is not sufficient to protect households from catastrophic expenditures and economic hardship. The ACTION study showed that despite having some form of health insurance, rates of financial catastrophe and economic hardship remained high (60% and 39%, respectively). This may be explained by the limitations of benefit packages available through health insurance programmes in some of the participating countries. Furthermore, non-medical costs such as transportation, accommodation, and childcare costs also increase household expenses for health care. Early diagnosis followed by prompt treatment remains the hallmark of an effective cancer control strategy resulting in less invasive treatment, better health outcomes, and, thus, potentially lower household economic burden. Policymakers, payers, and healthcare providers in low- and middle-income countries have to work towards making the best use of available resources to provide timely access to optimal cancer treatment (6). In addition, it is crucial for governments to create social safety nets and put in place programmes to improve welfare support for cancer (e.g. income support, access to short-term credit, and disability insurance) and public transport services, which are beyond the scope of health care systems, per se. In conclusion, breast cancer must be recognized, prioritized, and seen as a cross-governmental issue affecting households, society, and the economy, rather than merely health.

Key Messages

- Approximately three in four new breast cancer patients in South-East Asia experience financial catastrophe or die within one year after diagnosis.
- An advanced stage at diagnosis and living in lower socioeconomic status are significant risk factors for these poor outcomes.
- There is an urgent need for more resources to aid early detection
- Policies should aim to provide adequate financial protection from the costs of cancer.

References

1. Essue B et al. We can't afford my chronic illness! The out-of-pocket burden associated with managing chronic obstructive pulmonary disease in western Sydney, Australia. *J Health Serv Res Policy* 2011;16(4):226–231.

2. Kimman M et al. Socioeconomic impact of cancer in member countries of the Association of Southeast Asian Nations (ASEAN): the ACTION study protocol. *Asian Pac J Cancer Prev* 2012;13(2):421–425.
3. ACTION Study Group. Policy and priorities for national cancer control planning in low- and middle-income countries: lessons from the Association of Southeast Asian Nations (ASEAN) Costs in Oncology prospective cohort study. *Eur J Cancer* 2017;74:26–37.
4. Jan S et al. Financial catastrophe, treatment discontinuation and death associated with surgically operable cancer in South-East Asia: results from the ACTION Study. *Surgery* 2015;157(6):971–982.
5. Kimman M et al. Catastrophic health expenditure and 12-month mortality associated with cancer in Southeast Asia: results from a longitudinal study in eight countries. *BMC Med* 2015;13:190.
6. Horton S, Gauvreau CL. Cancer in low- and middle-income countries: an economic overview. In Gelband H, Jha P, Sankaranarayanan R, and Horton S, editors, *Cancer: Disease Control Priorities*, 3rd ed., vol. 3. Washington DC: International Bank for Reconstruction and Development/World Bank; 2015.

29

Moving from a 'One Size Fits All' to Personalized Follow-Up in Breast Cancer Survivors—Connecting Patient-Reported Outcomes with Economic Considerations

The Dutch Experience

Carmen D. Dirksen, Merel Kimman, Manuela Joore, and Liesbeth Boersma

Introduction

In the Netherlands, one out of seven women is faced with the diagnosis of breast cancer during her lifetime (1). In most European countries, these women, following primary treatment, are invited to attend frequent follow-up visits in the hospital, generally every 3–4 months in the first 2 years, every 6 months from year 3 to year 5, and annually thereafter (2). The aim of these follow-up examinations is not only to detect local disease recurrence, a second primary breast cancer, or detection and registration of side-effects of treatment, but also to provide information and psychosocial support. Yet the need for frequent follow-up visits with clinical examination in these patients remains an issue of debate, because studies have convincingly shown that it does not contribute to improved survival and may induce stress and anxiety because of the (perceived) risk of detecting a recurrence, and may fall short on meeting the needs of breast cancer patients in terms of physical and psychosocial support (3). At the same time, intensive follow-up is associated with a significant financial burden due to the growing number of breast cancer survivors on the one hand, and limited health care resources on the other. Less intensive and specialized follow-up strategies have therefore been investigated, for example, performed by specialized breast care nurses, general practitioners (GPs), or by telephone instead of hospital visits. Clinical trials investigating such strategies have not identified differences in terms of timeliness of recurrence detection, overall survival, and health-related quality-of-life (HRQoL) outcomes compared to traditional hospital visits (4).

In the Netherlands, two studies were performed to investigate not only the effectiveness of several alternative follow-up strategies in terms of patient-reported outcomes (HRQoL and satisfaction), but also to address economic considerations in breast cancer follow-up care. First, a pragmatic multicentre randomized controlled trial (RCT) was performed to compare traditional hospital follow-up with three alternative follow-up strategies that aimed to better address HRQoL and psychosocial needs of patients in the first one to two years after primary treatment. In addition, in order to investigate whether offering alternative follow-up strategies provides value for money and reduces the financial burden to society, the costs and effects of the four follow-up strategies were additionally compared in an economic evaluation (5). Second, a large patient preference study among Dutch breast cancer survivors was performed to identify patients' preferences for follow-up in terms of the frequency and type of contact, health care provider, and psychosocial support, since women's attitudes towards less intensive and less specialized follow-up strategies are key indicators for successful implementation. Results were combined with cost estimates so as to investigate potential cost consequences of introducing personalized follow-up in breast cancer care (6).

The MaCare Trial

Between 2005 and 2008, 320 eligible females who had completed curative breast cancer treatment were recruited into the MaCare trial and randomly assigned to one of four follow-up arms for the first 18 months after primary treatment:

1. Hospital follow-up as usual with five hospital visits at 3, 6, 9, 12, and 18 months including a mammography at 12 months.
2. Nurse-led telephone follow-up with a mammography at 12 months combined with a hospital visit and four telephone consultations by a breast care nurse (BCN) at 3, 6, 9, and 18 months.
3. Arm 1 plus an educational group programme (EGP).
4. Arm 2 plus an EGP.

The newly developed EGP consisted of two interactive group sessions of 2.5 h each and was attended by the patient and her partner (if possible/applicable) within three months after finalizing treatment. The BCN provided information on possible treatment side-effects (fatigue in particular), signs and symptoms of a possible recurrence, and prostheses. A health care psychologist addressed psychological and social consequences of breast cancer and psychological coping strategies. The telephone follow-up was performed by a BCN familiar to the patient and was guided by a semi-structured questionnaire which included screening for physical, especially locoregional and psychosocial symptoms, and compliance to hormonal therapy. Furthermore, the BCN informed about general wellbeing of the patient, her family life, social relationships, and work reintegration. The study protocol and detailed description of the follow-up strategies can be found elsewhere (5).

Patient-Reported Outcomes

The primary outcome in the MaCare trial was HRQoL as assessed by the global health subscale of the EORTC QLQC30 at 12 months after randomization. Although patients' HRQoL significantly improved over time, at 12 months there was no significant difference in HRQoL between nurse-led telephone and hospital follow-up nor between follow-up with or without an EGP. Secondary outcomes were emotional and role functioning (EORTC QLQ-C30 subscales), anxiety (State–Trait Anxiety Inventory), and perceived feelings of control (Mastery Scale). These all improved over time, but the study did not reveal significant differences between the follow-up strategies (see Table 29.1 for summary descriptions of the results) (7).

To assess patient satisfaction, the Dutch version of the validated Ware's Patient Satisfaction questionnaire III (PSQ III) was used, focusing on satisfaction with interpersonal aspects, technical competences of staff, access to care, and general satisfaction. For the purpose of the patient satisfaction study, hospital follow-up (arms 1 and 3) was compared with telephone follow-up (arms 2 and 4). Patient satisfaction scores were high in all subscales of the PSQ III, and no meaningful differences were found between the two types of follow-up (8,9).

Cost-Effectiveness

An economic evaluation was performed which compared the four follow-up strategies in terms of effects and costs over a 12-month period following study inclusion. A societal perspective was taken, meaning that all health care costs (e.g. diagnostic procedures, hospital visits/admissions, telephone consultations, GP visits, and medications) were taken into account as well as costs outside the health care sector such as out-of-pocket costs to patients, informal care, and productivity losses due to absence from work. The quality-adjusted life-year (QALY) was chosen to represent health gain in the cost-effectiveness analysis, which is a measure of life expectancy weighted by HRQoL. The EuroQol-5D instrument was used to capture each patient's health state and associated HRQoL. By dividing the difference in costs between study arms by the difference in QALYs, incremental cost-effectiveness ratios (ICER) were calculated. Hospital follow-up plus EGP yielded the most QALYs, but was also the costliest follow-up strategy. The ICER of hospital follow-up plus EGP versus the next best alternative—telephone follow-up plus EGP—amounted to €235.750/QALY. As this ICER exceeds the maximum acceptable threshold value of €80.000 per QALY in the Netherlands, this follow-up strategy was not considered cost-effective. Hospital and telephone follow-up without EGP were both costlier and returned less QALYs than telephone follow-up plus EGP, and these were judged inferior. Telephone follow-up plus EGP had the highest probability of being the most cost-effective follow-up strategy irrespective of the threshold value (see Figure 29.1) (9). It may be speculated that a combination of frequent contacts with a BCN together with comprehensive education about signs

Table 29.1 Patient-reported outcome scores (means) by study group at baseline and 12 months

	HRQoL[a]		Emotional functioning[a]		Role functioning[a]		Anxiety[b]		Feelings of control[c]	
	Baseline	12 mo	Baseline	12 mo	Baseline	12 mo	Baseline	12 mo	Baseline	12 mo
Telephone follow-up	67.2	78.4	77.7	81.7	62.6	83.4	40.9	37.8	2.6	2.5
Hospital follow-up	70.5	77.7	69.9	82.6	68.6	82.9	39.3	37.9	2.6	2.6
EGP	70.5	78.9	75.8	82.4	67.2	84.6	39.0	37.1	2.5	2.5
No EGP	67.3	77.2	71.8	81.9	64.0	81.7	41.2	38.6	2.6	2.6

EGP, Educational Group Programme; HRQoL, health-related quality of life; mo, months.

[a]Scores range from 0 to 100, a higher score indicating better HRQoL or functioning.

[b]Scores range from 20 to 80, a higher score indicating greater anxiety.

[c]Scores range from 0 to 5, with higher scores representing higher perceived feelings of control.

Adapted with permission from Kimman ML et al. 'Nurse-led telephone follow-up and an educational group programme after breast cancer treatment: results of a 2 × 2 randomised controlled trial'. *European Journal of Cancer.* Volume 47, Issue 7, pp. 1027–36. Copyright © 2011 Elsevier Ltd. DOI: 10.1016/j.ejca.2010.12.003

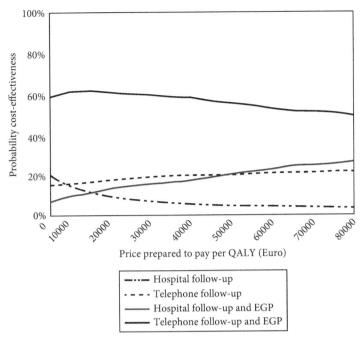

Figure 29.1 Cost-effectiveness acceptability curves for four follow-up strategies after treatment for breast cancer (base case analysis). EGP, educational group programme; QALY, quality-adjusted life-year.

Adapted with permission from Kimman ML et al. 'Economic evaluation of four follow-up strategies after curative treatment for breast cancer: results of an RCT'. *European Journal of Cancer.* Volume 47, Issue 8, pp. 1175–85. Copyright © 2011 Elsevier Ltd. DOI: 10.1016/j.ejca.2010.12.017

and symptoms of possible treatment side-effects and recurrence may have led to fewer contacts with (more specialized) health care professionals, and this could explain the lower costs of this strategy compared to follow-up without an additional educational programme.

Patient Preferences, a Discrete Choice Experiment

Patient preferences were investigated by means of a discrete choice experiment (DCE). In a DCE, respondents are asked to choose the preferred alternative from a set of two or more hypothetical scenarios (10). The scenarios are described by key characteristics of follow-up ('attributes') and the levels of these key characteristics. Responses to a DCE provide valuable insight into which characteristics of follow-up are most important to patients and reveal whether they would be willing to accept alternative follow-up options. The study was performed between May and July 2008 among 359 Dutch breast cancer patients who had finished curative treatment. The attributes and levels comprised 'attending an EGP' (yes; no), 'frequency of visits' (every 3 months; every 4 months; every 6 months; every 12 months), 'waiting time in minutes' (5; 30; 60; 90), 'contact mode' (face-to-face; telephone), and 'health care provider' (medical specialist; BCN; GP; BCN and medical specialist alternating). Respondents were asked in a series of 16 hypothetical pairwise choice tasks to select their preferred follow-up. An example of a choice task can be found in Figure 29.2.

Follow-up by the medical specialist was generally preferred to follow-up performed exclusively by a BCN or GP. Respondents preferred to have more frequent visits per year, a reduction of waiting time, and they strongly preferred face-to-face contact to telephone contact. Respondents were generally indifferent between a medical specialist performing the follow-up or alternating visits between the medical specialist and a BCN, and also to whether an EGP was part of the follow-up. Overall, 'healthcare provider' and 'contact mode' were the most important attributes to respondents, whereas 'frequency of visits', 'health care provider' and 'waiting time' were least important (11). Our study population, however, included relatively few respondents who had experienced telephone follow-up, follow-up by a nurse or GP, or the EGP, and it is known that people tend to prefer what they know best or have experienced. The results indicated that there was indeed a tendency for patients to prefer what one had personally experienced, although a considerable heterogeneity in patients' preferences was observed. This suggests that a personalized approach to follow-up based on patients' individual preferences would be a promising strategy in order to maximize patient satisfaction,

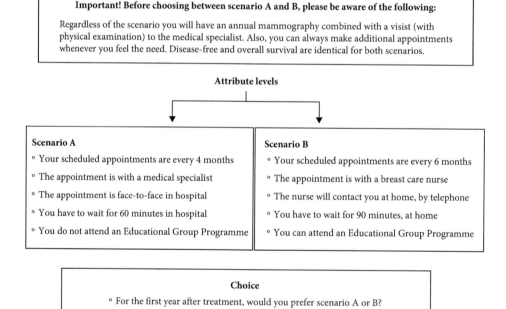

Figure 29.2 Example of a choice task in the DCE.

rather than a 'one size fits all' approach. Most heterogeneity was seen on the attributes 'EPG' and 'health care provider'. To illustrate, even though the medical specialist was preferred overall (i.e. in the aggregated results), one in four respondents preferred follow-up by a BCN. Similarly, almost half of the respondents were positive about attending an EGP. By contrast, just 5% of respondents preferred telephone follow-up over face-to-face contact.

To explore the potential economic impact of a fully personalized approach to follow-up, i.e. an approach in which patients can choose their own strategy, individual preferences from the 359 participants of the DCE were combined with a cost estimate of their preferred strategy. Hospital and EGP cost estimates were based on the cost analysis performed in the MaCare trial. The results of this analysis showed that offering a fully personalized follow-up yields the highest total patient satisfaction and is less costly than offering everyone the standard, hospital-based 'one size fits all' follow-up strategy (6).

Discussion

Results of the two studies performed showed that nurse-led telephone follow-up after breast cancer does not compromise patients' outcomes in terms of HRQoL, levels of anxiety and feelings of control, and satisfaction with the process of care, and thus may be an acceptable alternative to hospital follow-up. Furthermore, nurse-led telephone follow-up combined with additional psychosocial support and information through an educational group programme was the most cost-effective out of four different follow-up strategies. A great challenge is to replace the traditional hospital-based follow-up by a medical specialist with alternative (nurse-led) follow-up methods in a cost-effective manner and one that is also in line with breast cancer survivors' preferences. To this end, we investigated how changes in breast cancer follow-up would affect patients' preferences or utility (i.e. satisfaction). The discrete choice experiment showed that patient satisfaction would not differ significantly if patients have follow-up alternating between the medical specialist and the BCN instead of the medical specialist alone. And although face-to-face visits were generally preferred over telephone consultations, an EGP may be a good option to address psychosocial needs for many survivors. In summary, results of the clinical trial and patient preference study performed in the Netherlands seem to suggest that a personalized approach to follow-up, including the options to attend an EGP or have a nurse-led telephone consultation based on patient's individual preferences, would be a promising strategy in order to maximize patient satisfaction. To this it can be added that providing patients with the follow-up strategy of their choice has the potential to reduce costs compared to traditional follow-up.

Despite the patient and economic benefits, in many countries follow-up still tends to focus on scheduled hospital visits with the medical specialist. The results of our studies and those of others increasingly underscore the importance of assessing current clinical practice guidelines for breast cancer follow-up. Already in 2009, one of the key recommendations of the UK National Institute for Health and Care Excellence guidance for early and locally advanced breast cancer was that patients should have a choice in their method of follow-up (11). In 2012, the Dutch guidelines for follow-up care after primary treatment for breast cancer were adapted to reflect the increasing evidence for alternative, more cost-effective, follow-up strategies and wider acceptance of personalized follow-up. Breast cancer patients in the Netherlands currently receive an annual physical exam and mammography to check for recurrences with additional appointments in case of hormonal treatment (Nabon, 2012, see http://www.oncoline.nl). To screen for side-effects and psychosocial problems, however, health professionals and patients are encouraged to make a shared decision regarding the most suitable care for the individual patient. The guidelines do not specify by whom, or in what format, this support should be provided. While the studies described in this chapter focus on nurse-led (telephone) follow-up and a group programme for screening of side-effects and psychosocial support, there are several other evidence-based options available, most evidently follow-up provided by the GP (4). Furthermore, an increasing number of e-health applications in follow-up care are being developed and tested. For example, a Dutch web-based self-management intervention using cognitive behavioural therapy was found to reduce distress in breast cancer patients in the first months after treatment. To promote uptake of more personalized follow-up, and provide appropriate information to patients about their options, a patient decision aid was recently developed in the Netherlands. Such a tool can help patients understand their own preferences and make decisions regarding their health care based on these preferences. Use of the decision aid appears promising in terms of positive effects on shared decision-making, choice evaluation, follow-up care choice, and costs (12). Finally, a research team from the Netherlands has recently developed a prediction model (i.e. the Influence nomogram; http://www.utwente.nl/mira/influence) to obtain insight in the personal risk for a recurrence, based on data from the Netherlands Cancer Registry (13). Although follow-up is performed not only to detect a local recurrence, but also to detect a secondary primary tumour, this personal risk—based on patient, tumour, and treatment factors—could be combined with the patient's preferences to further support decision-making on follow-up care (13). In conclusion, considering the available evidence for several alternative follow-up strategies, it would be beneficial to revisit current clinical practice guidelines for breast cancer follow-up so as to acknowledge the patient's voice and the expressed need for a more personalized approach to follow-up care.

Key Messages

- There is increasing evidence that follow-up after breast cancer treatment can take many forms (e.g. performed by breast cancer nurses, by telephone, or with additional psychosocial support) without compromising patient outcomes or increasing the costs to society.
- In many countries follow-up still tends to focus on scheduled hospital visits with the medical specialist.

- It would be beneficial to revisit current clinical practice guidelines for breast cancer follow-up so as to acknowledge the patient's voice and the expressed need for a more personalized approach to follow-up care.

References

1. van der Waal D et al. Breast cancer diagnosis and death in the Netherlands: a changing burden. *Eur J Public Health* 2015;25(2):320–324.
2. Senkus E et al. ESMO Guidelines Working Group. Primary breast cancer: ESMO Clinical Practice Guidelines for diagnosis, treatment and follow-up. *Ann Oncol* 2013;24 Suppl 6:vi6–23.
3. Kimman ML et al. Follow-up after curative treatment for breast cancer: why do we still adhere to frequent outpatient clinic visits? *Eur J Cancer* 2007;43:647–653.
4. Moschetti I et al. Follow-up strategies for women treated for early breast cancer. *Cochrane Database Syst Rev* 2016;27(5):CD001768.
5. Kimman ML et al. Improving the quality and efficiency of follow-up after curative treatment for breast cancer—rationale and study design of the MaCare trial. *BMC Cancer* 2007;7:1–7.
6. Benning TM et al. Combining individual-level discrete choice experiment estimates and costs to inform health care management decisions about customized care: the case of follow-up strategies after breast cancer treatment. *Value Health* 2012;15(5):680–689.
7. Kimman ML et al. Economic evaluation of four follow-up strategies after curative treatment for breast cancer: results of an RCT. *Eur J Cancer* 2011;47(8):1175–1185.
8. Kimman M et al. Patient satisfaction with nurse-led telephone follow-up after curative treatment for breast cancer. *BMC Cancer* 2010;10:174.
9. Kimman ML et al. Nurse-led telephone follow-up and an educational group programme after breast cancer treatment: results of a 2 × 2 randomised controlled trial. *Eur J Cancer* 2011;47(7):1027–1036.
10. Kimman ML et al. Follow-up after treatment for breast cancer: one strategy fits all? An investigation of patients' preference using a discrete choice experiment. *Acta Oncol* 2010;49(3):328–337.
11. Harnett A et al. Diagnosis and treatment of early breast cancer, including locally advanced disease—summary of NICE guidance. *BMJ* 2009;338:b509.
12. Klaassen L et al. A novel patient decision aid for aftercare in breast cancer patients: a promising tool to reduce costs by individualizing aftercare. *Breast* 2018;41:144–150.
13. Witteveen A et al. Personalisation of breast cancer follow-up: a time-dependent prognostic nomogram for the estimation of annual risk of locoregional recurrence in early breast cancer patients. *Breast Cancer Res Treat* 2015;152(3):627–636.

PART 9

PATIENTS, PHYSICIANS, AND THE MEDIA

30

Who Controls the Message?

*Deanna J. Attai, Johanna Pas, Kwanele Asante-Shongwe, Liz O'Riordan,
Carol Benn, AnneMarie Mercurio, Diane M. Radford, Gary Schwitzer,
and Anna Wagstaff*

Introduction

After the initial shock of hearing the words 'you have breast cancer', a patient is faced with many decisions. Often, there is ample time to obtain the opinions necessary for deliberative decision-making. However, from a patient perspective, the reaction seems to be universal: remove the cancer immediately. There is a sense of urgency in that moment, and decisions may be guided by fear rather than by knowledge or a full understanding of the options.

It is imperative that patients are aware of all available options and the opinion from the multidisciplinary team. Each decision has associated risks and benefits. Patients who face a diagnosis of breast cancer may find it challenging to wade through all of the media messages that swirl about them as they try to make treatment decisions and to weigh quality-of-care concerns.

Traditionally, physicians controlled the healthcare message. There was relatively limited information, and treatment options were limited. Thus, patients relied heavily on the advice of their physician (1,2).

Currently, although treatment recommendations are often made with the assistance of evidence-based guidelines (for example, guideline-recommended post-lumpectomy radiation therapy or endocrine therapy for oestrogen receptor-positive breast cancer), patients should still be invited to participate in the decision-making process. In an era of patient-centred care, it is important to recognize that every patient is different. Some still prefer to have their clinicians tell them what to do and where to seek information, but many patients try to understand everything and immediately turn to the Internet for information. In small communities or in remote areas or environments underserviced by multidisciplinary teams, gathering accurate information may be challenging. In certain cultures, diagnosed patients may be expected to make decisions based upon decades old 'traditions' or are not expected to make decisions on their own behalf.

"I stumbled upon conversations among women trying to find answers to very basic questions that I felt should have been answered by their physicians. Some women were truly uninformed, but many were simply overwhelmed."

Deanna Attai MD

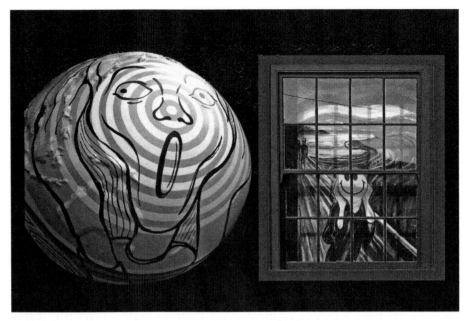

Figure 30.1 The cry: US and UK version.
Robert Paridaens (with permission).

Internet and Television

As of 2014, 87% of the US population had accessed the Internet, and 72% of Internet users had searched for health information online. According to the European Commission, six out of ten Europeans go online to look for health information, and more than 75% think that the Internet is a good way of finding out more about their health (3).

The volume of information has also increased significantly over the years. A google Internet search using the phrase 'breast cancer' reveals more than 150 million sites. Searching for 'shared decision making in cancer' yields 2.3 million results.

With the Internet giving patients instant access to information, the breast cancer specialist may sometimes have less information than the patient. Now that information flows freely through multiple channels, the physician is no longer the information gate-keeper (1,2). However, given that there are multiple sources of information competing for a patient's attention, it can be challenging for a newly diagnosed patient to know where to turn for reliable information. Patients, physicians, and the media all play a role in healthcare messaging and what information is available.

One of the first things that many patients do after receiving a breast cancer diagnosis is to reach for their phone and look up their illness on the Internet. A 2015 evaluation of 45 unique breast cancer information websites noted that most had unbiased and relevant information. However, only a few sites had prompts encouraging patients to examine options in context of their thoughts, feelings, fears, and goals. Therefore, most sites were felt to be inadequate for informed decision-making (4). Others have found that the quality of online health information varies considerably.

Reputable medical institutions such as the Mayo Clinic and Cleveland Clinic have a robust online presence. Twenty-six per cent of hospitals in the USA participate in social media (5). Non-profit sites where the content is physician-reviewed, such as breastcancer.org and Breast360.org, are also seen as reputable sources of information. Patients tend to look at many different sites searching for the answers to all of their questions and are unlikely to stop with their own hospital or physician's web site when researching treatment options. Wallner and colleagues (6) found that women who were frequently online appraised their decision-making more positively, were more likely to report a deliberative decision, and were more likely to report high decision satisfaction. Physicians can play an important role in terms of directing patients to credible web sites as well as forums and blogs that are factually correct and non-threatening instead of telling patients to stay offline.

Whereas a growing number of patients obtain health information online, some medical television shows are very popular. Korownyk and colleagues analysed the quality of healthcare information on two popular internationally syndicated medical television shows. They concluded that the recommendations often lacked adequate information on specific benefits or the magnitude of these effects, that approximately half of the recommendations either had no evidence or were contradicted by the best available evidence, and that potential conflicts of interest were rarely addressed (7). In 2014, Dr Mehmet Oz, a cardiothoracic surgeon who is also host of the popular Dr Oz television show, was called to testify before the US Congressional Subcommittee on Consumer Protection, Product Safety and Insurance, regarding false advertising related to weight loss products (8). Nevertheless, these shows do remain on the air and are very popular.

Peer-to-Peer Support

As patients are becoming experts in their own disease, they are often seeking out their peers for information. Online discussion forums such as breastcancer.org are popular sources of information and support. Both open and closed (private) Facebook groups exist for many different breast cancer subpopulations, including BRCA gene carriers (see Chapter 22), ductal carcinoma in situ, metastatic breast cancer, reconstruction type, and lack of reconstruction. Twitter is home to two robust breast cancer support communities: #BCSM (Breast Cancer Social Media) and #BCCWW (Breast Cancer Chat Worldwide). These Twitter communities were founded by breast cancer patient advocates as sites for patients to gather and discuss evidence-based information and issues related to breast cancer diagnosis, treatment, and survivorship. Both communities benefit from regular physician participation, and, in the case of #BCSM, participation in the group chats has been shown to improve patient education and decrease anxiety (9).

However, there are some cautions in directing patients to online information sources. Newly diagnosed patients need to understand that accessing information, especially in a peer-to-peer setting, does not ensure that the information is evidence-based or even applicable to themselves. This situation may be exacerbated by individuals (media, medical, or other) who drive traffic to their websites in order to sell or to promote ideas or thoughts that may not be well-researched or credible. Patients should be encouraged to bring information found online to the attention of their physician and to discuss whether the information actually pertains to them.

Role of the Journalist

Journalists, public relations professionals, and social media messengers play a key role in disseminating information, shaping opinions, and holding accountable those with powerful and influential voices in health care. The media are not uniform entities. They take many forms and address different audiences, who are looking for different things—from factual news-led reporting, to opinion and comment, or gossip, celebrity items, and entertainment. They also now encompass the huge world of social media, which is an enormously important platform for disseminating and commenting on health and medical issues. But even the best health, medical, and science journalists are challenged by the complexity of the information they write about in the midst of scientific uncertainty. Many strive to do their best in an environment of staff cutbacks and declining resources for background research and training.

The media have an important role as a 'watchdog' of the public interest, 'holding to account' powerful people and organizations, including the health care providers that their audiences rely on. Carrying out this role responsibly and effectively is a core role for journalists, but it can be a challenge given the complexity of healthcare, stretched resources within news media, and pressures to maximize audiences. A constructive relationship between doctors and journalists, with understanding on both sides about their respective roles and responsibilities, can help promote good-quality health journalism that is accurate and fair but also investigative and independent.

Health journalists and their editors working in mainstream media generally take very seriously their professional and ethical responsibilities to be accurate and fair in their reporting. But healthcare is a complex field, and, despite good intentions, journalists do not always get things right. The digital age has impacted health journalism in a number of ways, both good and bad. Free access to online sources of information has disrupted traditional news media business models, and the consequent downsizing of newsrooms means the position of dedicated health reporter is disappearing, particularly from local news media. Thus, health stories are often covered by reporters who have little specialist knowledge.

How to Avoid Drowning in the Tsunami of Health Care News

Media messages about health care interventions may influence patients' individual decision-making, their encounters with their physicians, and even public policy. HealthNewsReview.org was a US-based non-profit organization that reviewed and critiqued medical news stories and press releases that included a claim of efficacy about a specific treatment, test, product, or procedure. They ceased publication at the end of 2018.

For 13 years, the HealthNewsReview.org project analysed media messages that included claims about interventions. Information about breast cancer in many news stories and public relations news releases was among the most problematic (Table 30.1).

There is a clear and troubling pattern of imbalanced messages that may mislead and harm those who read them and accept them as definitive:

- emphasis on, or exaggeration of, potential benefits of interventions; minimizing or even ignoring potential harms of interventions;
- failure to independently vet claims or to evaluate the quality of the evidence;
- framing screening as a mandate rather than an as an informed, shared, decision-making choice;
- preliminary results from early-stage drug trials being promoted as breakthroughs, game-changers, and possible new standards of care;
- stories detailing celebrity breast cancer experiences with media giving undue weight to what these individuals did in circumstances that may not match or have relevance to readers' experiences.

Table 30.1 Report card on more than 2,600 news stories 2006–2018

Criteria—Does the story . . .	% graded unsatisfactory
Adequately discuss the costs of the intervention?	69%
Adequately quantify the benefits of the intervention?	66%
Explain/quantify the harms of the intervention?	63%
Evaluate the quality of the evidence?	62%
Avoid disease-mongering?	19%
Use independent sources and identify conflicts of interest?	48%
Compare the new approach with existing alternatives?	53%
Establish the availability of the intervention?	25%
Establish the true novelty of the approach?	24%
Appear to rely solely or largely on a news release?	9%[a]

[a]This grade may appear at first glance to be very positive, but the fact that 9% of 2,600—or nearly 200—news stories, which are expected to independently vet claims, were instead judged to be influenced solely or largely by a public relations source is troubling.

Powerful Platforms Provided for Problematic Breast Cancer Messages

Media messages about celebrities' breast cancer treatment decisions may bias public opinion (10). Analysts have pointed to 'strong biological, psychological, and social bases for people's adoration of celebrities and trust in their medical advice,' suggesting that health professionals 'can counter the negative influences of celebrities by speaking to their patients about the validity of the celebrities' advice and sources of reputable health information, especially when patients ask about the latest celebrity endorsement'.

Through patient interviews, HealthNewsReview.org has examined how conflicting news stories make it more difficult for patients to make decisions regarding their own care. In addition, they detail other issues that influence the accuracy and credibility of information including:

- researcher-authors who submit journal manuscripts which put their findings in the most positive light and sometimes exaggerate the potential impact;
- journal editors or peer reviewers who do not address this spin or hype;
- writers of public relations news releases from the journal or from the researcher's home institution who further promote the exaggerated claims;
- industry sources, who stand to benefit, add more fuel to the flames of hype;
- journalists who fail to independently investigate the claims.

Gary Schwitzer, founder of HealthNewsReview.org, states: 'Why does this matter? Because women trying to make difficult, complex decisions about screening or treatment may be given inaccurate, imbalanced, incomplete information that will lead them to make uninformed choices. It also matters that the credibility and integrity of scientists, clinicians, and those who communicate with the public about science and medicine is threatened. Professions that deserve and rely on public trust may lose that trust.'

The Role of Health Professionals

Some national and regional health authorities (both in the UK and in the USA) are now moving towards putting more data on quality and safety of individual treatment centres into the public domain as part of their audit and quality control efforts, and as a service to patients, to help them make informed choices about where to go for treatment.

The medical profession has tended to favour 'self-regulation' and is wary about making data on quality and safety publicly available. The worry is that it presents a partial and inaccurate picture and exposes professionals and institutions to the risk of being unfairly judged. There is also a fear that it could skew clinical decision-making; surgeons may, for instance, feel the need to turn down more risky procedures to protect their complication and mortality track record, even if the decision runs counter to the best interests of the patient.

In practice, it is true that stories in the mass media about quality of care often appear in the form of 'health care scandals', framed as isolated instances of serious malpractice or mismanagement taking place within a health system that is implicitly assumed to be otherwise reliable and well-functioning: a rogue surgeon, who has been using a technique that has no evidence base; a radiotherapy, radiology, or chemotherapy unit that has put patient safety at risk through unique and catastrophic failures to do things right.

It is arguable, however, that far from encouraging these sorts of stories, making more data on quality and safety publicly available would help raise the level of reporting and public discourse. Access to comparative data makes it possible for journalists to put the story within the wider context of the safety and quality record of that hospital, see how it compares with similar institutions, ask questions about why some places do better than others, and consider what can be done to improve quality and safety across the board.

The question is whether news media can be trusted with data on quality and safety. The digital age is also opening up new ways to gather, report, and disseminate data, which means that so-called 'data journalism' is now also becoming a core journalistic skill. Interestingly, Florence Nightingale is often cited as a pioneer of data journalism, because of the innovative infographics she developed in 1858 to present data on the causes of mortality among British soldiers fighting in the Crimean war.

Digital media are also opening up new opportunities for niche journalism and for special interest groups, such as patient advocacy groups, to disseminate their own information and analysis and feed into and comment on mainstream media, which can play a positive role in raising the level of informed discussion and debate.

Good and Bad Practices

When journalists get health stories wrong, it can be very damaging. When they get things right, however, the media can play a valuable role in informing the public, holding health care providers and policymakers to account, and opening up informed discussion on how to improve standards of health care. Examples of both are presented below.

The *Toronto Star*'s 'A wonder drug's dark side' story (5 February 2015, now removed from their website), is a prime example of inaccurate and damaging journalism that misused data to tell a story that was not backed up by evidence. It built a story about the purported dangers of the cervical cancer vaccine Gardasil, using publicly accessible data on reported adverse events, and then focusing on the impact of serious health problems that had developed in some teenage girls at around the time they received the vaccination; they did not present any epidemiological, medical, or other evidence that there was a causal connection.

Less than two weeks later, the *Star* retracted the story, accepting that, even though they had stopped short of claiming proof of a link, 'the weight of the photographs, video, headlines, and anecdotes led many readers to conclude the *Star* believed its investigation had uncovered a direct connection between a large variety of ailments and the vaccine'. The paper defended as legitimate, however, its attempts 'to sift through data in which the red flag of an undiscovered side-effect might be found.' (11)

Ben Goldacre, a medical doctor who runs a web site dedicated largely to exposing and challenging media misrepresentation of scientific and medical evidence (http://www.badscience.net), commented at the time, in a string of tweets to one of the journalists concerned, that 'reporting the raw data from an open adverse event reporting system in that manner ... is simply misleading, and an abuse. Where data is made openly accessible we all ... have a responsibility to reciprocate, and analyse/report on it competently.'

Responding to the reaction against the story, the paper's public editor commented that 'It's too bad there isn't a vaccination to prevent journalistic misstep. I suspect we'd all line up for that shot about now. The fallout here has been devastating for the newsroom.' Interestingly, one of the points she made was that the paper's health reporters had not been involved in that story, and that if they had been consulted, 'they could have explained the inherent land mines in not giving greater weight to scientific evidence in a story of such importance to public health.'

A more positive example of data-based reporting on cancer comes from the five-yearly Eurocare reports on comparative cancer survival rates in Europe, which started back in 1995 (12). Many governments were, and still are, less than enthusiastic about having their 'ranking' in terms of cancer survival made public. From the perspective of the public interest, however, it is now widely recognized that putting those data in the public domain has transformed the public and political conversation about cancer. The job of journalists is to ask questions. Those data made it possible to ask questions about the quality of cancer care at a national level, because they put a measurable value on the best survival outcomes that are currently achievable (for different types of cancer) and opened up discussions in countries with lower survival rates about what they are doing wrong, and how they can do better. Is the problem late detection, delays in treatment, too little radiotherapy capacity, a culture of undertreating older patients, inadequate supportive care, lack of team work and poor-quality decision-making, or poor-quality surgery?

Having those conversations in the public sphere gave them political traction. It is no coincidence that the two countries most shocked by their level of performance, the UK and Denmark, were the first to introduce national comprehensive cancer plans, which have since spread across the EU. Professor Sir Mike Richards, England's first national cancer director, or 'Cancer Tsar', has himself credited adverse media reports with helping his quest to improve services. 'If all the journalists stopped criticising and said cancer [care] is wonderful, my ability to move things forward would be diminished,' he said (12). His comment illustrates that a constructive relationship between the medical profession and journalists, with understanding on both sides about their respective roles, responsibilities, and challenges, can help promote good-quality health journalism that is accurate and fair but also investigative and independent.

Disparities

Many factors influence access to care, including geography, race, socioeconomic status, and health literacy. As many health organizations now expect patients to play an active role in monitoring their care, Internet literacy is also important. Over the past decade as the Internet has become a major source of health information, it has contributed towards a shift in emphasis on the patient as a more active consumer of health information. However, opportunity for all does not exist, and people with low literacy levels are less likely to benefit from the advances, since the content of the material is often at high reading level, and these patients are less likely to have access to technology. Seniors are also less likely to be comfortable using online tools for healthcare related issues (13). These factors impact the level of patient engagement in their care and how the information available or shared allows them to make treatment decisions. Access to information that cannot be translated, whether due to language or literacy barriers, poses its own dilemma. The role of the physician in a society that is not health-'educated' or aware is essential in ensuring early detection, awareness, and access to health services. Promotion of sensible healthcare education resources, across different racial, ethnic, educational, and language barriers is also vital.

Reliable sources of information must be made readily available to all patients, regardless of where they reside, their level of literacy, or their ability to decipher what is being presented to them. Messaging by patient advocacy organizations, individuals, media medical, and allied professionals should come with a disclosure, so that understanding of the difference between opinion and guideline can be translated to the patient.

What Can Physicians Do?

Physicians, nurses, and other caregivers may find it challenging to answer the questions of patients who are influenced by media messages about breast cancer. Some may view any dealings with journalists as conflicts to be avoided rather than as opportunities to educate and inform. Physicians need to truly understand that patients are receiving information from multiple sources. It is unrealistic to expect that patients will not search for information online as well as from friends and family members. Whereas physicians are not the only source of health information, they remain the most credible source. Therefore, physicians have a unique opportunity to impact patient education, but they must meet patients where they are, which most often is online. Physicians can direct patients to quality online information, can create content, and can participate in online discussion groups. Increased physician engagement can substantially improve patient experience for those patients actively seeking information and advocating on behalf of other patients with similar diseases (14).

One of the primary roles of a physician is to be a source of education and support to patients. Thackeray et al. studied the use of Twitter as an educational platform during Breast Cancer Awareness Month. The majority of users were individuals, though they found that organizations and celebrities posted more often and had the most re-tweets. Celebrity tweets primarily focused on fundraising, early detection, and diagnosis. Individuals primarily tweeted about wearing pink. This is an example of a missed opportunity by physicians to promote health literacy (15). Physicians engaging in various social media platforms have a unique opportunity to provide credible medical information, support, and guidance to a large audience that is thirsty for this sort of information. Physicians have a responsibility to use the available tools to engage this growing segment of the population.

An often-overlooked aspect of physician participation in social media and engaging with patients in online forums is the benefit that physicians receive from these interactions. The current authors have all noted that participation in interactive online patient communities adds a much deeper level of appreciation for what patients are going through, and they also feel that their in-person patient interactions have benefited (changing the way they ask questions and gaining a better understanding of the patient experience). Perhaps even more important, by engaging on social forums, physicians may better learn what questions patients are asking when they are not sitting in examination rooms.

Key Messages

- Physicians can play an important role in terms of directing patients to credible web sites as well as forums and blogs that are factually correct and non-threatening, instead of telling them to stay offline.
- Patients should be encouraged to bring information found online to the attention of their physician and to discuss whether the information actually pertains to them.
- A constructive relationship between doctors and journalists, with understanding on both sides about their respective roles and responsibilities, can help promote good-quality health journalism that is accurate and fair but also investigative and independent.
- When journalists get health stories wrong, it can be very damaging. When they get things right, however, the media can play a valuable role in informing the public, holding health care providers and policymakers to account, and opening up informed discussion on how to improve standards of health care.
- Physicians need to truly understand that patients are receiving information from multiple sources. It is unrealistic to expect that patients will not search for information online as well as from friends and family members.
- Physicians can direct patients to quality online information, can create content, and can participate in online discussion groups.

References

1. Vartabedian B. The case for new physician literacies in the digital age. 2012. Available from: https://33charts.com/new-physician-literacies/
2. Attai DJ. What are we missing? *Ann Surg Oncol* 2016;23(10):2088–92.
3. European Commission. Europeans becoming enthusiastic users of online health information | Digital Single Market. 2014. Available from: https://ec.europa.eu/digital-single-market/en/news/europeans-becoming-enthusiastic-users-online-health-information
4. Bruce JG et al. Quality of online information to support patient decision-making in breast cancer surgery. *J Surg Oncol* 2015;112:575–580.
5. ReferralMD. 30 facts and statistics on social media and healthcare. Available from: https://getreferralmd.com/2017/01/30-facts-statistics-on-social-media-and-healthcare/
6. Wallner LP et al. Use of online communication by patients with newly diagnosed breast cancer during the treatment decision process. *JAMA Oncol* 2016;2(12):1654–1656.
7. Korownyk C et al. Televised medical talk shows—what they recommend and the evidence to support their recommendations: a prospective observational study. *BMJ* 2014;349:g7346.
8. Christensen J, Wilson J. Congressional hearing investigates Dr. Oz "miracle" weight loss claims. CNN Online; updated 19 June 2014. http://www.cnn.com/2014/06/17/health/senate-grills-dr-oz/
9. Attai DJ et al. Twitter social media is an effective tool for breast cancer patient education and support: patient-reported outcomes by survey. *J Med Internet Res* 2015;17(7):e188.
10. Sabel MS and Cin SD. Trends in media reports of celebrities' breast cancer treatment decisions. *Ann Surg Oncol* 2016;23:2795.
11. *Toronto Star*: A note from the publisher. 20 February 2015. Available from: https://www.thestar.com/news/2015/02/20/a-note-from-the-publisher.html
12. McIntry P. How bad news can be good news for cancer services. *Cancer World* 2012;50:46–49.
13. Levine DM et al. Trends in seniors' use of digital health technology in the United States, 2011–2014. *JAMA* 2016;316(5):538–540.
14. An LC et al. Online social engagement by cancer patients: a clinic-based patient survey. *JMIR Cancer* 2016;2(2):e10.
15. Thackeray R et al. Using Twitter for breast cancer prevention: an analysis of breast cancer awareness month. *BMC Cancer* 2013;13:508.

31

Medicolegal Aspects

Robert Mansel

Introduction

There are well-established principles in the law of civil negligence (tort). First, the doctor must have a duty of care for the patient, i.e. she is responsible for treating the patient. Second, the doctor must fail to give the correct treatment, and this failure is judged by her peers (a body of doctors who are specialists in the same field). This is known as breach of duty. Third, the patient has to show that he/she has been harmed in a measurable way, such as earlier death, increased pain and suffering, or financial loss. This is known as causation. If causation is proved, then the court can award financial compensation to the patient with the aim of restoring the individual to the position they would have been in, if the breach of duty had not occurred.

In the UK, there have been cases where the negligence has been so severe that an alternative charge of criminal negligence, which carries a penalty of imprisonment, has been brought against the doctor. This has been a controversial charge when applied to medicine, and recently two doctors have overturned their convictions in the Appeal Court, and currently the use of criminal negligence charges in relation to medicine is being reviewed and may be abolished.

In this chapter, the more usual civil charge of negligence (malpractice) will be discussed.

There are major differences in the judicial structures between countries, and different cultures exist regarding suing doctors, such that negligence claims are very common in some countries and almost unknown in others.

The procedure is that the claim is submitted by the patient's lawyers to the hospital or insurers, and expert reports are obtained by the claimant and the defence lawyers acting for the doctor or hospital. This is followed by discussions between the two sides and often between the experts. In the UK system, it is rare for the case to be heard in court, because the costs of trial are very high, and most cases are settled out of court.

Some countries prefer to pursue a 'no blame' system, where the patient is compensated from public funds, and costs are reduced by avoidance of the legal adversarial system.

Breach of Duty—Diagnosis

The most common allegations of breach of duty in breast cancer are the failure to diagnose the tumour early by imaging, and this relates to both screening and symptomatic cases. In general, screening issues are easier to defend, since most screening programmes double-read the mammograms and have extensive quality and review schemes in place. A breach of duty would be established if a peer reviewer, usually a radiology expert hired by lawyers, gives an opinion that a body of radiologists would have picked up the cancer on the original mammograms. There are well-known 'difficult to diagnose' cancers on imaging, such as lobular cancers or very lateral cancers, which cannot be imaged with conventional mammographic views. Reports from both the UK and US colleges of radiology show that claims have been escalating against radiologists in recent years (1,2). Halpin reported that failure to diagnose breast cancer was the most common allegation in delayed diagnosis claims against UK radiologists, and 37% of the claims resulted in damages being paid to the patient, with the largest payment being £464,000 (1).

Similarly, the US College of Radiologists reported that between 2008 and 2012 one-third of claims resulted in a mean pay-out of US$481,000 per claim (2).

Halpin also noted that claims in the UK were increasing with more than 30 claims per annum in 1995–1998 and 48–60 claims per annum in 2001–2005. Harpwood reported that in the UK National Health Service (NHS) in 1978 total claims were 500 per annum and this had risen to 9,321 per annum in 2005 (3). The 2017/18 report of the NHS Litigation Authority (now known as NHS Resolution) showed that 10,686 new claims were received for England alone, and the total payments increased from the previous year from £1.7 billion to £2.23 billion. Only 33% end up in active litigation, and less than 1% proceed to a court hearing (https://practicebusiness.co.uk/legal-claims-against-nhs-continue-to-rise/).

Figure 31.1 illustrates the resolution of 17,338 claims settled in 2016/17 by the NHS (4).

By contrast, a report from China cited 1087 claims notified to the Center for Legal Information of Peking University between 1998 and 2011, and 76% resulted in a mean pay-out of US$1,224 (5). It is clear that the number of claims relative to the population is extremely small when compared to the UK or USA. The authors did note that the number of claims was increasing each year. This highlights the rarity of medical negligence litigation in some countries.

Other common claims for breach of duty relate to failure of the clinician to appreciate the significance of the clinical signs of a cancer. Palpation is an inaccurate method of detection, particularly for small cancers as well as for some lobular cancers which do not form a typical hard mass in the breast and are easily mistaken for benign changes. Palpation is part of the well-accepted method of triple assessment

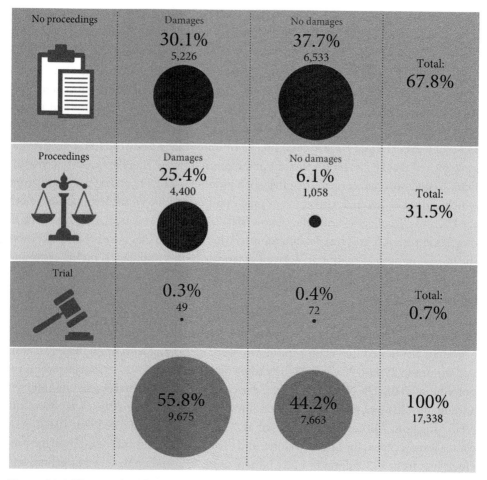

Figure 31.1 How 17,338 claims were settled in 2016/17.

consisting of clinical examination, imaging, and pathology biopsy. The key to the successful application of triple assessment is multidisciplinary working and the integration of all three elements. There must be agreement between all three elements, such that all point to normal/benign before it can be concluded that no cancer is present. However, no test is 100% accurate, and the patient must be informed that, even if the current assessment shows no evidence of cancer, this does not rule out the possibility of future development of cancer, and that new or persistent symptoms should prompt further investigation.

If triple assessment has been carried out properly and any discordant results have been discussed in a multidisciplinary meeting with the conclusion that there is no evidence of cancer present, this process, if fully documented, will be a solid defence against any claim of failure to diagnose.

Breach of Duty—Treatment

Allegations of breach of duty in treatment are less common than failure to diagnose and principally relate to failure to prescribe appropriate treatment, e.g. not giving radiotherapy after a lumpectomy or not administering hormones in hormone receptor-positive tumours. There are a large number of guidelines for the appropriate treatment of all subtypes of breast cancer, and following such guidelines would provide a defence for claims against allegations of failing to provide correct treatment. It should be pointed out that most guidelines are written by and for economically advanced nations. The Breast Health Global Initiative has developed guidelines for poorer countries in order to give the best clinical outcomes at the lowest cost (see Chapter 9). In the global context, it should be remembered that economic constraints will determine availability of more expensive treatments such as third-generation chemotherapy agents or HER 2 therapies.

A growing area of litigation relating to treatment is the new field of oncoplastic surgery, where new techniques and new materials such as acellular dermal matrices (ADMs) have been developed to support implant-based reconstructions. Problems often arise from the very high expectations of patients, who may find the results of their reconstruction are not as good cosmetically as their normal breast. This is compounded by the inadequate information that many patients receive prior to their operation, as well as the choice and complexities of the numerous techniques now available. The problem is further complicated by the poor evidence available on the ADM techniques, where numerous small uncontrolled trials of personal experience are the main publications available. In the UK, a recent ruling by the Supreme Court known as the 'Montgomery judgment' has completely changed the issue of informed consent by making the patient the person who determines what information the doctor should give in order to achieve informed consent. The implication is that the doctor must ascertain what information each individual would want in their personal circumstances to make a proper decision on whether to proceed with surgery. Claimant lawyers can therefore argue breach of duty if comprehensive oral and written information adjusted for each individual has not been given and fully documented in the medical record. This has meant that several extensive consultations are needed on each occasion informed consent is sought from the patient. If the detail of the information and discussion have not been fully documented in the notes, it is difficult to mount a defence that informed consent has been properly obtained, and breach of duty will then be proved.

Causation

Once breach has been established, the claimant will need to prove that the failure has resulted in measurable damage to the patient. Such damages could be the cost of additional treatments or the cost of additional care, and the cost of psychological treatments as a result of psychological injury.

The usual argument is that the breach of duty has made the patient's prognosis worse, resulting in shortening of her life. The court system usually works on the 'balance of probability', which means if the claimant can show that it was 51% true that the breach caused a measurable loss, then she will win the causation argument and will be compensated. But if the claimant has a survival greater than 50% there is no basis for a claim for loss of life even if an omitted treatment reduces survival from 85% to 65%. This poses considerable problems in regard to prognosis—an individual patient's cancer cannot be put into neat compartments and percentages, because the survival rates refer to cohorts of patients rather than to individuals. This means that somewhat arbitrary decisions may be made as to the prognosis in an individual case. Prognostic tools such as Adjuvant Online (currently not available), Predict in the UK, or Life Maths in the USA may give an indication of likely prognosis in a cohort of patients similar to the claimant and taking into consideration tumour factors and treatments.

Since adjuvant treatments have continued to give better results, and in developed countries tumour sizes on diagnosis have become smaller, the resulting prognostic calculations often give 10-year survivals better than 51%, and the claimant can find it difficult to prove any loss under the legal definition of causation. The argument that the claimant has lost years of life has generally not found favour in the courts, if the overall survival is better than 51%.

Once any loss has been demonstrated, the value of the loss is quantified by the lawyers, and the patient can be compensated.

Key Messages

- Breast cancer is a leading source of malpractice claims for radiologists. Other disciplines are concerned, including surgeons, pathologists, radiotherapists, medical oncologists, and reconstructive surgeons.
- The importance of breast imaging in screening and diagnosis means that breast radiologists are in the frontline for medicolegal actions.
- Once a breach of duty has been established, the claimant must prove the measurable damage to the patient.
- All doctors present at the multidisciplinary breast cancer meeting and contributing to the decision-making process are accountable for decisions related to their area of expertise.
- A greater awareness of the responsibility of all disciplines will optimize outcome for patients and limit exposure of doctors to legal liability.

References

1. Halpin SFS. Medico-legal claims against English radiologists: 1995–2006. *Br J Radiol* 2009;82:982–988.
2. Harvey HB et al. Radiology malpractice claims in the United States from 2008 to 2012: characteristics and implications. *J Am Coll Radiol* 2016;13(2):124–130.
3. Harpwood VH. *Medicine, Malpractice and Misapprehensions*. London: Routledge–Cavendish; 2007. Available from: https://www.taylorfrancis.com/books/9780203940457
4. NHS Resolution. 2016. Available from: https://www.gov.uk/government/publications
5. Li H et al. Claims, liabilities, injuries and compensation payments of medical malpractice litigation cases in China from 1998 1998 to 2011. *BMC Health Serv Res* 2014;14:390.

PART 10

THE ROLE OF GOVERNMENTS AND EXECUTIVES

32

European Perspective

Lieve Wierinck, Benjamin Baelus, Emilie Hoogland, Donata Lerda,
Robert Mansel, Cary S. Kaufman, and Luzia Travado

Introduction

Cancer is a major health concern in the EU, which is one of the most developed regions in the world and has a rapidly ageing population. After heart and cardiovascular diseases, cancer is the second most common cause of death in the EU; 26.4% of the annual deaths in 2014 were caused by various types of cancer. One estimate for the total societal cost of cancer in the EU amounted to €126 billion for 2009. Of this cost, approximately €50 billion (40%) was accountable to direct health care-related costs such as treatment and medication, and the remainder consisted of indirect effects such as lost productivity due to early deaths, lost working days, and informal care. Moreover, trends over the last two decades indicate an increasing direct cost of cancer healthcare, especially with cancer drugs becoming increasingly expensive (1).

Given the significant impact of cancer on European society, it should not be surprising that, both on European and national levels, policymakers have devoted much attention to the battle against cancer. However, health is a policy area in which the EU has only limited competence conferred to it by the Treaties, and, consequently, it is mainly limited to complementing national policies through coordination or information sharing (Table 32.1) (2). By providing a framework for cooperation between national entities, the EU promotes efficient research and development, propagates best practices regarding cancer prevention and treatment, encourages information exchange, and regulates the use of carcinogenic substances. Throughout this chapter, the EU's fight against cancer is discussed on three dimensions:

- coordination and cooperation;
- research and development;
- regulation of carcinogenic chemicals and oncology medicines.

A short introduction to each of these topics is provided, while real-life examples and measures illustrate what the EU does in practice.

Table 32.1 Competences of the European Union on health policy

Institution	Competences
European Union	Complement national policies by: • Assisting EU governments in achieving shared objectives; • Generating economies of scale by pooling resources; • Helping EU countries tackle shared challenges such as pandemics, chronic diseases or the impact of increased life expectancy on healthcare systems.
EC (DG SANTE)	• Leadership on EU health-related policies. • Works with Member States in the management of funds in the health sector. • Supports dialogue between Member States.
Member States	• Full competence in health care delivery. • Decide, define, and implement health sector investments.
European Medicines Agency (2)	The Agency's main responsibilities are authorizing and monitoring medicines in the EU. It does so by: • facilitating the development of medicines and access to them; • evaluating applications for marketing authorizations; • monitoring the safety of medicines throughout their life cycle; • providing information to health care professionals and patients.

Coordination and Cooperation

Through ensuring better coordination and cooperation, the EU aims at achieving synergies and avoiding duplication of efforts or inefficient actions confined to single Member States. By bringing together stakeholders from all over Europe through a more efficient information exchange, economies of scale can be utilized to ensure a more efficient fight against cancer. In this light, coordination is understood as: (i) bringing stakeholders together, (ii) harmonizing national policies, and (iii) promoting information exchange.

Bringing Stakeholders Together

By lowering barriers between different stakeholders such as oncologists, patient organizations, the pharmaceutical industry, and research institutions from all over Europe, the EU encourages better coordination and cooperation in the fight against cancer. In doing so, it provides a forum for these stakeholders to advise on legislation, involves them in cancer-related projects, and facilitates access to policymakers.

One of the main channels for stakeholders to interact is through the EU Health Policy Platform. It is based on cooperation and communication between health interest groups and the European Commission (EC). It also tries to improve the communication among these organizations (3).

The Breast Cancer Network is one of the stakeholders with whom the EC works. This is the first international network of clinical centres exclusively dedicated to the diagnosis and treatment of breast cancer. It is a project of the European School of Oncology with the aim of promoting and improving breast cancer care in Europe and throughout the world (4).

Another example is the European Society of Mastology (EUSOMA), which was founded in 1986 by a group of European breast cancer specialists including Professor Veronesi. In 2003, the EUSOMA requirements of a specialist breast unit were recognized by the European Parliament in the resolutions of 2003 and 2006 (see Chapter 4).

The Commission Expert Group on Cancer Control (CANCON) was a forum consisting of a broad array of stakeholders who advised and assisted the Commission in its cancer-related policies. For example, it assisted in drawing up legal instruments, policy documents, and guidelines; it advised on the implementation of EU actions and suggested improvements thereof; it facilitated coordination and exchange of information between Member States. CANCON was established in 2014 in light of the Partnership Programme and replaced a previous advisory committee for cancer prevention. However, membership was rather exclusive, since it consisted of a limited number of representatives: one for each of the member states' competent authorities, and only ten representatives of the major stakeholder associations. The main outcome of this Joint Action was the 2017 publication of a European guide on quality improvement in cancer care (5). The new Innovative Partnership for Action Against Cancer (iPAAC) Joint Action (2018–2020) was selected for EU funding (80%) and seeks to build on the CANCON guidelines (6).

The European Partnership for Action Against Cancer 'Joint Action' initiative was a notable example of active engagement of stakeholders which engaged different stakeholder groups in the realization of the European Partnership Programme between 2009 and 2013. Most of these projects were funded through the EU's Third Health Programme, as administered by the Consumers, Health, Agriculture and Food Executive Agency.

Harmonizing National Policies

Since the EU has limited leverage regarding cancer healthcare in member states, European policy harmonization efforts are likewise restricted. Exceptions to this rule are the harmonization of cancer screening programmes and the adoption of national cancer control programmes. However, it should be noted that these measures are not legally binding, meaning that Member States are not obliged to comply. Although there are still large policy differences between the different EU Member States, especially along the East–West divide, these initiatives have nonetheless succeeded in bringing Member States' practices closer together.

The Council Recommendation on Cancer Screening (2003) prompted Member States to organize and implement population- and evidence-based screening for breast, cervical, and colorectal cancers. Targeted measures by Member States in line with this recommendation helped in achieving a substantial improvement of the number of the abovementioned cancer screening programmes in the EU. The Commission estimates that more than 500 million screenings will have been performed between 2010 and 2020. Furthermore, the Council Recommendation proposed minimum standards for registering and managing screening data: data systems for screening programmes should be centralized, all persons of a targeted population should be invited, and the data gathered should be protected according to relevant data protection laws.

The 50–69-year age range is recommended as target for breast cancer screening and is common to most of the European programmes. According to data gathered by the EC, out of approximately 32 million women in the EU in this age group, nearly 25 million have been invited to mammography screening, and 16 million were screened in 2013. The coverage by the breast cancer screening tests across different Member States is shown in Figure 32.1 (3).

Going a step further than the Council Recommendations, Member States have been adopting National Cancer Control Programmes (NCCPs) within the framework of the Commission's Partnership Programme. The Commission defines these NCCPs as public health programmes designed to ensure the centrally managed implementation and monitoring of evidence-based strategies for prevention, early detection, diagnosis, treatment, rehabilitation, palliation, and research. Regarding the quality standard of these NCCPs, the aforementioned EPAAC Joint Action has published standardized guidelines and best practices to assist the member states in creating these. As of November 2016, all but one of the Member States had adopted such a programme.

Another initiative to harmonize national policies was made by the EC, which asked the Joint Research Centre (JRC)—the EC's in-house science and knowledge service—and the EC's Directorate General for Health and Food Safety (DG SANTE) to act after the resolutions in the European Parliament. The JRC is coordinating the EC Initiative on Breast Cancer (ECIBC), which develops European guidelines for breast cancer screening and diagnosis ('European Breast Guidelines'), provides a platform of guidelines for all other stages of care, develops a quality assurance scheme to facilitate implementation in the member states, and develops a digital mammography training template (3). To ensure that all stakeholders, professionals, patients, and citizens remain informed, all these aforementioned activities are published on the ECIBC web hub (http://www.ecibc.jrc.ec.europa.eu) and shared directly with some 1,100 existing ECIBC contacts.

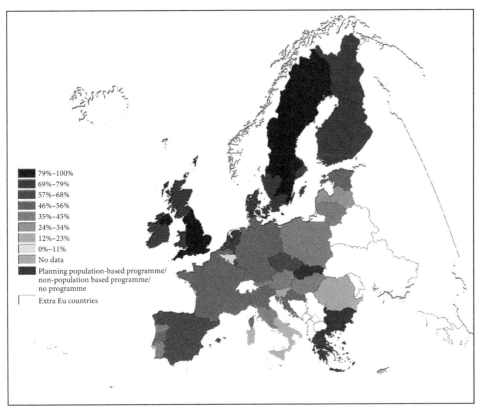

The legend in the map reads:

79%–100%
69%–79%
57%–68%
46%–56%
35%–45%
24%–34%
12%–23%
0%–11%
No data
Planning population-based programme/
non-population based programme/
no programme
Extra Eu countries

*The estimates do not take into account opportunistic screening

Figure 32.1 Breast cancer screening programmes in the EU (2017): examination coverage for the 50–69-year age range. In 2007 more than 59 million women in the EU were of the target age for breast cancer screening based on mammography specified in the Council Recommendation (50–69 years) (7). Data (last update July 2018) from the European Health interview survey Wave II—breast cancer screenings.

Reproduced with permission from Cancer Screening in the European Union (2017): Report on the implementation of the Council Recommendation on cancer screening. Available from: https://ec.europa.eu/health/sites/health/files/major_chronic_diseases/docs/2017_cancerscreening_2ndreportimplementation_en.pdf

Promoting Information Exchange

The EC promotes a better flow of information to avoid duplication of efforts, disseminates best practices, and creates more encompassing datasets. Two aspects are discussed here: databases centralizing European information and the dissemination of guidelines and best practices.

The EU supports multiple cancer-related databases; the most important are the European Network of Cancer Registries (ENCR) and the European Cancer Registry-based study on survival and care of cancer patients (EUROCARE). ENCR and EUROCARE have both been launched within the framework of the 1985 Commission Programme. For ease of access, the data from both these databases can be consulted through EUROSTAT (7).

A more recent achievement is the new European Cancer Information System, launched in February 2018, bringing together institutions and resources dealing with cancer information and data to provide the knowledge to optimize cancer control activities. ECIS provides the latest information on indicators that quantify cancer burden across Europe (8). It permits the exploration of geographical patterns and temporal trends of incidence, mortality, and survival data across Europe for the major cancer entities. It is developed and coordinated by the EC's Joint Research Centre (JRC) in association with the ENCR. This new European Cancer Information System lays down the foundation for a framework for interoperability of all European cancer registries. Hence, it regulates access of all users to updated high-quality cancer data at European level.

The Commission also encourages the development and dissemination of European guidelines and best practices, mostly by granting tenders to stakeholder associations. Some examples are:

- various screening guidelines regarding breast cancer;
- a policy statement on multidisciplinary cancer care;
- a training strategy to improve psychosocial and communication skills among health care providers.

Of special notice is the European Code Against Cancer, jointly developed by the World Health Organization's International Agency for the Research on Cancer (IARC) and the EC. This regularly updated guide provides 12 recommendations to citizens to reduce their risk of cancer. Many are self-evident such as on tobacco use or sun/ultraviolet light exposure, but others also refer to hormonal therapy or pollutants.

Research and Development

The EU supports research and development of new methods to fight cancer, primarily through the funding of research performed mostly in universities and research centres. It has different frameworks which enable funding of projects, and most of these are on a tender basis. The Commission regularly launches calls for projects within a certain scope, for example within the present EU Research and Innovation programme called 'Horizon 2020' and the future Framework Programme called Horizon Europe. Two other relevant EU instruments that support innovation are the Innovative Medicines Initiative (IMI) and the European Research Council (ERC), both of which have links to Horizon 2020.

Currently, the most important European tool to assist cancer-related research is Horizon 2020. It is the seventh and largest EU research and innovation programme with a total budget of nearly €80 billion. It is a flagship initiative of the Europe 2020 growth strategy covering 2014–2020. As of April 2016, it has funded 272 cancer-related projects for a total budget of €415 million. The EC maintains a website listing cancer-related Horizon 2020 projects and publishes an extensive funding guide to the programme to assist (potential) participants (9).

Funded for half of its budget by Horizon 2020, IMI is a collaboration between the EC and the European innovative pharmaceutical industry as represented by the European Federation of Pharmaceutical Industries and Associations. It is the world's biggest public–private partnership in the life sciences with a budget of €3.3 billion for the period 2014–2024. Some examples of its cancer-related projects are: CANCER-ID, which researches cancer treatment and monitoring through identification of circulating tumour cells and tumour-related nucleic acids in blood; MARCAR does research on biomarkers and molecular tumour classification for non-genotoxic carcinogenesis; PREDECT develops new models for preclinical evaluation of drug efficacy in common solid tumours.

The European Research Council is one of Horizon 2020's own flagship components. It enables researchers to conduct ground-breaking fundamental research. Contrary to most other funding instruments within Horizon 2020, it is not tender-based. Instead, researchers' proposals for projects are judged on their merit by a scientific council.

Regulation of Carcinogenic Chemicals and Cancer Medicines

The EU's most far-reaching competence regarding the fight against cancer is the aspect of regulation of cancer-related chemicals including both carcinogenic substances and medicines. Due to the existence of the European single market, goods produced or traded in the EU have to adhere to high environmental and health standards to ensure the safety of consumers, employees, and the environment. Correspondingly, risks concerning carcinogenic substances have to be minimized, and medicines must be safe for patients' use. Charged with medicine authorization, the European Medicines Agency (EMA) is another important institutional actor in the EU.

Pharmaceutical companies that want to market new cancer medicines containing novel active substances must have them reviewed by the EMA. In this agency, the Committee for Medicinal Products for Human Use assesses whether the medicine meets the necessary quality, safety, and efficacy requirements, that it has a positive risk–benefit balance, and it grants marketing authorizations for the EU. To perform this assessment, it reviews the results of clinical trials conducted at the national level. Besides this authorization function, EMA also facilitates development and access to medicines, monitors the safety of medicines across their life cycle, and provides information to healthcare professionals and patients (10).

Quality and Equality in Breast Cancer Screening and Care: The EC Initiative on Breast Cancer

In Europe, breast cancer incidence, prevalence, mortality, and survival rates data suggest that there might be substantial differences in the quality of breast cancer care

(11–13). Data from 2012 show that the estimated age-standardized mortality rate ranged from 15 to 29 women out of 100,000 dying of breast cancer (an almost two-fold range!) across the 27 countries of the EU. Although in some local areas higher mortality rates may reflect higher incidence, in other countries higher mortality rates might be due to lower survival of women with breast cancer caused also by inequalities in breast care delivery. These inequalities may be caused by several factors, such as differences in epidemiology of other fatal diseases, genetics, socioeconomic status, exposure to risk factors, health policies (e.g. presence/absence of screening programmes), or the effective delivery of cancer control measures among these appropriate breast cancer care services.

The EU does not engage in the organization and provision of health services and medical care. Instead, its action serves to complement national policies and to support cooperation between member states in the field of public health. The EU works for better health protection through its policies and activities within the remit of Article 168 of the Consolidated Treaty of the EU. It is within this spirit that in 2008 the Council of the EU invited the Commission to initiate the ECIBC, a new initiative to develop a European quality assurance scheme for breast cancer services supported by evidence-based guidelines.

The Council Conclusions of 2008 on reducing the burden of cancer invited the Commission to 'explore the potential for the development of voluntary European accreditation schemes for cancer screening and appropriate follow-up of lesions detected by screening, such as a European pilot accreditation scheme for breast cancer screening and follow-up based on the European guidelines for quality assurance in breast cancer screening and diagnosis.' ECIBC has the ultimate goal of developing a European quality assurance scheme for breast cancer services (European QA scheme) which will facilitate implementation within countries.

The scheme's requirements and indicators are being designed on the basis of the evidence provided by the European Guidelines on breast cancer screening and diagnosis (European Breast Guidelines) and a platform of guidelines for all other processes of care (Guidelines Platform). Both guidelines and platform are part of the ECIBC.

Differences in the Quality of Breast Cancer Services in Europe

Differences in the quality of healthcare services exist across European countries. More than ten different quality assurance schemes for breast cancer services coexist (14). This puzzle, while proving the effort of many relevant entities in improving care, makes it impossible for policymakers to compare service quality and to efficiently evaluate quality indicators. It also limits a patient's ability to make informed care decisions.

A common set of benchmarking quality requirements will harmonize and improve the quality of care in breast cancer services throughout Europe.

How is the European QA Scheme Being Developed?

To ensure that all stakeholders including patients and citizens are continuously informed, all ECIBC activities are published on the ECIBC web hub (http://ecibc.jrc.ec.europa.eu), and dedicated news alerts are sent directly to approximately 1,100 ECIBC contacts.

The Council Recommendations of 2008, signed by all EU countries, made it clear that the quality assurance (QA) scheme has to be based on evidence.

In 2013–2014, the EC's Joint Research Centre (JRC) met all stakeholders and ran surveys and studies to acquire the necessary knowledge base. These studies focused on breast cancer care organization in Europe, existing projects, QA schemes, and the accreditation and conformity assessment activities in breast cancer care.

The JRC ensures independence of all private, commercial, and national interests and works in a fully transparent way under the auspices of the Directorate General of Health and Food Safety (DG SANTE). Throughout this initiative, public calls for feedback are published online to ensure that all stakeholders are involved. On the ECIBC web hub, all relevant documents and information on working group members, methodologies applied and developed are published and updated.

In 2013, the respective 34 national authorities appointed ECIBC National Contacts (one per country). While the JRC continued to meet and exchange with the relevant stakeholders, the Quality Assurance Scheme Development Group (QASDG) and the Guidelines Development Group (GDG) were nominated by the EC in July 2015 to support the initiative. The QASDG met for the first time in September 2015. Since then, the QASDG has met four times per year. The members of the group work on a voluntary basis and are committed to act independently and in their best expert knowledge. The commitment they have signed and their declarations of interests are publicly available online as well as the policy for the management of the conflict of interest and the minutes of all meetings.

Breast Cancer Pathway and Organizational Modules

The methodology for selecting the clinical requirements (indicators) implies defining quality potentials along which to prioritize evidence-based requirements and then score them along relevance and clinical feasibility during Delphi-like rounds. The first two rounds have been run, and another four are foreseen to cover the entire pathway. Afterwards, the methodology foresees a key role for countries in defining

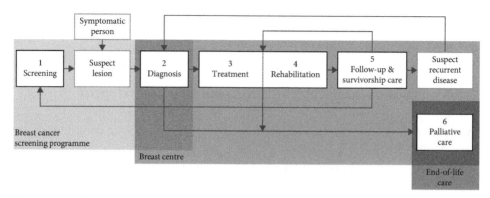

Figure 32.2 Organization of breast cancer care services in Europe.
Reproduced from *European Quality Assurance Scheme for Breast Cancer Services, Scope.* 2016. European Commission Initiative on Breast Cancer. Available from https://ecibc.jrc.ec.europa.eu/quality-assurance

the organizational and structural feasibility of the selected requirements/indicators (Figure 32.2).

Future Efforts

The Manual of the QA scheme is being developed for the piloting phase based on a variety of requirements (e.g. clinical and organizational, frequency of audits, format of the pre-assessment, etc.).

In 2019, the European QA scheme will be piloted, and this pilot will serve as a test of the robustness of the European QA scheme. Agreed criteria will be used to select a maximum of 15 breast cancer services across Europe which had responded to the online call for expression of interest for participating in the pilot.

The JRC and the QASDG collaborate towards implementation, on a full schedule of calls for feedback, dialogue between countries, and events participation to ensure that all countries are informed, involved, supported, and, in view of the call for expression of interest, to participate in the pilot.

How Will the European QA Scheme Work?

In substance, the European QA scheme is person-centred and includes survivorship and rehabilitation, psycho-oncology, and a multidisciplinary approach (in line with previous EC Joint Actions (EPAAC and CANCON) findings), while directly involving individuals, patients, and patient organizations from the development phase through implementation and beyond (15).

The European QA scheme plans to use the pre-existing infrastructure of National Accreditation Bodies (one per country) and follow a specific workflow (Figure 32.3).

Relation between NAB, CB and BCS (incl. testing and examination)

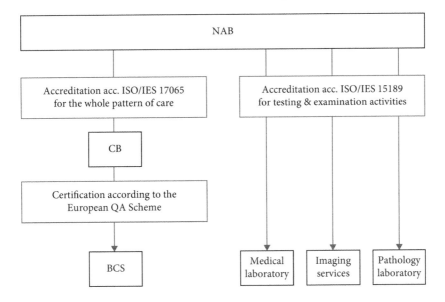

NAB: National Accreditation Bodies
CB: Certification Bodies
BCS: Breast Centre Service

Figure 32.3 Projection of European QA scheme in the future.
Reproduced from *European Quality Assurance Scheme for Breast Cancer Services, Scope.* 2016. European Commission Initiative on Breast Cancer. Available from https://ecibc.jrc.ec.europa.eu/quality-assurance

What's Next?

The European context implies greater complexity than national/local schemes both for development and for implementation.

The European QA scheme is, by definition, voluntary, but to demonstrate its impact, a consistent number of breast cancer services complying with the scheme would be crucial. For this reason, the ECIBC and notably its subgroup, the QASDG, is applying diverse communication strategies to target stakeholders, professionals, patients, and citizens.

The QA scheme manual may be fine-tuned to incorporate feedback from the piloting. Subsequently, the European QA scheme will be available to all stakeholders, breast cancer services, conformity assessment and certification bodies, national accreditation bodies and countries.

Key Messages

- The EU has a rather limited leverage in the treatment of breast cancer.
- It facilitates coordination and cooperation by bringing stakeholders together and harmonizing cancer policy between Member States.

- It promotes information exchange through databases and the dissemination of guidelines.
- It assists research and development through different funds, the most important of which are Horizon 2020, the European Research Council, and the Innovative Medicines Initiative.
- It regulates cancer-related substances, both carcinogenic chemicals as well as new cancer medicines.
- Europe chooses evidence-based quality of care.
- Equal access to care that improves outcomes is to be granted across the borders.

References

1. Leungo-Fernandez R et al. Economic burden of cancer across the European Union: a population-based cost analysis. *Lancet Oncol* 2013;14(12):1165–1174.
2. European Medicines Agency. Available from: https://www.ema.europa.eu/
3. Public Health Europe—European Commission—EU. Available from: https://ec.europa.eu/health/
4. Breast Centres Network, the first international network of Breast Cancer Centres. Available from: http://www.breastcentresnetwork.org/
5. Cancon: a joint action to improve cancer control in Europe. Available from: https://cancercontrol.eu/archived/
6. iPAAC. Available from: https://www.ipaac.eu/
7. Eurostat. Available from: https://ec.europa.eu/eurostat
8. European Commission. European Cancer Information System. Available from: https://ecis.jrc.ec.europa.eu
9. European Commission. Research and innovation. Available from: https://ec.europa.eu/info/research-and-innovation_en
10. European Parliament and the Council of the European Union. Regulation (EU) No 536/2014 of the European Parliament and of the Council 16 April 2014 on clinical trials on medicinal products for human use, and repealing Directive 2001/20/EC. The European Parliament and the Council of the European Union; 2014. Available from: https://ec.europa.eu/health/sites/health/files/files/eudralex/vol-1/reg_2014_536/reg_2014_536_en.pdf.
11. Ferlay J et al. Cancer incidence and mortality worldwide: sources, methods and major patterns in GLOBOCAN 2012. *Int J Cancer* 2015;136(5):E359–E386.
12. Allemani C et al. Breast cancer survival in the US and Europe: a CONCORD high-resolution study. *Int J Cancer* 2013;132(5):1170–1181.
13. De Angelis R et al. Cancer survival in Europe 1999–2007 by country and age: results of EUROCARE-5—a population-based study. *Lancet Oncol* 2014;15(1):23–34.
14. Lerda D et al. Report of a European survey on the organisation of breast cancer care services: supporting information for the European Commission initiative on breast cancer. EC Publications Office; 2014. Available from: https://ec.europa.eu/jrc/en/publication/eur-scientific-and-technical-research-reports/report-european-survey-organisation-breast-cancer-care-services-supporting-information.
15. Travado L et al. Psychosocial oncology care resources in Europe: a study under the European Partnership on Action Against Cancer [EPAAC]. *Psychooncology* 2017;26(4):523–530.

33

Perspectives on the Governance and Management of Breast Care Services in the USA

Lee F. Tucker and Teresa Heckel

Introduction

Access to affordable, high-quality breast care is a public health priority in the USA shared by national and state governments, third-party payors, health care professionals, advocacy groups, and patients alike. Breast cancer is the most commonly diagnosed non-cutaneous malignancy of women in the USA with an estimated 246,660 newly diagnosed cases in 2016 and 40,450 deaths (1). The last three decades have witnessed new legislation aimed at improving patient access, privacy, safety, and affordability. Patient advocacy groups and professional societies have contributed significantly to the education of those in elected office charged with enacting legislation at the local and national level (see Figure 33.1). In addition, national professional organizations have been pivotal in developing clinically relevant, actionable performance metrics.

Legislative Initiatives

The federal and state governments have enacted a variety of laws specific to breast care. The Mammography Quality Standards Act of 1992 was intended to improve the quality of mammographic screening by regulating mammographic screening at the federal level. Under this law, mammography facilities are subjected to annual inspections, and individuals interpreting screens are required to meet minimum professional qualification and continuing education requirements (2). The influence of this legislation has been felt nationwide, and the overall accreditation pass rate increased from 88.1% in 1987–1991 to 98.2% in 2003. The Health Insurance Portability and Accountability Act of 1996 applies to health care providers, medical facilities, insurance companies, and, in effect, virtually anyone in possession of protected health information. It regulates how entities and individuals can view and disseminate individually identifiable information about a person's health. This well-intentioned legislation imposes stiff penalties for non-compliance and has met with controversy. One study reported a 72.9% reduction in accruals to clinical trials and a threefold increase in recruitment costs.

The federal government has enacted legislation to require insurance coverage for breast care in select circumstances. In 1998, The Women's Health and Cancer Rights

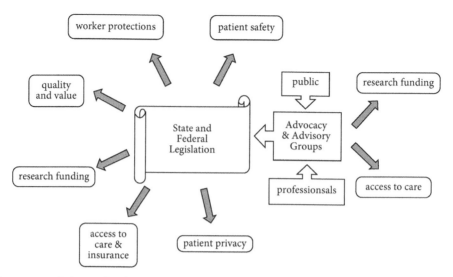

Figure 33.1 Relationship between government and advocacy in the development of health policy, access, and funding in the USA.

Act became federal law (3). The Women's Health and Cancer Rights Act requires health insurance plans to provide coverage for reconstructive surgery, prostheses, and certain physical complications of surgery such as lymphoedema, if the insurer included mastectomy among covered services. In 2014, the state of Ohio followed with the 'Lizzie Byrd Act', which requires that prospective mastectomy patients be offered preoperative referral to a reconstructive surgeon. This legislation is the first example of a state law requiring compliance with a performance standard of a voluntary accreditation programme, specifically the National Accreditation Program for Breast Centers. The Genetic Information Non-discrimination Act of 2008, enacted by the US Congress, prohibits health insurers from denying insurance coverage to otherwise healthy persons based solely on knowledge of genetic risk for disease. Employers cannot use genetic status when hiring, firing, or promoting employees (4). Individual states have enacted laws requiring written notification of women who have undergone a screening mammogram of the limitations of mammography in the detection of breast cancer in mammographically dense breasts. Collectively known as 'breast density laws', a total of 28 of the 50 states, beginning with Connecticut in 2009, have passed legislation to date. Legislation is currently pending in several other states.

Advocacy and Advisory Initiatives

Meaningful legislation is accomplished through the combined efforts of numerous advisory and advocacy organizations. It is beyond the scope of this chapter to enumerate them all; however, a discussion of several key organizations will illustrate their complex and necessary role of informing legislators, policymakers, and third-party payors in the relevant aspects of access, affordability and value in the delivery of breast care services. Additionally, advocacy and advisory groups serve as a valuable resource to health care executives and breast centre leaders.

Advocacy and advisory organizations in the USA are exceedingly varied in terms of mission, funding, and reporting accountability. Many are funded through volunteer contributions, whereas others receive significant public funding. The American Cancer Society (ACS) is one example of an organization with far-reaching influence on public policy that also serves as a resource for breast centre management professionals and the lay public. Since 1913, the ACS has relied on volunteer contributions, volunteer lay-persons, and clinicians to pursue a mission of patient and professional support, education, research funding, and early detection. The ACS Cancer Action Network is a non-partisan advocacy affiliate of the ACS that works at the state and federal level to improve funding for cancer research and to preserve and enhance funding for screening mammography and early breast cancer diagnosis. Founded in 1991, the National Breast Cancer Coalition (NBCC) is an example of a breast-specific volunteer advocacy effort. A diverse collaboration of advocacy groups, survivors, and professionals from across the nation, the NBCC has worked successfully to maintain and enhance research funding for breast cancer treatment and prevention. For the past 30 years, the Komen Foundation has served as one of the largest breast cancer philanthropy and advocacy groups in the USA. With over 120 affiliates across the country, Komen works in collaboration with local, state, and federal policymakers to increase access to affordable, high-quality breast services. A primary vehicle for the organization's fundraising has been the Komen Race for the Cure, a 5 km race first held in October 1983 in Dallas, Texas. In 2015, Komen affiliates held 154 race events globally, raising US$86.4 million. At least 20% of the annual fundraising is earmarked for breast cancer research, totalling US$889 million in breast cancer research funding as of 2015. In addition, Komen supports patients with breast health information, a breast care hotline, access to low-cost mammography, and financial assistance information (5).

By contrast, The US Preventive Services Task Force (USPSTF) serves in an advisory capacity only. The USPSTF was formed in 1984 as an independent, volunteer group of experts in evidence-based medicine and disease prevention to make recommendations regarding clinical preventive services (6). The task force has published recommendations for age and frequency of mammographic screening on three occasions since 2002. These guidelines, although intended to provide clarity to the debate, have been controversial among the professional community. The federal Patient Protection and Affordable Care Act of 2010 required the USPSTF to report annually to Congress areas where clinical evidence is deemed insufficient to support use of a clinical preventive service, presumably to prioritize future research funding. The USPSTF has identified three research gaps in breast care, centred on the utilization of breast imaging (7).

Performance Management

National professional societies representing clinical disciplines engaged in breast health have developed voluntary quality management programmes with measures of professional performance or clinical outcomes. Two examples of specialty-specific programmes designed to provide individual and peer practitioner comparisons include the Quality Oncology Practice Initiative of the American Society of Clinical Oncologists (8) and the Mastery of Breast Surgery programme of the American Society of Breast Surgeons (9). Increasingly, breast programme leaders have recognized that measures such as these can form the core of a data-driven quality management culture. In addition, several interdisciplinary breast-focused organizations have achieved national prominence by virtue of accreditation and quality management initiatives. These organizations serve as a valuable resource to leadership at all levels from national policy decision-makers to those management professionals in individual breast centres. The National Accreditation Program for Breast Centers (NAPBC), founded in 2005, is a voluntary accreditation programme of the American College of Surgeons based on 28 standards covering the spectrum of breast care from screening through survivorship (10). With more than 600 accredited programmes in the USA, NAPBC emphasizes performance improvement through data collection and process development. The National Cancer Database (NCDB), a collaborative effort of the American College of Surgeons and the American Cancer Society, is another resource available to breast programme leaders. It consists of a clinical oncology database derived from the cancer registry of individual hospitals that can be used to track patients following a diagnosis of malignancy. The NCDB compiles data from more than 70% of cancer diagnoses in the USA each year.

Clearly defined and actionable performance metrics are of interest to third-party payors and policymakers alike who envision a transformation of breast care reimbursement from a claims-made model to one that incorporates a value quotient (11). The Physician Quality Reporting System (PQRS) was the product of a decade-long initiative of the Centers for Medicare & Medicaid Services to improve health care quality through accountability and public disclosure of performance. The programme uses performance measures provided by the professional societies themselves with ten of the more than 300 measures specific to breast care. The PQRS began as a system of penalties and rewards for the reporting of performance with a reimbursement penalty levied for non-reporting. The data submitted are also used to calculate a 'value modifier' based on reported quality of care and cost data. The value modifier is used to further adjust practitioner payments. The evolutionary Medicare Advanced Alternative Payment Model and Merit-Based Incentive Payment System (MIPS) add an outcomes perspective to these concepts, with MIPS programme quality indicators adopted from the PQRS programme (12).

The implications of these programmes should be obvious to all clinical and administrative leaders of breast programmes in the USA. Reimbursement for breast care services provided to those patients in the Medicare programme and aligned third-party payors is maximized by reporting performance under the applicable measures and potentially diminished by adverse value modifiers or MIPS performance. Further, informed decision-making by patients and their families might include review of published performance and value data. Continuous review of a core dataset should be a priority for breast programme leadership. A high-value solution available to breast care leaders is the National Quality Measures for Breast Centers (NQMBC) programme, launched in 2005 as a voluntary web-based certification process to monitor breast centre performance. Using more than 30 individual breast measures, NQMBC tracks service attributes, professional performance, and clinical outcomes across disciplines from screening, diagnosis, treatment, and survivorship. The NQMBC offers breast centres the ability to measure and compare individual and peer performance over time against filtered subsets of programmes (13). As of February 2016, 539 breast centres had submitted data with more than six million patient data-pool entries.

The Role of Health Executives and Management: Challenges of Breast Programme Leadership

Leadership models for breast care services vary considerably across the USA reflecting the geographic and economic diversity of the nation. Clinical care delivery sites range from independent not-for-profit hospitals and associated outpatient clinics to for-profit hospitals, multispecialty clinics, solo physician-owned practices, government-owned and military facilities, for-profit treatment-only centres, and integrated health systems. Some breast care is provided by affiliations with a medical school, but 93% of hospitals in the USA do not claim an academic affiliation. Therefore breast care services vary in how they are delivered, the degree to which services are integrated, and how they are managed. In most cases, management models for breast care services are derived from the business structure and ownership of the health facility, not the other way around. Even though most practitioners acknowledge that interdisciplinary coordination of clinical care is essential in the modern era of breast care, business models and management paradigms have been slow to embrace an interdisciplinary breast-centric model. An individual clinic, hospital, or health system may purport to offer a comprehensive breast centre, yet closer inspection reveals fragmented care delivery. Part of the problem stems from the organizational structure of the hospital itself. For example, in many hospitals including academic medical centres, operating budgets, staffing, strategic goals, and reporting accountabilities are all defined by 'cost centers' in the traditional departments of surgery, radiology, oncology, pathology, and nursing rather than in a coordinated breast-centric model. Although at least 75% of hospitals now have at least a basic electronic health record (EHR), many records exist in a private physician practice environment without being shared. Commonly, restrictive third-party payor contracts direct diagnostic services such as biopsy interpretation away from the programme to non-affiliated practitioners.

Oncologic care may be provided by multiple, competing medical and radiation oncology practices. Individual physicians may vary in the degree to which they support the breast centre, evidenced by sporadic participation in leadership activities and pretreatment planning conferences or non-adoption of evidence-based evaluation and management guidelines. Care and reimbursement are viewed as episodic events, not as a continuum of a chronic disease process. Restrictive payor contracts contribute to care fragmentation by directing patients along a care path outside the influence, and often knowledge, of an individual breast programme. Leadership is confronted with a difficult choice between leveraging a hospital or health system's market presence to negotiate inclusion in a payor's network or persuading out-of-network practitioners to align with their programme. Alignment would include many of the attributes expected of practitioners supportive of a breast centre including acceptance of evidence-based evaluation and management guidelines, conference participation, and shared recordkeeping. Neither approach by leadership is a guaranteed success; however, specific leadership skills are required to bring alignment to out-of-network practitioners in the interest of improving patient care. Skilled leaders may languish if management is non-supportive. Internal competition among traditional hospital departments creates conflict in capital prioritization, operating budgets, and resources including staff. These conflicts may lead to under-allocation or over-allocation of the resources necessary to deliver high-value breast care.

These are but a few of the many management challenges facing today's breast programme leaders. Furthermore, the effectiveness of programme leadership is made more difficult by a changing regulatory and reimbursement environment. Despite these obstacles, successful breast programme leadership in the USA has evolved around two basic strategies: evolution toward an interdisciplinary management model and development of skilled physician leadership.

Attributes of Successful Breast Programme Leaders

To optimize the care continuum in a consistent fashion, breast health leaders must first understand the diversity of existing challenges and identify the resources available to resolve them. Health care institutions in the USA, and breast programmes specifically, have benefited greatly from pioneering leadership developments in the corporate realm. The principles of 'emotional intelligence' described by Goleman in *Primal Leadership* emphasize self-awareness, self-management, social awareness, and relationship management as essential qualities of leaders. These qualities are as applicable to health care leaders as they are to industry. Stoller et al. make the case for physicians as executive leaders in hospitals and cite the Cleveland Clinic and the Mayo Clinic as among the best US examples (14). The limitations faced by physician leaders, Stoller et al. write, are imposed upon them by training as independent clinicians. Valuable in diagnostic medicine, independent behaviours are often counter-productive in leaders who must be trained in the management principles of teambuilding, conflict

resolution, and emotional intelligence (Figure 33.2). Examples of successful management training programmes for physicians include those at Yale Medicine pioneered by
CEO Paul Taheri and The Cleveland Clinic. Evidence is mounting of a correlation between physician leadership and improved hospital performance and patient care. Many
of the best-performing US hospitals are now led by physicians (15).

Although the physician-CEO is becoming more common in the USA, physician-
only management of breast programmes is unusual. The traditional non-clinical administrative leadership of breast programmes is being rapidly replaced with a dyad
leadership model which pairs a physician with a non-clinical manager. In the most mature iteration, the relationship is mutually supportive with clearly defined responsibilities and accountabilities drawn from the specific strengths of each leadership partner.
Integration of physicians into health care leadership has been limited not only by a lack
of physician leadership training, but by physician perception of hospitals as partners.
In a 2010 survey of 1,009 US physicians, 60% believed that physicians and hospitals
had competing goals, 56% said there was insufficient physician leadership or representation on the hospital board, and 56% believed incentives were not aligned. An appropriate degree of accountability and responsibility of breast programme leadership to
the parent organization and medical staff is one requirement for accreditation by the
National Accreditation Program for Breast Centers.

Increasingly, employment is viewed as a means of achieving alignment of physician
goals with 63% of US physicians reporting status as an employee in 2015. Practitioner
employment is the norm in academic institutions and some non-academic environments. In the private sector, many breast programmes have taken the step of creating
employment positions for physician medical directors or other key practitioners such
as breast surgeons and imagers. In positions of programme leadership, it is preferable
to create compensated positions supported by detailed job descriptions; too often the
critically important task of leadership is relegated to a busy clinician to the end of a
work day. Compensated, job description-supported, physician management in health
care is a growing trend; however, this employment model by itself does not guarantee

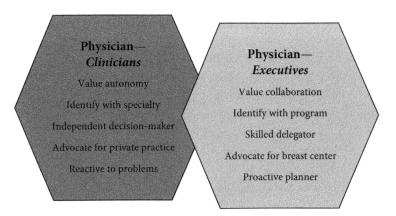

Figure 33.2 Attributes of physicians versus leaders.

desired practitioner performance in a breast programme. It is incumbent on the hospital executive leadership as well as on the breast centre medical director to recognize the importance of including the attributes of acceptable alignment in the practitioner's employment contract, subject to at least annual review. Some breast programmes have developed 'participation agreements' for non-employed private practitioners to delineate expected performance as a condition of inclusion in the programme's roster of service providers.

Effective Breast Care Organizational Models

The full potential of talented breast care leaders is only achieved when the organizational model and reporting structure are optimized to deliver interdisciplinary breast-focused care. Breast patients are high users of health care resources, and they arrive with high expectations for service and quality. The surge in breast advocacy has empowered women to take control of their disease and treatment. Breast cancer patients are more likely to seek the quality of care and services that will optimize their chance of survival as well as quality of life. Medical expenditures associated with breast cancer in the USA were projected to reach US$16.5 billion in 2010. It is estimated that the number of breast cancer survivors will rise to 4.5 million by the year 2026, and this will challenge breast health leaders to provide better value and management of the psychological and physical effects of breast disease.

Traditional oncology service lines focus primarily on outpatient cancer treatment, providing ample opportunity for fragmentation among practitioners with poor coordination of care, waste, and inefficiency. Beginning with breast cancer, 'tumour site programmes' or cancer-specific 'centres of excellence' have rapidly grown in the USA as a strategy to overcome the limitations of traditional service lines and clinical departments. Many successful breast programme directors have developed a performance-based management structure spanning disciplines and departments resulting in defragmentation of the patient's care and subjective experience. Breast centres remain the most prevalent tumour site programme today. The organizational structure of a tumour site programme facilitates a comprehensive approach to cancer care by coordinating the specialists, technologies, and support services that are needed across the care continuum. Such integrated programmes can address the full spectrum of interventions from prevention, early detection, diagnosis, and treatment through survivorship or end of life. In a 2015 survey conducted by the Advisory Board Company, 90% of responding cancer leaders reported having a fully or partially developed breast programme. In a survey of oncology leaders, respondents reported a perceived 86% increase in cancer programme competition, highlighting the urgency to develop care delivery models that appeal to both patients and physicians. Although becoming a centre of excellence does not guarantee programme growth, programmes that commit to a standards-focused, outcomes-driven approach differentiate themselves in a market by offering measurable, high-quality care. In this era of accountability, they are more likely to become the providers of choice for physicians and patients.

Health System Coordination of Care

Hospital merger and affiliation activity affords unique opportunities to influence breast health across broad segments of the US population. In 2014 alone, 100 mergers or acquisitions occurred among hospitals across the USA totalling US$62 billion; 65% of these involved non-profit hospitals. In some cases, affiliations appear to prevent closure of vulnerable rural hospitals, thereby maintaining access to clinical services. In 2016, the largest non-profit health systems in the USA were Ascension Health and Catholic Health Initiatives with 141 and 104 hospitals, respectively. Among the for-profits, Hospital Corporation of America (169 hospitals) and Community Health Systems (158 hospitals) are the largest.

By leveraging information technology, management talent, and capital resources, health systems are beginning the process of coordinating access to screening, diagnostic and treatment services, identifying gaps in provider coverage and socioeconomic barriers, while reducing redundancy in clinical services. Health systems such as Kaiser Permanente, California, Catholic Health Initiatives, Colorado, and Inova Breast Care Institute, Virginia are examples of systems that have developed interdisciplinary breast or oncology care management models to coordinate care across their enterprise. The composition of these system-wide management teams varies, but typically they consist of a designated physician director and executive partner with medical directors and management staff representing the individual breast units, system-wide information technology support, quality management and cancer registry staff, and, frequently, clinical research, strategic development, and marketing professionals. System-wide breast health committees have the resources to conduct robust, market-specific service and performance analyses, identify loci of care variation, and establish programmatic priorities across a diverse socioeconomic patient base.

Key Messages

- Recent legislation aims to improve patient safety, privacy, and access to care.
- Advocacy and advisory groups serve a vital function informing government, payors and breast programme leaders of public access, affordability, and research funding priorities.
- Breast programme leadership is becoming more breast-specialized and interdisciplinary.
- Breast-specific performance measures are increasingly utilized by leadership to inform management decision-making and strategic planning.

- Value-quotient performance management remains uncommon and poorly understood by most.
- Poor definitional standardization of breast quality metrics limits peer performance benchmarking.
- Robust health system merger and acquisition activity facilitates coordination of breast care across broad geographies and populations.

References

1. American Cancer Society. *Cancer Facts & Figures 2016.* Available from: http://www.cancer.org/research/cancer-facts-statistics/all-cancer-facts-figures/cancer-facts-figures-2016.html

2. US Food and Drug Administration. *MQSA National Statistics.* Available from: https://www.fda.gov/RadiationEmittingProducts/MammographyQualityStandardsActandProgram/FacilityScorecard/ucm113858.htm

3. United States Department of Labor. *Fact sheet: Women's Health and Cancer Rights Act.* Available from: https://www.dol.gov/agencies/ebsa/laws-and-regulations/laws/whcra

4. Equal Opportunity Employment Commission [US]. *The Genetic Information Nondiscrimination Act of 2008.* Available from: https://www.eeoc.gov/laws/statutes/gina.cfm

5. Susan G. Komen Foundation. *Our Mandate at Susan G. Komen˚.* Available from: http://ww5.komen.org/WhatWeDo.html

6. US Preventive Services Task Force. *About the USPSTF.* Available from: https://www.uspreventiveservicestaskforce.org/Page/Name/about-the-uspstf

7. US Preventive Services Task Force. *Fifth Annual Report to Congress on High-Priority Evidence Gaps for Clinical Preventive Services.* Available from: https://www.uspreventiveservicestaskforce.org/Page/Name/fifth-annual-report-to-congress-on-high-priority-evidence-gaps-for-clinical-preventive-services

8. American Society of Clinical Oncology. *Quality Oncology Practice Initiative (QOPI˚).* Available from: http://www.instituteforquality.org/quality-oncology-practice-initiative-qopi

9. American Society of Breast Surgeons. *Mastery of Breast Surgery*ˢᴹ. Available from: https://www.breastsurgeons.org/mastery/background.php

10. American College of Surgeons. *National Accreditation Program for Breast Centers.* Available from: https://www.facs.org/quality-programs/napbc

11. Porter ME. *Redefining Health Care: Creating Positive-Sum Competition to Deliver Value.* 2005. Available from: https://www.hbs.edu/faculty/Pages/item.aspx?num=46805

12. Centers for Medicare and Medicaid Services. *Quality Payment Program.* Available from: https://qpp.cms.gov/mips/overview.

13. Tucker L. *National Quality Measures for Breast Centers.* National Consortium of Breast Centers, Inc.; 7 September 2015. Available from: https://www.youtube.com/watch?v=EUrAeqBiM1E

14. Stoller JK. Why the best hospitals are managed by doctors. *Harvard Business Rev.* 27 December 2016. Available from: https://hbr.org/2016/12/why-the-best-hospitals-are-managed-by-doctors

15. Goodall AH. Physician-leaders and hospital performance: is there an association? *Social Sci Med* 2011;73(4):535–539.

34

Perspective from Latin America

Eduardo L. Cazap and Gilberto Schwartsmann

Introduction

The world is facing a critical health care problem: in the next few decades cancer will become a leading global public health problem disproportionately increasing in low- and middle-income countries. Breast cancer is a high priority within the global cancer problem (1).

In the USA, 60% of breast cancer cases are diagnosed in the earliest stages, whereas in Brazil only 20% and in Mexico only 10% are diagnosed at an early stage. The all-cancer mortality-to-incidence ratio for Latin America is 0.59, compared with 0.43 for the EU and 0.35 for the USA. In practical terms, the risk of dying from breast cancer in Latin America is double that in the USA (2).

A study done by our group in 2006 obtained, through a 65-question telephone interview with 100 breast cancer experts from 12 Latin American countries (LAC), preliminary information about the state of breast cancer care at that time. The methodology was employed to obtain fast qualitative information about breast cancer in the region, due to the lack of hard data at that moment (3).

With respect to epidemiological characteristics, the incidence of breast cancer in Latin American countries was lower than that in more developed countries, whereas the mortality rate was higher. These differences probably are related to differences in screening strategies and access to treatment. The authors agreed that population-based data were urgently needed to make informed decisions. It was also reported that more than 90% of countries had, at that time, no national laws or guidelines for mammography screening, and that the access rate to mammography was around 50%. However, diagnostic testing for hormone receptors and biomarkers was available at most centres (>80%), and overall nearly 80% of patients started treatment within 3 months of diagnosis. In most Latin American health systems, doctors work both at academic institutions and public hospitals, therefore the subjective interpretation of these data may be inaccurate. Alternative data collection strategies for better understanding the state of breast cancer care in developing countries could help to identify areas for improvement (3).

Some of the relevant conclusions of the study are summarized in Table 34.1.

A subsequent study published in 2010 compared expert perceptions with medical care standards through a systematic review of the norms, recommendations, and guidelines considered as medical care standards for breast cancer in 12 Latin American countries

Table 34.1 Conclusions from the 2008 study on breast cancer in Latin America (3)

1. Lack of epidemiological data

2. Lack of political commitment

3. Low rate of mammographic screening

4. Hormone receptor and molecular markers not available for all patients

5. High percentage of mastectomy

6. Surgery done by gynaecologist or general surgeon in a significant number of cases

7. Clinical–epidemiological and basic research were insufficient

8. Short interval between diagnosis and treatment in some countries

9. Adequate palliative care for patients (chemotherapy, hormonotherapy, and morphine)

10. Good level of education among specialists treating breast cancer

(4). Information related to medical care standards was requested from governmental health authorities, cancer institutes, and national scientific and professional societies. The documents received were reviewed by breast cancer experts from each country. Additionally, three key survey questions from our previous 2006 study on early detection and diagnosis were reprocessed to provide information related to the implementation practice of existing medical care standards. We concluded that all countries included in the study had medical care standards whether published by governmental authorities, national professional or scientific associations, cancer institutes, or through the adoption of international medical care standards. The results were reported at the centre level (mainly private institutions) or at the national level (public hospitals). For diagnostic suspicion of breast cancer, 80% of experts considered that the diagnostic suspicion at a national level came from patients compared to 50% from breast centres. About 30% of patients waited more than 3 months for a diagnosis at the national level compared to 7% at the centre level. All countries in the study reported the use of similar medical care standards for breast cancer care. The reported difference between care practised at national level versus centre level suggests that the challenge is not in generating new medical care standards, but in implementing policies and control mechanisms for compliance with existing medical care standards and guaranteeing their applicability and access to all populations (4).

Our study published in 2013, performed by the Karolinska Institute, the Stockholm School of Economics, the Pan American Health Organization, the American Cancer Society, and the Latin-American and Caribbean Society of Medical Oncology analysed in more detail the picture of the disease according to several aspects (5).

We summarize below some conclusions about different aspects of breast cancer control. This was the most recently published and most comprehensive information produced by our group. The study was based on a review of the scientific literature and public database, and a survey of clinical experts and patient organizations. The literature review, focusing specifically on treatment patterns and costs of breast cancer in each study country, was conducted on Medline, LILACS, and SciELO but also included grey literature targeting data and information on the epidemiology of the disease and its outcomes in the region as well as treatment guidelines, cancer control plans, and documentation on the cost of breast cancer.

The study faced a number of limitations mostly due to the lack of data. Perhaps the most important to bear in mind when interpreting this information is the publication bias. Many factors influence the research and intellectual production in the countries under study, resulting in highly diverse volumes of evidence, and, whereas for some countries rich materials and data have been identified, for others only a few and scattered articles were found. Nevertheless, this is one of the few comprehensive data sets available today regarding breast cancer in Latin America.

Epidemiological Burden

Breast cancer is the most common form of cancer in women in the region. Each year, approximately 115,000 women are diagnosed and 37,000 die due to breast cancer, and incidence and mortality are increasing. Unlike in Europe or the USA, both incidence and mortality rates in LACs are on the rise, and mortality is expected to double in less than 20 years.

Ageing is the main risk factor; it will cause an increase in breast cancer cases and is recognized as the main risk factor of developing breast cancer.

LACs today have a relatively low mean age, but this is bound to change. The demographic profile of Argentina and Uruguay may offer a look into the future of the region: mean age is 5–10 years above and breast cancer crude mortality rates are five to six times higher than present LAC averages. In some countries, Brazil being one, breast cancer cases are expected to increase rapidly and reach epidemic proportions.

Limited by the availability of comparable data, the only significant correlations with the LAC incidence rates of breast cancer risk were their wealth and women's educational level (Table 34.2).

Clinical Burden

The survival rate in LACs is considerably lower than the EU benchmark that achieves 5-year survival rates >80%. Enhanced treatments and earlier diagnosis explain progress made over past years. The available data show a 5-year survival rate in LACs that fluctuates around 70%. This difference in survival is mainly caused by late stage at diagnosis, which is an important predictor for overall survival. The benchmark for detection of early breast cancer in the EU is 90%, while the LAC average is between 60% and 70%. In countries such as Peru, Colombia, or Mexico, around 50% of detected breast cancer cases are in advanced stages. Late stage at diagnosis negatively impacts survival rate and notably increases per case health expenditures.

Table 34.2 Relationship between breast cancer incidence and some reproductive, socioeconomic, and lifestyle factors from the 2013 study (5)

Country	Age-standardized incidence rate per 100,000 person-years	Births, women aged <30 years	Childbearing mean age (years) (1)	Fertility rate (1)	Overweight and obesity (%)[a]	Alcohol consumption (L)[b]	Women's life expectancy (years)	Per-capita GDP 2008 (US$) (6)	Female education (%)[c]
Uruguay	90.7	64.96%	27.7	2.1	73.48	12.7	79.9	8,161	96.3
Argentina	74.0	65.83%	27.9	2.2	77.28	7.6	79.1	9,885	93.3
Costa Rica	42.9	75.00%	26.6	1.9	74.16	7.8	81.3	5,189	74.4
Venezuela	42.5	75.24%	26.8	2.5	74.30	–	76.8	5,884	75.7
Brazil	42.3	76.58%	26.9	1.8	68.40	10.6	76	4,448	89.4
Chile	40.1	65.74%	28.0	1.9	76.66	8.2	81.6	6,235	82
Peru	34.0	63.53%	28.5	2.5	78.88	5.6	75.9	2,924	89.9
Colombia	31.2	72.51%	26.5	2.4	70.41	4.7	76.7	2,983	80.9
Ecuador	30.8	72.25%	27.4	2.5	62.75	33.4	78.1	1,745	–
Panama	29.2	74.86%	26.6	2.5	65.66	–	78.3	5,688	83.5
Mexico	27.2	71.79%	26.8	2.2	79.95	17.3	78.7	7,092	79
Correlation coefficient		–0.4849	0.3779	–0.3091	0.2188	–0.1880	0.3248	0.6878	0.6786
P-value		0.1306	0.2519	0.355	0.5181	0.6281	0.3298	0.0193	0.0310

GDP, gross domestic product.

[a]Estimated overweight and obesity (body mass index ≥25 kg/m²) prevalence, females, aged ≥30 years, 2005.

[b]Female per-capita consumption of pure alcohol, aged ≥15 years; drinkers only.

[c]Combined gross enrolment ratio in education, 2007 (%).

Modified with permission from Justo N et al. 'A Review of Breast Cancer Care and Outcomes in Latin America'. *The Oncologist*. Volume 18, Issue 3, pp. 248–256. Copyright © 2013 John Wiley & Sons. DOI: 10.1634/theoncologist.2012-0373

Social and Economic Burden

The costs of breast cancer are directly related to stage of diagnosis, and yearly healthcare cost for a patient with stage IV breast cancer in LACs has been shown to be three to four times the cost of treating a patient with stage I breast cancer (6). The increased morbidity and mortality of metastatic patients greatly increase overall expenses throughout the healthcare system, i.e. by also affecting primary care facilities or emergency care while also depriving society of productive years.

In addition, the majority of women are diagnosed when still in working age, so productivity losses due to younger age at death are exacerbated by the increased morbidity due to younger age at diagnosis. Due to insufficient funding, patients are undiagnosed, unattended, untreated, and uncared for, while others receive suboptimal treatment. General healthcare expenditure in LACs is far below European and US standards, not only in absolute but also in relative terms. Yearly expenditure per breast cancer case in Europe is around $40,000 while in LACs, e.g. Brazil, depending on insurance type, values can vary from $4,800 in the Sistema Único de Saúde-Unique Health System to $16,400 in a private facility (7).

Access to Treatment and Framework of Care

Healthcare Coverage is Expanding, Although Not Across All Dimensions

Health access in LACs has improved continuously over the years driven by reforms towards more universal health access and a growing participation of the private sector. Of the three dimensions to universal health access, expansion has been made mainly in terms of the population that is covered. To prevent financial hardship, impoverishment, and social inequity, expanding depth of services and proportion of costs covered are critical for catastrophic conditions such as breast cancer.

There are Vast Differences in Access to Care

Nevertheless, there are vast differences in access to breast cancer care across LACs that depend mainly on insurance type and geographical location. Even within a particular insurance type or country, great differences in access can exist depending on the wealth of the region (i.e. state or province, municipality, etc.) and the willingness to invest in breast cancer care.

As examples, Brazil assigns different levels of resources to breast cancer care depending on the type of insurance. Inequalities exist based on insurance type.

In Argentina, the Compulsory Medical Plan guarantees 100% public coverage for oncology drugs. However, the type and quality of provided treatments vary in different provinces or districts, causing geographical inequalities, whereas in Peru, 64% of the population depends on the public health insurance, which covers breast cancer diagnosis, but no treatments. Not surprisingly, health outcomes in Peru are far below average and among the lowest in the region. It is important to mention that this situation has improved in recent years.

Absence of National Cancer Control Programmes

National Cancer Control Programmes (NCCP) are recommended by the World Health Organization (WHO), because they are the blueprint for a holistic cancer control strategy and play a vital role in optimizing health care systems and reducing the burden of cancer. The function of an NCCP is to define critical processes in cancer control such as overall national strategy, priorities, governance, financing, service delivery, monitoring, and continuous improvement. Several LACs do not have a formal NCCP in place, and basic elements of an NCCP, such as population-based cancer registries, are missing or implemented only with a limited scope.

Treatment Guidelines Exist—the Challenge is Implementation

Evidence-based treatment guidelines are published in most countries by governmental authorities, cancer institutes, or scientific associations (Chapter 9). The challenge is the implementation of policies and mechanisms to ensure consistent compliance with these guidelines across the entire population (Box 34.1).

Box 34.1 Treatment and guidelines

- Treatment guidelines exist—the challenge is implementation
- Evidence-based treatment guidelines are published in most countries by governmental authorities, cancer institutes, or scientific associations.
- The challenge is, again, the implementation of policies and mechanisms to ensure a consistent compliance with these guidelines across the entire population.

Diagnosis and Treatment

Generally speaking, there is low commitment to mammography screening. In LACs, most breast cancer cases are detected when women seek care after having noticed a breast lump. Early detection is an opportunity for improvement in the region, and there is no consistent strategy for breast cancer prevention or detection that could be recognized. Actions are being taken in countries such as Mexico, Costa Rica, Argentina, Uruguay, and Brazil, where population-based programmes have been or are being implemented.

Hormone receptor and biomarker determination are common practice. Contrary to the low commitment to mammographic screening, post-diagnostic screening with hormone receptor and biologic marker determination seems to be widespread in the region. Some questions arise in terms of the differences found in HER2+ overexpression, which leads us to conclude that:

a. there is a need to standardize criteria for immunohistochemistry assay interpretation;
b. it is not clear whether HER2+ overexpression has been consistently tested.

Concerning medical therapy, all systemic treatments are licensed, but budget considerations limit the use of some effective treatments. Adjuvant chemotherapy reduces the relative yearly risk of death by almost 40% for women aged <50 years and by 20% for women aged 50–69 years. Endocrine therapy with tamoxifen in oestrogen receptor-positive patients results in a more than 30% relative risk reduction of mortality.

One year of adjuvant therapy with trastuzumab in women with HER2+ breast cancer leads to 50% reduced risk of recurrence. Usage of modern drugs greatly differs from country to country and insurance type. Chemotherapy treatments with anthracyclines are widely accepted, as is tamoxifen for patients with oestrogen receptor-positive tumours. However, new-generation hormonal treatments such as aromatase inhibitors and the biological therapy trastuzumab are not accessible for all women.

In metastatic breast cancer, medical treatment is the most important consideration. Access to modern drugs is vital, but not yet a reality. Targeted therapies trastuzumab or pertuzumab are important treatment options for the advanced breast cancer patients. Access to these drugs follows similar restrictions as in early breast cancer, leaving patients with few therapeutic alternatives, uncontrolled disease progress, and consequently poor outcomes.

An Example from Brazil: Assessing Value for Money

Over the last two decades, the decrease in mortality due to infectious and cardiovascular diseases placed cancer as the leading health-care challenge in various LACs. In

Brazil, cancer became the number one cause of patient morbidity and mortality in various geographic regions. Providing these patients with appropriate health care is limited by inequity in the distribution of resources, personnel, and equipment as well as in access to health care, especially for patients in socioeconomic, ethnic, or geographically disadvantaged areas (8).

The access to surgery, radiation, and medical therapy for Brazilian cancer patients is more limited for the three out of four patients relying exclusively on the National Health System (NHS). As an example, the impact of access to anti-HER2 therapy for women with advanced breast cancer was analysed by Debiasi et al. (9). The authors estimated that about 2000 women were diagnosed with advanced HER2+ breast cancer in Brazil in the year 2016. Only 40% of them were projected to be alive in the year 2018, if they received only chemotherapy as offered by Brazilian NHS guidelines (9).

However, the bar would rise to about 70%, if they had the opportunity to receive chemotherapy plus anti-HER2 therapy (i.e. trastuzumab), as offered to women with private insurance. This prpoportion would increase to about 75% if the reference standard would be chemotherapy plus trastuzumab and pertuzumab. Notably, trastuzumab was added to the WHO list of essential anticancer medications several years ago, but Brazilian health authorities delayed its introduction in the armamentarium against advanced HER2+ breast cancer until recently. Health care authorities should dedicate their efforts to reduce disparities in cancer care, especially in less developed countries, as well as in more vulnerable populations not covered with adequate health insurances in any country, making overall cancer care more affordable to all patients.

Palliative Care

Quality of life during end of life is poor in LAC patients, and symptoms such as pain, fatigue, nausea, physical impairment, and sleeplessness have been found to be persistent problems. Studies show that care is fragmented, suffering is uncontrolled, communication between professionals, patients and families is poor, and a great burden is placed on patients, families, and caregivers. The main barriers to optimal pain control are inadequate staff knowledge of pain management (70%), inability to pay for services or analgesics (57%), inadequate pain assessment (52%), and excessive regulations for prescribing opioids (44%).

Breast Cancer in Young Women in Latin America

Breast cancer among LAC women is a growing burden throughout the region. The increased proportion of breast cancer cases in young women is important, because their diagnoses and tumour behaviour are usually more aggressive than in their older counterparts. The findings of a recent study reveal that there is scarce information regarding this matter in LACs, especially concerning the particular effects and complications that this group of women faces during and after treatment. Also, there are no specific clinical or educational programmes that focus on this population. A call to action from health policy planners, medical providers, researchers, breast cancer patients, families, and the community in general is needed to address this emergent challenge (10).

Role of Executive Leadership, Organizations and Governments

Latin American countries are experiencing a continuous growth in cancer control activities and partnerships during recent years.

One example is of all National Cancer Institutes working together under the umbrella of the Network of National Cancer Institutes. This body is also the operating structure for cancer of UNASUR Health, the Union of South American Nations, and they have breast cancer regional programmes and quality control of mammography (11).

The International Agency for Research in Cancer (IARC) has a hub in Buenos Aires, Argentina, as part of the Global Initiative for Cancer Registry Development, an international partnership that combines technical support, training, and advocacy to ensure that population-based cancer registries are developed across the world. The improvement of data collection is fundamental to establish better breast cancer control programmes (12).

The Latin-American and Caribbean Society of Medical Oncology has an important programme for research in breast cancer with several original publications providing new information on breast cancer in the region.

The Latin-American Federation of Mastology is the leading organization for breast diseases and gathers most of the Latin American Mastology Societies.

Key Messages

- Breast cancer is the most frequent cancer and kills more women than any other cancer in LACs.
- In most countries, incidence and mortality are increasing. The number of deaths from breast cancer is expected to double by 2030, and ageing is the principal risk factor.
- The economic burden is also significant, and countries today allocate insufficient resources to tackle the disease.
- Women go undiagnosed, uncared for, or treated with suboptimal therapies.
- Universal health-care coverage is still not the rule in LACs.
- Vast inequities in access to breast cancer health translate into unequal results in breast cancer outcomes.
- Data on survival are scarce and fragmented, but outcomes have improved over the past decade.

- The majority of breast cancer cases are detected when women seek care following symptoms onset. Initiatives to increase the awareness of breast cancer are very important.
- No one-suits-all prevention strategy is feasible given the outstanding epidemiological contrasts in terms of disease occurrence, risks, and available resources both across and within countries.
- Population-based mammography has been shown to improve outcomes, but, in some LACs with limited resources and low incidence, the best screening strategies differ.
- Prevention plays a fundamental role, but several additional measures such as health education and behaviour modification, breast self-awareness, and clinical breast examination should be considered.
- The challenge in LACs is to implement policies and control mechanisms to ensure compliance and their applicability to the entire population.
- Latin American patient groups fulfil an important task, where healthcare systems cannot, or do not sufficiently, assist breast cancer patients.

References

1. Cazap E et al. Implementation science and breast cancer control: a Breast Health Global Initiative (BHGI) perspective from the 2010 Global Summit. *Breast* 2011;20Suppl 2:S1–2.
2. Goss PE et al. Planning cancer control in Latin America and the Caribbean. *Lancet Oncol* 2013;14(5):391–436.
3. Cazap E et al. Breast cancer in Latin America: results of the Latin American and Caribbean Society of Medical Oncology/Breast Cancer Research Foundation expert survey. *Cancer* 2008;113(8 Suppl):2359–2365.
4. Cazap E et al. Breast cancer in Latin America: experts perceptions compared with medical care standards. *Breast* 2010;19(1):50–4.
5. Justo N et al. A review of breast cancer care and outcomes in Latin America. *Oncologist* 2013;18(3):248–256.
6. Teich N et al. Retrospective cost analysis of breast cancer patients treated in a Brazilian outpatient cancer center. *J Clin Oncol* 2010;28(Suppl):Abstract 11026.
7. Knaul FM et al. The health care costs of breast cancer: the case of the Mexican Social Security Institute. *Salud Publica Mex* 2009;51(Suppl 2):s286–s295.
8. Goss PE et al. Planning cancer control in Latin America and the Caribbean. *Lancet Oncol* 2013;14(5):391–436.
9. Debiasi M et al. Estimation of premature deaths from lack of access to anti-HER2 therapy for advanced breast cancer in the Brazilian Public Health System. *J Glob Oncol* 2016;3(3):201–207.
10. Villarreal-Garza C et al. Breast cancer in young women in Latin America: an unmet, growing burden. *Oncologist* 2013;18(12):1298–1306.
11. RINC (Red de Institutos Nacionales de Cáncer), Sobre la RINC. Available from: http://www2.inca.gov.br/wps/wcm/connect/RINC/site/home/sobre
12. Global Initiative for Cancer Registry Development. Available from: http://gicr.iarc.fr/

35

Perspective from India

Improving Breast Health Care

Raghu Ram Pillarisetti

Introduction

The incidence of breast cancer in India has been rising steadily over the past decade. With 155, 000 new cases being diagnosed in 2018, the incidence of breast cancer has overtaken cervical cancer to become the commonest cancer affecting women (1). Some 75,000 women succumb to the disease every year—for every two women newly diagnosed with breast cancer, one dies (2).

There are several worrying trends in the country:

- Rising incidence in young women—as opposed to the west, where the vast majority present aged >50 years, most breast cancers present in younger women (peak incidence: 40–50 years).
- More than 60% present in advanced stages due to lack of awareness and absence of an organized population-based screening programme.
- Higher incidence of triple-negative breast cancers (27%) when compared to the west, with consequent poor prognosis in this subgroup (3).
- The 5-year survival rate is around 60% as opposed to more than 80% in the west.
- India currently spends only 1.2% of its GDP on publicly funded health care. This is considerably less than most other comparable countries.

There is a huge discrepancy in the availability, quality, and reporting of breast imaging and pathology across the country. The vast majority of breast cancers is managed by general surgeons rather than by surgical oncologists. Breast surgery is not a distinct subspecialty in the country, and only a small fraction of women presenting with breast cancer are assessed by a comprehensive multidisciplinary team. There is very little effort directed towards empowering people about the importance of early detection of breast cancer, and counselling patients is not considered to be an important component of breast cancer care. Breast-conserving surgery is not routinely offered, and axillary radiotherapy is routinely given to many patients due to inadequate axillary surgery. Due to the enormous costs, many do not complete their course of chemotherapy. Most patients who are Her2 positive simply cannot afford trastuzumab. While few cancer centres offer care comparing with the best centres across the world, by and large, cancer care in India is a 'lottery' with some getting excellent care, while most do not. That there is huge variation in the survival of patients with breast cancer across the country is an understatement.

Cancer displays a significant socioeconomic gradient in India. Out-of-pocket expenditure is among the highest in any ailments. The out-of-pocket spending on inpatient care in private clinics is about three times that of public facilities. Treatment of about 40% of cancer hospitalizations is financed mainly through borrowings, sale of assets, and contributions from friends and relatives. Figure 35.1 shows the percentage of cancer patient households reporting distressed financing by wealth quintiles in public and private sector treatment. Although important differences are observed, a lot of households in all categories report distress (4).

Four aims were created to improve the delivery of breast healthcare in India:

1. Establish a dedicated centre for breast health.
2. Establish a breast cancer foundation.
3. Implement a population-based breast cancer screening programme reaching out to the underprivileged community.
4. Establish breast surgery as a subspecialty in India.

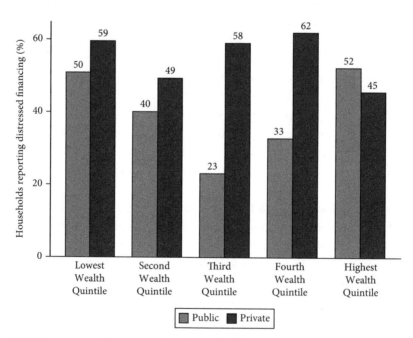

Figure 35.1 Percentage of cancer patient households reporting use of distressed financing as a major source, by wealth quintiles and public and private sector treatments, India, 2014.

Reproduced from Rajpal S, Kumar A, Joe W. 'Economic burden of cancer in India: Evidence from cross-sectional nationally representative household survey, 2014'. PLoS One. Volume 13, Issue 2: e0193320. Copyright: © 2018 Rajpal et al. DOI: 10.1371/journal.pone.0193320. Available under the Creative Commons Attribution 4.0 International License. http://creativecommons.org/licenses/by/4.0/

Three out of these four aims have been completed, and the path for the fourth one has been paved.

A Dedicated Centre for Breast Health

South Asia's first free-standing, purpose-built, comprehensive Breast Health Centre was conceived and designed in Hyderabad (2007). Krishna Institute of Medical Sciences (KIMS)–Ushalakshmi Centre for Breast Diseases was established under the auspices of KIMS hospitals, one of the largest corporate hospital groups in South India (5). It was designed and based on the best aspects of the Royal Marsden, Cardiff, and Nottingham, breast centres in the UK. KIMS–Ushalakshmi Centre for Breast Diseases is a unique set-up in India, where clinical assessment, breast imaging, breast biopsy, and counselling are all done in a purpose-built unit that is dedicated to the management of all types of breast disease, both benign and malignant, by a committed multidisciplinary team. This landmark initiative has brought about a revolutionary change— the 'breast centre' concept in the Indian subcontinent.

One of the essential roles in delivering a state-of-the-art breast health service is a good breast radiologist. Breast radiology services were in their infancy, in India. The consultant radiologist at KIMS Hospitals in Hyderabad travelled to the UK to obtain training at St George's Breast Screening Centre in London. A breast radiologist and members of her team at the Jarvis Screening Centre in Guildford (UK) came to India to train the radiographer and to quality-assure the first 950 screening mammograms. Mobile screening began in 2007 in Hyderabad. It was the first initiative of its kind in India. In 2012, a national organization, The Breast Imaging Society of India, was formed, inspiring many radiologists across India to take up breast radiology as a career.

Establish a Breast Cancer Foundation

The Ushalakshmi Breast Cancer Foundation was established in 2007 (6). Working closely with Breast Cancer Care UK, Britain's only UK-wide charity providing breast care, the Foundation printed and distributed some 100,000 information booklets that provide information about every aspect of breast health in English and the local regional language (Telugu). The author developed the world's first mobile phone breast app (Figure 35.2). This novel digital application provides information about every aspect of breast cancer and benign disease in 12 languages. The aim of the app is to counsel, guide, and educate women across the nation about various aspects of breast health.

The Foundation championed a one-of-a-kind, large-scale breast cancer awareness drive across the southern Indian states of Telangana and Andhra Pradesh. A number of unique and innovative events have been organized in urban and rural regions with many celebrity breast cancer survivors from India and abroad lending their support to

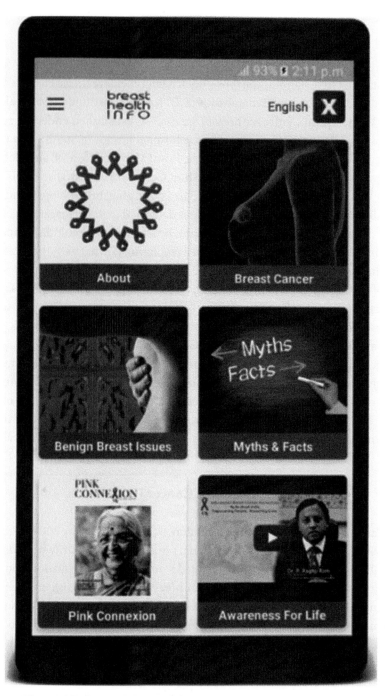

Figure 35.2 The world's first mobile phone breast app.

this worthy cause. Over the past decade, the campaign has addressed more than 1,000 organizations across India and abroad, has appeared in several television programmes, and has been featured in more than 100 full-page articles in major newspapers and magazines.

Implement a Population-Based Breast Cancer Screening Programme Reaching out to the Underprivileged Community

Due to the absence of a nationwide population-based screening programme, more than 60% of breast cancers present in advanced stages in India. Mammography is not a viable option for population-based screening in India. The reasons are the enormous costs, early age at diagnosis (<50 years), huge variation in mammographic reporting, and issues relating to quality assurance. However, there is considerable evidence regarding the efficacy of clinical breast examination (CBE) in detecting small breast cancers when performed by trained healthcare workers in the community setting.

Between 2012 and 2016, some 200,000 underprivileged women between the ages of 35 and 65 years across 4,000 villages in 15 districts of Telangana and Andhra Pradesh were screened for early signs of breast cancer with CBE. The programme used the services of 3,750 healthcare workers, employed by the government, who were trained under the auspices of the Foundation to perform CBE. Cancers detected through this initiative are treated free of charge through the State Government-funded Aarogyasri scheme. In 2017, The Ministry of Health, Government of India incorporated clinical breast examination into the National Cancer Screening Guidelines. Since 2018, the national cancer screening programme for breast, cervical, and oral cavity has been rolled out across the nation. In the fullness of time, this landmark screening programme would hopefully make a significant impact on ensuring early detection and reducing the burden of advanced cancers in the country.

Establish Breast Surgery as a Subspecialty in India

Breast surgery is not a recognized subspecialty in India. Moreover, until 2011, there was no dedicated Surgical Society in India focused exclusively upon issues surrounding breast disease. Recognizing the need for a paradigm shift in delivery of breast health care in India, the Association of Breast Surgeons of India (ABSI) was formed in 2011, the first and only organization in South Asia representing general surgeons, surgical oncologists, and plastic surgeons treating patients with breast disease. The Association has been established along similar lines to those of the Association of Breast Surgeons in the UK and the American Society of Breast Surgeons. The formation of ABSI is in many ways the first step towards developing breast surgery as a distinct subspecialty in India (7).

A nationwide ABSI Training Module was developed as a structured breast surgical training programme in many cities and towns across India to instruct trainees and surgeons in every aspect of breast health in a simple, easy-to-understand format. An ABSI Overseas Fellowship Programme was established to enable breast surgical trainees from India to obtain 'hands on' one-year oncoplastic surgical training in preselected centres of excellence in the UK. Since 2016, three trainees from India completed subspecialty training in the UK. They have since returned to India and are practising the art and science of breast surgery in the country.

Key Messages

- The rising incidence and mortality coupled with age shift and late stage of presentation is a cause for great concern.
- Breast cancer advocacy can transform breast cancer from a 'taboo' issue to a more commonly discussed one.
- There is a need for a paradigm shift in the management of breast cancer and indeed breast health care in India.
- The concepts of breast cancer advocacy, breast centre, breast specialists, and the subspecialty of breast surgery are all bound to improve the delivery of breast healthcare in India in forthcoming years.

References

1. Asthana S et al. Breast and cervical cancer risk in India: an update. *Ind. J Public Health* 2014;58:5–10.
2. Global Comparison of Breast Cancer. Available from: http://www.breastcancerindia.net/statistics/stat_global.html
3. Dikshit R et al. Cancer mortality in India: a nationally representative survey. *Lancet* 2012;379:1807–1816.
4. Rajpal S et al. Economic burden of cancer in India: evidence from cross-sectional nationally representative household survey, 2014. *PLoS One* 2018:13(2):e0193320.
5. KIMS–Ushalakshmi Centre for Breast Diseases. Available from: http://www.breastcancerindia.org/
6. Ushalakshmi Breast Cancer Foundation. Available from: http://ubf.org.in/
7. ABSI—The Association of Breast Surgeons of India. Available from: http://www.absi.in/

36

Perspective from South Africa and sub-Saharan Africa

Carol Benn

Looking at the Data

According to South Africa's National Cancer Registry, in 2011 breast cancer was the most commonly diagnosed cancer among women with an age-adjusted incidence rate of 31.4 per 100,000 women and a lifetime risk of 1 in 29. In 2012, 9,815 women were diagnosed with breast cancer, and 3,848 died from the disease. Non-radiological and 'lower-cost' but personal time and training-dependent methods of breast disease detection, which can be taught and made available, include breast self-examination and clinical breast examination by a healthcare provider. Screening programmes based on clinical breast examination, although recommended as promising for the early detection of breast cancer in low- and middle-income countries (LMICs), still require research. Whereas the presentation of breast cancer remains with more locally advanced breast cancers (LABCs) and more palpable disease, clinical assessment remains a useful screening tool as effective as mammography every 2 years in reducing mortality in limited-resource areas.

Although the US Preventive Task Force concluded that breast self-examination does not contribute additional benefits to preventing breast cancer mortality where routine mammographic screening is commonplace, breast self-examination may be of value in low-income settings, where population-level mammographic screening is not available. In Egypt, women who practised breast self-examination presented earlier and with smaller tumours than women who did not practice self-examination (1). Self-examination teaching usually includes the signs of breast cancer, greater awareness of breast conditions, addresses cancer stigma, and provides information about where to receive care. In addition to self-examination and clinical breast exams, ultrasound of the breast can be used for exploring the characteristics of palpable and impalpable breast lesions, particularly in dense and young breasts. It is used to guide breast biopsies for diagnostic purposes. Ultrasound can be as good as mammography in detecting invasive cancer, particularly when breast cancer presents as a palpable mass, although this comes with slightly higher false-positive rates. Understandably, ultrasound is not a recommended test for early-stage population screening due to the lack of sensitivity and specificity in detecting ductal carcinoma in situ, operator variability, and resource intensity. It should be understood that South Africa classifies as an upper middle-income

country and not as a 'very low-resource setting'. Technically, South Africa has significant disparities in health care access and treatment, not unlike many LMICs.

Access to Care

Historically as well as currently, access to breast cancer screening and treatment in
South Africa is characterized by regional and socioeconomic disparities. These differences, as in many LMICs, often start with the relatively low levels of knowledge of the
disease in certain geographic areas and within certain communities around issues such
as 'how breast cancer presents' with the resultant late presentation at health facilities.
A continent-wide review of surgical management of breast care in Africa described a
disproportionate number of black African patients presenting with locally advanced
and metastatic disease (stage 3 or 4). Only 25% presented with early-stage disease
(stage 1 or 2) (2). Since then, a change in awareness and access to care has doubled the
percentage of women presenting with stage 2 cancer or lower to 46%. Still, significant
disparities and barriers to accessing services persist in comparison to the USA, where
82% of women are diagnosed with stage 2 cancer or lower.

Delay regarding access to health care services is due to both patient- and provider-
driven factors. The global trend to understanding barriers to health care has become less
vertical with doctor–patient factors being listed (e.g. patient (mis)beliefs and cultural
factors) to a more horizontal interplay between economic, geographical, psychosocial,
cultural, financial, and medical influences affecting delays in patient presentation.
Investment in breast cancer research and treatment in LMICs should be a global health
priority (3).

Medical influences more commonly understood as 'provider delay' (defined as the
structural or provider-dependent factors which impact negatively on time from the
first presentation to a healthcare practitioner to receiving primary treatment, be that
surgical or non-surgical) contribute to limitations in accessing health care in many
LMICs. For example, in South Africa, restrictions to healthcare system access and delays in service delivery mechanisms will most positively affect the outcome regarding
diagnosis, management, and, ultimately, cancer survival. Data suggest that patients
presenting with advanced disease with a delay of more than 60 days from tissue diagnosis to primary treatment may have an adverse impact on mortality. A meta-analysis
studying delay from surgery to adjuvant therapy found that a backlog of more than 4
weeks to chemotherapy as well as delays to radiation adversely affected patient outcomes (4). These delays are often seen in LMICs. An important study in LMICs is that
of service delivery models and how they impact the results. For South Africa, given
the large proportion of women who present with clinically detectable, later-stage
cancer, clinical breast examinations conducted in primary health clinics, for all symptomatic women and asymptomatic women aged >35 years, are a low-cost option for
population-level screening in the medium term. A service delivery model is needed
whereby trained primary care healthcare workers could immediately refer women with

suspected breast concerns to specialist centres where diagnostic radiology and/or an ultrasound and biopsy could be performed. If walk-in access was prioritized at specialist centres, women could also initiate their diagnosis process at the specialist centres directly, and this would reduce appointments and patient costs. Regardless, quick and coordinated referral would contribute to reductions in delays to treatment. Multilevel interventions will ensure access, availability, and affordability of a minimum standard of care in sub-Saharan Africa (5).

Service Delivery Models

Little is published about breast cancer services in LMICs. Although the South African model has undergone fundamental improvements to clinical care in some settings over the last 20 years, the need for further improvement remains. Training of primary care physicians and community-based patient navigators (often those from the community who have experienced breast cancer (either self or with close family) is vital. In most LMIC areas currently without specialist care, women with breast concerns would present to a primary care nurse with subsequent referral to a surgical outpatient clinic or emergency department of a nearby hospital. The doctors on duty would have a varying degree of clinical knowledge on breast health. Conventional methods of diagnosis would be no radiological aspiration of the breast mass(es) using palpation alone or a surgical biopsy. The specimen would be sent to the nearest laboratory service, and results turnaround could be anywhere between 2 and 6 weeks. This is further complicated by the possibility of not being able to send a definite diagnosis reliably to the patient, but rather the patient having to return to receive the result. An inadequate specimen would necessitate repeat aspiration, dependent on the patient returning and the clinician confirming this against the clinical picture. Alternatively, surgical excision of the mass(es) or mastectomy without confirmatory diagnosis may occur without any radiology. These approaches, although time-efficient and possibly providing a quicker initial treatment, are fraught with problems such as disfigurement of the patient without confirmed diagnosis as well as possible unnecessary or inadequate excision, which could potentially compromise oncological care.

Service delivery in South Africa, as in other LMICs, has progressed considerably in some cosmopolitan urban cities. In these public, non-privately funded, sector units, diagnosis now includes the global reference standard: triple assessment (i.e. clinical breast examination, imaging by ultrasound or mammography or both, and biopsy). A recent study in Zambia showed that a single-visit breast care algorithm is feasible with most clients receiving same-day counselling, early detection, and diagnostic services. Cancer patients were referred for further evaluation (6). The quality of the radiology and pathology services may vary, and thereby affect the efficacy and reliability of the triple assessment. A recent study in Kenya collected payment data on breast cancer from two public hospitals and private sector practitioners and hospitals (6). The breast cancer cost for stage III (curative approach) was about 1500 dollars in public facilities

Table 36.1 Patient costs of breast cancer treatment (2017 US dollars)

Breast cancer treatment[b]	Percentage of patients[a]	Public facility (US$)	Private facility (US$)
Stage I	7	1,340.38	10,914.45
Stage II	35	1,340.38	10,914.45
Stage III (curative approach)	19	1,542.58	11,862.36
Stage III (palliative approach) and Stage IV	40	675.35	8,569.87
Palliative care[c]		169.20	752.43

[a]Distribution of patients by stage was obtained from the Nairobi Cancer Registry.

[b]Hormonal therapy would follow the initial breast cancer treatment, depending on the tumour profile and patient characteristics. Tamoxifen cost was US$0.10 per day.

[c]Palliative care includes pain and symptom management as well as psychosocial support to the patents and their families. Patient payments for an average duration of 6 months are presented.

Reproduced from Subramanian, S. et al. 'Cost and affordability of non-communicable disease screening, diagnosis and treatment in Kenya: Patient payments in the private and public sectors'. *PLoS One*. Volume 13, Issue 1. e0190113. © 2018 Subramanian et al. DOI: https://doi.org/10.1371/journal.pone.0190113. Available under the Creative Commons Attribution 4.0 International License.

and more than 7500 dollars in the private facilities. Many Kenyans aged 15–49 years do not have health insurance, which makes cancer services unaffordable for most people given the overall high cost of services relative to income (average household expenditure per adult is 413 dollars per year). Table 36.1 shows a substantial variation in patient cost between public and private sector. The cost represents a very substantial economic burden. The development of a national strategy for the prevention and control of non-communicable diseases between 2015 and 2020 provides a road map for improving (breast) cancer care and the quality of life of all Kenyans (7).

Multidisciplinary Meetings and Care in LMICs

Multidisciplinary patient care is widely regarded as the international reference standard. True multidisciplinary care requires the acceptance of clear multidisciplinary unit guidelines and the need for particular disciplines being represented at the multidisciplinary meeting (MDM). Numerous breast cancer specialist centres have been developed in South Africa, usually by interested clinicians and receptive hospitals. Patients access these services through a variety of sources. Medical sources include primary healthcare facilities, district hospitals, general practitioner or radiology referrals, and patient-based referrals such as 'word of mouth', the internet, and in some cases 'self-referral'. Most multidisciplinary breast cancer teams include medical and radiation oncologists, surgeons, radiologists, pathologists, nurses, and counsellors in various numbers. Correct documentation and audit probably occur in very few South African multidisciplinary units.

Collaboration within multidisciplinary teams facilitates expedient diagnosis and referral and is likely to be the most significant driver of multidisciplinary units in LMICs. It thus improves the navigation of patients from diagnosis to treatment options. Whether this is an LMIC modification on MDM and considered a true MDM, where treatment options and order are determined, documented, and audited, may be debated. In some multidisciplinary units, breast cancer advocacy groups, comprising survivors and other interested parties, play an integral part of the team and contribute to improvements or assistance with transportation, translation of treatment decisions, as well as overall education for patients in the disease management process. Advocates also assist in raising awareness of survivorship issues such as prosthesis following surgery, compliance on accessing medication and treatment, as well as psychosocial support, grants, and social welfare access.

Breast Cancer Management in South Africa

In South Africa, and other LMICs, the first screening goal is to reduce late presentation and late-stage disease through community-based population-level screening combined with open access to health care services for any women with breast symptoms.

After diagnosis, cancer management and treatment in South Africa varies. Some excellent private and government facilities offer full multidisciplinary care, whereas other facilities offer disjointed care with no coordination both in the private and government sectors.

Diagnosis of breast cancer cannot be based on purely clinical grounds in limited-resource settings, even when locally advanced breast cancers are the usual presentation. Diseases such as tuberculosis and HIV-related lymphoma can clinically mimic the visual and clinical presentation of advanced breast cancer. Therefore, excellent pathology services are critical.

Pathology diagnostics often require central laboratory services that, even with the use of international interpretation of specimens, may lack safe collection and processing systems, and this can result in an inaccurate correlation between sample and patient and translate into misdiagnosis and mismanagement.

Treatment limitations in most resource-poor environments revolve mainly around oncological services such as lack of radiation facilities and access to oncology drugs.

Due to the large numbers of patients presenting with LABC, and when using the 2013 guidelines to determine which patients require radiation therapy, the lack of radiotherapy services in LMICs means that most patients requiring radiation therapy may not receive the treatment. Overburdening of radiation resource due to patient numbers may also result in extensive delays in time to radiation treatment or the need to shorten the course of therapy. The high incidence of cervical cancers experienced in some of these countries further increases the burden on these few units. The setting up of an Advisory Group on increasing access to radiotherapy technology in LMICs in 2009 under the Programme of Action for Cancer Therapy, with the technical support of the International Atomic Energy Agency's Division of Human Health and Division of Radiation, Transport and Waste Safety, has resulted in an increased awareness of the radiotherapy resource problem (8).

Treatment is offered in centralized oncology units in select facilities in both regional or centralized teaching hospitals. Access to most of these units requires a referral, which is a common delivery model for specialist care globally. When added to the provider-driven delays in the diagnosis process, this results in South African women experiencing significant delays, frustrations, and unnecessary progression of the disease before treatment.

Currently access to trastuzumab is not available in the government setting; however, the minister of health has sanctioned that it will become available.

Oncology drugs may be obtained on tender, and certain endocrine therapies are available in some government settings but not in others.

Regarding access to surgery, most regional units offer mastectomies with axillary lymph node dissections. Some specialized units offer breast conservation surgery, oncoplastic surgery, and sentinel lymph node biopsies. Breast-conserving surgery has become the reference standard, but only in cases where there is easy access to radiation facilities. In South Africa, breast surgery has progressed from being the bread and butter of the general surgeon to currently being considered as a recognized subspecialty.

In South Africa, access to diagnostic, treatment, and surgical services are not homogeneous. Late-stage presentation of disease continues to prohibit individual management approaches such as breast-conserving therapy, and there is a lack of treatment facilities and specialists capable of performing these procedures in the public sector.

Finally, palliative care for patients experiencing life-threatening and terminal illnesses of all kinds requires a multidisciplinary service, from pain management to psychological and spiritual counselling and support. Palliative care is currently available in South Africa, often through community- and home-based structures.

Access varies due to geographic location, and service disparities are further complicated by lack of facilities and inadequate referral structures. Facilities for patients with lymphoedema are few and far between, and huge differences exist between public and private access to palliative treatments.

Survivorship is a relatively new specialty in South Africa, and it is not routinely offered to patients post breast cancer care. Surveillance for cancer recurrence is often approached in a non-multidisciplinary manner. This is further complicated by cancer survivors using the public health systems while having comorbidities such as HIV, tuberculosis, and other non-communicable diseases.

Strategies for Progress

A national-level policy document on breast cancer screening and treatment has just been drafted and launched in South Africa. The policy document addresses options for improving access to breast cancer-related services, and looks at the current environment regarding breast cancer-related care. Barriers to the implementation of equitable access, including perceived costs, are discussed, and health delivery models which could help achieve South Africa's goals are suggested (9).

In Nigeria, the Breast Cancer Association alerted more than one million people about prevention and lifestyle with a special programme during the 2018 World Cancer Day. Their strategies included seminars, sending out materials via mails, and reaching people via social media sponsored advertisements http://www.brecan.org (10). In addition, there is an urgent need to train the necessary medical professionals, and the available radiotherapy machines must be operated by trained engineers to avoid breakdown soon after their acquisition. The aim is to decrease current provider-dependent delays. Increased availability of multidisciplinary teams functioning in specialist centres should improve access. The policy document hopes to improve patient access and improve communication between regional and central units with more timely access to all treatment modalities.

Specialist centres would take responsibility for the regional, local primary health clinics, and district hospitals in their areas regarding staff training and more appropriate referral times. Community-trained counsellors would coordinate patient-based education and support activities through navigation from diagnosis to treatment and survivorship.

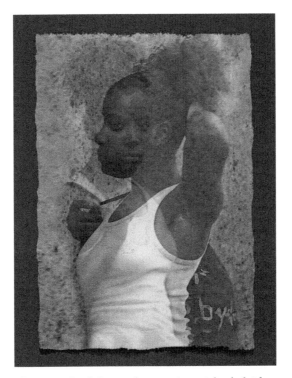

Figure 36.1 South Africa is indeed the rainbow nation with a kaleidoscope of care. A few driven clinicians across the country, as unique as each rainbow colour strive daily towards the pot of gold of true excellent patient care ensuring an integrated, education orientated, multidisciplinary approach to treatment; with cost effective service delivery and high quality patient care. (Carol Benn, Paris, 2 August 2013)

Attempts to improve service delivery are largely clinician-driven. Planning and piloting of national health insurance is currently underway, and improved outreach at the primary health care service level has contributed to a more efficient community-level service delivery (11).

Key Messages

- Improve education and awareness on breast health, including signs of breast cancer, and breast self-examination.
- Increase the number of breast specialist centres nationwide and ensure that they are staffed with multidisciplinary teams.
- Re-train primary health care nurses on how to perform clinical breast examinations and begin screening of asymptomatic women aged >35 years (in addition to offering to screen for all symptomatic women).
- Population-level mammographic screening is not recommended for insufficient resource settings.
- Strengthen existing referral systems including facilitated patient transport systems.
- Maximize the use of mammography and ultrasound for diagnosis by ensuring that the machines are placed in breast specialist centres with trained personnel.
- Increase support for, and links to, patient advocates and counsellors in communities and within breast specialist centres to ensure comprehensive, full-spectrum care.
- Leadership involvement is sparse but strong in places.

References

1. Sharaa H. Beliefs and reported practices related to breast self-examination among sample of Egyptian women. *Academic J Cancer Res* 2013;6(2):99–110.
2. Sutter A et al. Surgical management of breast cancer in Africa: a continent-wide review of intervention practices, barriers to care and adjuvant therapy. *J Glob Oncol* 2017;3(2):162–168.
3. Pace L and Shulman L. Breast cancer sub-Saharan Africa: challenges and opportunities to reduce mortality. *Oncologist* 2016;21(6):739–744.
4. Xiaofang H et al. Risk factors for delay of adjuvant chemotherapy in non-metastatic breast cancer patients: a systematic review and meta-analysis involving 186982 patients. *PLoS One* 2017;12(3):e0173862.
5. Grosse Frie K et al. Why do women with breast cancer get diagnosed and treated late in sub-Saharan Africa? Perspectives from women and patients in Bamako, Mali. *Breast Care* 2018;13:39–43.
6. Pinder L et al. Leverage of an existing cervical cancer prevention service platform to initiate breast cancer control services in Zambia: experiences and early outcomes. *J Glob Oncol* 2018;(4):1–8.
7. Subramanian S et al. Cost and affordability of non-communicable disease screening, diagnosis and treatment in Kenya: patient payments in the private and public sectors. *PLoS One* 2018;13(1):e0190113.
8. Ministry of Health. Kenya national strategy for the prevention and control of non-communicable diseases: 2015–2020. Available from: www.health.go.ke

9. Zubizarreta E et al. Need for radiotherapy in low and middle income countries—the silent crisis continues. *Clin Oncol* 2015;27(2):107–114.
10. Department Health, Republic of South Africa. Breast cancer control policy (June 2017). Available from: www.health.gov.za
11. *Nigerian Daily Trust* (newspaper). Editorial. 10 May 2018. Available from: http://www.dailytrust.com.ng

37

Optimization of Breast Cancer Management in Low- and Middle-Income Countries

Catherine Duggan, Benjamin O. Anderson, Eduardo L. Cazap,
Paul A. El-Tomb, and Nagi S. El Saghir

Optimization of Breast Cancer Management in LMICs

Breast cancer mortality can be decreased by increasing awareness, improving access to early detection and screening programmes, and providing advanced care, as long as appropriate infrastructure and properly trained health care professionals are available. Clinicians, radiologists, and pathologists are needed for diagnosis, and well-trained surgeons, radiation oncologists, and medical oncologists are needed to guide and perform treatment (1).

Low-income countries face many challenges, including spreading community awareness that breast cancer is a treatable disease, and that it is potentially curable when discovered early enough and with the presence of basic pathology services and treatment options. Both low- and middle-income countries (LMICs) share these challenges, although middle-income countries fare better, due to higher rates of health expenditure and better investments in health care infrastructure including programmes that prioritize breast cancer control. All LMICs healthcare systems face challenges including lack of national or regional data registries for breast cancer, which makes it difficult to measure the impact of changes in breast cancer control policies. Alternative data collection systems could be an intermediate step for this problem. Quantitative, qualitative, and cost-effective research programmes with reference to the already published work could guide the development of pragmatic solutions in developing countries. In addition, LMICs also suffer from poor infrastructure and low financial capacities that make it more difficult to obtain the appropriate equipment, drug acquisitions, training for health care professionals, and accreditations (1).

Establishing national data on health care resources, including information about the number and distribution of radiation oncology centres, trained surgeons, and ultrasound and mammography machines, medical oncologists would help countries create a national cancer plan, where patients are triaged and referred to specialty centres when needed. These centres would be capable of handling advanced disease cases and could offer suitable treatment options to patients—options that are not present in rural areas. This emphasizes the key role of trained primary care physicians in the triage process. Systematic approaches to patient navigation, which guide patients and primary care providers to appropriate available services, are becoming an increasingly important part of timely referral pathways within the health systems of high-income countries, but these have not been developed to scale in middle-income countries and are mostly absent in low-income countries. Crucial workforce issues, such as an insufficient number of nurses, are experienced globally and limit access to care. Investments in training programmes for medical personnel in LMICs are needed (1). In addition, better patient care and quality can be improved by advancing multidisciplinary management tumour boards at hospitals that treat cancer patients (2).

Many international organizations have sought ways to improve breast cancer care and outcome in LMICs. Their focus was on the establishment of 'resource-stratified guidelines' that identify cost-effective, evidence-based plans to detect, diagnose, and treat patients in LMICs and taking available resources into account. From 2002 to 2012, the Breast Health Global Initiative (BHGI) published a series of resource-stratified guidelines, where resources are divided into four categories based on the resource availability and its impact on clinical outcome: basic, limited, enhanced, and maximal (3,4). In later meetings, the BHGI updated the guidelines and was concerned about obstacles to their implementation as well as issues of supportive and palliative care (5,6).

The National Comprehensive Cancer Network (NCCN) published the most recent available resource-stratified guidelines in April 2018 (7). The NCCN framework includes three levels of resources: basic, core, and enhanced resources. It follows the principle of cost-effective interventions in improving disease outcome.

Another way to improve breast care, particularly in middle-income countries, is to scale up existing breast cancer care resources to overcome structural barriers to diagnosis and treatment. This requires accurate estimates of the burden of the disease, identification of available treatment resources, and plans to overcome the obstacles. This will require a coordinated effort locally to address the financial, medical, and sociocultural roadblocks (8).

Our review of breast cancer control in low-, lower-middle-, and upper-middle- income countries identified common problems suggesting common solutions. However, specific differences exist both between and within countries, which suggest a need to look more closely at subpopulations within each country or region in order to understand better how to optimize breast cancer care for underserved women worldwide.

Key Messages

Recommendations developed by BHGI consensus panel for low-resource and middle-resource countries (5):

- Cancer registries are needed so that disease prevalence, stage, and treatment outcome can be measured.
- National cancer plans should define healthcare networks in which centres of excellence become connected through outreach to rural and surrounding areas for consultation and patient triage.

- Resource-adapted multidisciplinary cancer care models should be used to avoid system fragmentation and to facilitate consistent health-policy reform.
- Training for physician and non-physician staff should be linked to equipment acquisition and quality care initiatives that measure utilization and clinical outcomes.
- Public awareness that breast cancer outcomes are improved through early detection should be promoted in conjunction with the development of resource-appropriate early detection programmes.
- Clinical breast examination should be promoted as a necessary method for clinical diagnosis of breast abnormalities.
- Diagnostic services, surgical treatment, radiotherapy, systemic therapy, and palliative care should become integrated within coordinated multidisciplinary environments.
- Systems for coordinated tissue sampling and pathology services should be developed to optimize pathology practices for accurate diagnosis and effective treatment planning.
- Barriers to accessing cancer drugs need to be addressed in conjunction with the deployment of properly trained physicians and staff.
- Workforce issues should be addressed through resource-sensitive strategies that provide quality care but without limiting access.

References

1. Anderson BO et al. Breast cancer in low and middle income countries (LMICs): a shifting tide in global health. *Breast J* 2015;21(1):111–118.
2. El Saghir NS et al. Global practice and efficiency of multidisciplinary tumor boards: results of an ASCO survey. *J Glob Oncol* 2015;1(2):57–64.
3. Anderson BO et al. Overview of breast health care guidelines for countries with limited resources. *Breast J* 2003;9 Suppl 2:S42–50.
4. Anderson B et al. Breast cancer in limited-resource countries: an overview of the Breast Health Global Initiative 2005 Guidelines. *Breast J* 2006;12:S3–S15.
5. Anderson BO et al. Optimisation of breast cancer management in low-resource and middle-resource countries: executive summary of the Breast Health Global Initiative consensus, 2010. *Lancet Oncol* 2011;12:387–398.
6. Distelhorst SR et al. Optimisation of the continuum of supportive and palliative care for patients with breast cancer in low-income and middle-income countries: executive summary of the Breast Health Global Initiative. *Lancet Oncol* 2014;16(3):e137–e147.
7. National Comprehensive Cancer Network. Framework for Resource Stratification of NCCN Guidelines. Invasive Breast Cancer (Version 2.2017, April 2018). Available at: https://www.nccn.org/professionals/physician_gls/pdf/breast_basic.pdf
8. Cazap E et al. Structural barriers to diagnosis and treatment of cancer in low- and middle-income countries: the urgent need for scaling up. *Clin Oncol* 2016;34(1):14–19.

Conclusion

Didier Verhoeven, Cary S. Kaufman, Robert Mansel, and Sabine Siesling

Concluding Comments

Comprehensive breast cancer care requires an exchange of ideas among providers on a regular basis in order to fully identify the patient's unique clinical situation including their tumour characteristics, the patient's anatomy, the availability of resources, and the skillsets of the clinician team. A single excellent clinician focuses on his own discipline and may miss vital issues valuable for patient care. Moreover, the patient might prefer no treatment or a treatment with less clinical benefit than the preferred treatment from clinical/guideline perspective because of her own preference or social economic context.

This book demonstrates the complexity of care surrounding breast cancer and the difficulty in choosing the ideal treatment, especially when local resource issues intrude on the desired choices. High-quality breast cancer care requires constant communication among the treatment team with ongoing monitoring of the level of care the team provides. Excellent communication with the patient throughout her journey is needed in addition to a well-organized programme providing the broad spectrum of care necessary for a patient to receive optimal treatment in today's environment. Ten key messages were identified.

1. Breast cancer is the world's most common cancer in 140 of 184 countries. It is also the most significant cancer killer. The risk of breast cancer diagnosis varies widely by world region. Cancer registries provide insight on the burden of cancer by systematically recording data within a specific area.

2. Today's breast cancer care requires an integrated team approach by clinicians concentrated within a breast centre. The future only guarantees more complex decision-making. The best possible treatment is obtained by increasing availability and access to multidisciplinary teams. Integrated care with regularly scheduled meetings among the therapeutic group is needed to handle the wide scope of the health care services provided.

3. The breast cancer team is strongly influenced by both internal and external forces. A strong primary care presence is necessary to guide patients throughout the entire care pathway. The World Health Organization provides a list of minimally required medicines for all patients, while the choices require a collaborative approach.

4. Guideline adherence is associated with improved patient outcomes. Although many therapeutic guidelines have been widely available, implementation of those guidelines remains inadequate in many areas. Resource-stratified guidelines provide an approach for evidence-based treatments adapted to the local structures.

5. Clarity of the goals of treatment and informing the patients at all stages of disease is paramount to make decisions on the actions that will be taken. These decisions should be made together with the patient. Each individual may see the world differently, and patient-centred care should be the goal. Some women are truly uninformed, but many are simply overwhelmed. Information should be given at the right time and in the right amount. Communication among the care providers as well as with the patients and their families is necessary throughout the breast cancer journey.

6. Breast cancer research has led to constantly evolving therapeutic options mostly guided by molecularly targeted drug therapy. New tools of tailored treatment can also bring more uncertainty.

7. The level of care should be regularly monitored within the breast centre. Quality management of breast cancer should be part of daily practice and can be enhanced by accreditation programmes and better continuing education for doctors, nurses, and the entire breast care team. Local resources will influence the choices to be made. Although survival is a relevant endpoint, quality-of-life expectations are becoming increasingly important and support a more holistic approach.

8. In an age of increasing technologies, these should be harnessed to improve the care of the patient with breast cancer. New information technology can aid to improve treatment value as well as bringing treatment closer to the patient.

9. Breast cancer costs are increasing due to rising patient numbers coupled with increasing treatment costs. Health economic analysis can provide information to more efficiently organize the care. Overdiagnosis and overtreatment are important issues in developed countries. Accessibility and health coverage are most important in low- and middle-income countries (LMICs).

10. Government, local authorities, and national cancer plans are the most important components necessary to address the cancer burden and coordinate required actions. Efforts to engage local authorities to the needs of the patients with breast cancer require continuous attention. In LMICs healthcare networks should be defined in order to connect surrounding areas to centres of excellence. Awareness of breast cancer and understanding of the disease can help the fight worldwide.

Index

Tables, figures, and boxes are indicated by *t*, *f*, and *b* following the page number.

For the benefit of digital users, indexed terms that span two pages (e.g., 52–53) may, on occasion, appear on only one of those pages.